HEALTH CARE **AT RISK**

HEALTH CARE **AT RISK**

A CRITIQUE OF THE CONSUMER-DRIVEN MOVEMENT

TIMOTHY STOLTZFUS JOST

Duke University Press   Durham and London   2007

© 2007 Duke University Press

All rights reserved

Printed in the United States of America on acid-free paper ∞

Designed by Heather Hensley

Typeset in Linotype Sabon by Keystone Typesetting, Inc.

Library of Congress Cataloging-in-Publication Data appear
on the last printed page of this book.

To Allen and Reuben Stoltzfus

CONTENTS

The Problems Facing Our Health Care System, and the Consumer-Driven Solution

America's health care system is in trouble. The problems that it faces are described in detail in chapter 1, but that it is in serious difficulty is disputed by almost no one. There is little agreement, however, as to what to do about it. Half a century of debate about how to expand access to health care, control its cost, and improve its quality has brought about some major advances — access to health care for the elderly, disabled, and many poor children, for example — but has failed to yield anything approximating a comprehensive solution. Managed care, our latest health care policy nostrum, seemed to hold down cost escalation through the mid-1990s, but as we reach the end of the first decade of the twenty-first century, health care costs continue to grow while the number of uninsured is expanding, and we seem to be progressing only slowly in narrowing significant deficits in health care quality.

Advocates of the consumer-driven health care (CDHC) movement, sometimes called the consumer-directed health care movement, claim that they have found the solution to our dilemma. CDHC is currently being pushed very effectively by policy advocacy organizations such as the National Center for Policy Analysis and the Galen and Cato institutes; by academic economists; by business school gurus, notably Regina Herzlinger; by insurers, such as United, Aetna, and the Blue Cross plans, who market consumer-driven products; by some employers who see it as a way of saving money for employee benefits; and by a wide range of politicians spanning the political spectrum from conservative Republicans to moderate Democrats.

CDHC advocates propose the creation of medical or health savings accounts (MSAs or HSAs), coupled with high-deductible health plans (HDHPs).[1] Their idea is that consumers should be encouraged to save up for medical care, rely on these savings to cover routine medical expenses, and turn to insurance only to cover truly catastrophic medical events. They contend that insurance policies should have deductibles as high as $5,000 to $10,000. These advocates believe that if consumers are spending their own money on medical care, they will only purchase medical care with real value to them. Consumers will also shop around, finding the least expensive health care providers and bargaining to get lower prices. As consumers get used to shopping for health care services, they will also focus more on quality and thus encourage providers to improve the care that they offer. Finally, high deductibles will reduce the cost of health insurance by relieving insurers from processing small health care claims.

To make their proposals a reality, CDHC advocates push for federal and state tax subsidies for consumer investments in specially earmarked HSAs. Under recently adopted federal legislation, money deposited in these accounts is, up to certain limits, excluded or deducted from income for purposes of calculating income taxes, as is the investment income earned on these accounts.[2] Money from these accounts can be spent on a variety of health care products and services, including some not covered by traditional health insurance, but money withdrawn to pay for non-healthcare goods or services is subject to an excise tax as well as regular income taxation. Alternatively, funds can be accumulated in these accounts and withdrawn when the account holder reaches the age of sixty-five or dies, so there is some incentive not to spend the money simply because it is there. The tax benefit is only available, however, if the account holder also has a high-deductible insurance policy, with a deductible of at least $1,100 for individuals or $2,200 for families (in 2007). Deductibles as high as $5,500 (for families in 2007) are permitted, although the maximum for out-of-pocket exposure is $11,000 (for families in 2007) for those who purchase this form of insurance. CDHC advocates have also lobbied successfully for state tax subsidies and regulatory exemptions for HDHPs and HSAs. They have even achieved some success in advocating HSAs for Medicare and Medicaid recipients.

Is CDHC the miracle elixir that will cure the ailments of the American health care system? That is the subject of this book. It is not my intention to confirm or refute the claims of CDHC advocates. Rather, I intend to demonstrate the ineluctable complexity of what they attempt to simplify.

CDHC advocates begin with certain beliefs and stories — about the nature of human beings, economies, health care, and health care systems — and on the basis of these beliefs and stories propose a simple explanation of what is wrong with our health care system and a simple proposal to fix it. My contention is that their beliefs are contestable, their stories debatable, their empirical claims questionable, and their solutions at best partial.

Consumers do have a role to play in our health care system, and it is an important role. CDHC advocates offer useful ideas about how to engage consumers more effectively in addressing cost and quality issues in health care. They call for greater price transparency and more and better information on health care quality, for example. But providers also have an important contribution to make in solving the problems of our health care system, as do insurers. Above all, government must play a major role in solving problems, because only government can assure that all have access to health care.

Designing a Health Care System

In the final chapter of this book I suggest what I think a broader solution to the problems of our health care system could look like. But let us begin with basics. How does one begin designing a system to finance health care? What issues must be addressed? There are four primary considerations that one must take into account in building a health care financing system.

First, there is the remarkably skewed nature of health care costs. In any given year, a very small proportion of the population accounts for a very high proportion of health care costs: 1 percent of the population accounts for 27 percent of health care costs, 5 percent for 55 percent of health care costs, and 10 percent for nearly 70 percent of health care costs (Berk and Monheit 2001, 12). Half of the population, on the other hand, uses virtually no health care services, accounting for only 3 percent of the costs of health care. This skewed distribution holds not just for the population generally but for segments of the population, such as the employed and the elderly. Over a period of several years, and certainly over a lifetime, the distribution of costs becomes considerably less skewed. Individuals who incur high costs in one year may cost little two or three years later and vice versa. Even over a lifetime, however, significant discrepancies remain between some individuals who incur the highest costs and others who incur considerably lower costs (Roos, Shapiro, and Tate 1989).

It is difficult at any one time to predict precisely which individuals are going to fall at which point on the cost distribution scale. Generally persons with chronic diseases and the elderly are more likely to incur high costs than those who are young and healthy, but we all know that in an instant a life can be changed by an auto or skiing accident, and that apparently healthy people can fall victim to heart attacks or cancer and suddenly face catastrophic costs. We are all to a greater or lesser degree at risk.

The way we normally deal with capricious catastrophic risk is by purchasing insurance, and it is not surprising that in all developed countries health insurance, public or private, is ubiquitous. But in designing a health insurance system choices must be made: Should insurance be public or private? If it is public, should it be designed on a national health insurance or a social insurance model? If private, should premiums be community rated, or based on past or projected future experience? Is the goal of insurance to make everyone carry his or her own weight — is insurance essentially a form of savings, to even out the cost of health care over an individual's life? Alternatively, is insurance a means of sharing risk widely across a society? Is the goal of health insurance social solidarity?

These choices must take into account that the incidence of health care costs is to some extent predictable, a fact that encourages gaming on the part of both insureds and insurers. On the one hand, there is the well-known phenomenon of adverse selection: persons who have reason to believe that they are about to incur high health care costs are much more likely to purchase insurance than those who expect continued good health. This poses serious problems for private health insurers if the law requires them to accept all applicants and charge the same rate to all. On the other hand, if insurers are permitted to refuse coverage or to charge very high premiums to persons with medical problems, insurance may be unavailable to those most in need of it.

Second, there is the problem of the affordability of health care. Most of us pay for the majority of the goods and services that we consume — food, clothing, shelter, entertainment, transportation — from current income. When we purchase high-cost items such as homes or automobiles, we either save or borrow, or both. When we simply cannot afford something, we do without. Most (although not all) Americans can pay for routine health care — dental checkups, occasional primary care visits, new eyeglasses — out of current income. But few Americans are capable of covering very high-cost health care services such as heart transplants or chemotherapy for cancer out of current income (see chapter 1). One could attempt to save up for health care services. In fact, this is a central proposal of the CDHC movement. But unless a patient has accumulated a lifetime of savings, covering truly high-cost health care will be difficult. Finally, persons who need health care services could in theory borrow the money to pay for it, and recent research on consumer bankruptcy reveals that many Americans do so. Medical debt is one of the leading causes of bankruptcy in the United States, and much of this debt is hidden in credit card debt or home equity loans (Himmelstein, Warren, Thorne, and Woolhandler 2005). But borrowing for health care seems less realistic when we consider that health care costs are disproportionately borne by people who are disabled from gainful employment or who are nearing the end of life and thus are not good credit risks. Moreover, it would be difficult to obtain a security interest in most health care interventions (do you rip out the stitches if the patient doesn't make her payments?). Borrowing is not going to solve the problem of affordability.[3]

Again, insurance commends itself as the solution to this problem as well. When health insurance was introduced in the United States in the 1930s, it was sold as prepayment for health care, a means of saving ahead for future needs. Because health insurance pools risk, as well as allowing the accumulation of funds to cover risk, it solves the problem of high-end users who are not in a position, even over a lifetime, to save enough to cover their costs. Insurance also takes care of those who because of their health status are not in a position to borrow money to pay for health care. CDHC advocates almost all recognize that saving and borrowing are not an adequate solution to the problem of very high-cost care, and that catastrophic insurance is necessary to supplement HSAS.

But experience-rated insurance (with premiums based on the claims experience of the insured) will almost certainly be unaffordable to many of those who need it most, and even community-rated insurance (with all insureds charged more or less the same premium) will be unaffordable to many. Indeed, community-rated insurance may be even less affordable than experience-rated insurance to young, healthy individuals and families, because their premiums must be increased to cover the expenses of the unhealthy. It is an unfortunate fact that in our current global market, workers in the United States must compete with workers in India and China. This is particularly true for workers lacking education and special skills. In 2006 the average employer-sponsored health insurance policy in the United States cost $11,480 a year (Kaiser Family Foundation / Health Research and Educational Trust 2006, 1). Someone earning the legal minimum wage in the United States and working forty hours a week would earn $10,712 in a year. An employer who offers an average health insurance policy to an employee working for minimum wage must pay more for the policy than it pays in wages. Individual insurance policies tend to cost less, but their benefits are usually much less generous and they commonly include high cost sharing (America's Health Insurance Plans 2005b). If any significant cost sharing (coinsurance, co-payments, or deductibles) is imposed upon low-income workers, even insured services may become unaffordable.

Because health insurance is so expensive, every developed country makes available publicly subsidized health insurance, at least to some low-income people. Every country recognizes, at least implicitly, that access to health care is important, and should not be denied simply on the basis of income.

The third inescapable reality that the architects and administrators of every health care system must worry about is the supply side; they must figure out how to organize and pay for the delivery of health care products and services. In most sectors of the economy, the supply side takes care of itself (as does, for that matter, the demand side). A few industries, such as public utilities, are considered natural monopolies, and in many other industries some level of scrutiny under the antitrust laws is needed to forestall combinations in restraint of trade. But throughout most of the economy, businesses themselves determine their form of organization and set their own prices. In health care, however, organization of the supply side presents particularly difficult problems.

We have just noted that the natural response to the skewed nature of health care costs is health insurance, while the obvious response to the high cost of private health insurance is public health insurance. Even in the United States, the government pays for almost half of all health care, and in most countries the public share of health care costs is much higher. But if government is paying for health care, the obvious question is whether it should "make or buy." In many countries (including the United States), government runs some health care facilities. Private insurers can also own or employ health care providers, and in the United States some health maintenance organizations (HMOs), such as the Kaiser-Permanente system, do so.

It is common throughout the world, however, for insurers, public or private, to purchase services from professionals and institutional providers rather than to own or employ them. In particular, primary care providers, doctors, optometrists and opticians, and pharmacists usually work in the private sector. Drugs and devices are also almost universally provided privately, as are the services of alternative and complementary medical providers. Public and private insurers must therefore figure out how to pay for their services. Are services purchased on a fee-for-service, fee-per-case, capitation, or negotiated budget basis, or some combination? Each approach to payment creates its own incentives, and each offers opportunities and problems.

Another issue is how to produce enough information about the cost and quality of medical products and services to permit their efficient purchase. Regardless of who pays for services and products, enough must be known about them for an appropriate payment rate to be set or negotiated. Accurate information is also needed to make sure that products and services purchased are worth their cost.

Fourth and finally, every health care finance system must struggle with the problem classically called moral hazard. By its very nature, insurance dramatically lowers the price of health care to the immediate consumer. Absent cost sharing, insurance lowers the price of health care to zero. The demand for a valued good or service that is offered wholly without cost, however, could expand infinitely. If the only cost of health care services is the time and discomfort incurred in consuming them, the demand for health care products and services is potentially very large. Moral hazard is a problem with respect to virtually all kinds of insurance (and indeed is an issue whenever the possibility exists for the costs of production or consumption to be externalized — that is, for someone other than the consumer to be incurring them). But it is in particular a problem with respect to health insurance because the need for many health care services is determined by professionals who also provide the services. There is, therefore, considerable opportunity in health care for providers to induce demand for their own services. If these services are free to consumers, however, consumers have no reason to constrain their use of services. They will also have no reason to question the prices charged for services. Indeed, physicians are likely to not discuss prices with patients (and perhaps not even to know or to consider the prices of the services that they recommend).

While insured services are free to consumers, however, insurers must still pay market prices for them. If consumers do not constrain the utilization and price of health care products and services, there is a danger that the costs paid by insurers for health care will expand uncontrollably. But if insurers attempt to constrain demand either through their own utilization controls or through provider incentives, it is likely that rationing will result, either by the insurers, the providers, or both. Moreover, if health care is free, consumers may forgo taking measures like eating properly, exercising, and refraining from smoking, knowing that insurance will always pay to repair the damage later after they experience the health consequences of their bad behavior.

Health policy experts generally agree that moral hazard is a problem, but disagree as to how serious a problem it is. Some experts believe that it is not a major problem. People rarely consume health care services unless they really need them. Other experts believe that the real problem is not consumer demand but rather demand induced by providers, and that there are ways of controlling this short of imposing cost sharing on consumers. Still others believe that insurance-induced demand is a problem, but that cost sharing, at least if it exceeds certain limits, is more of a problem than a solution because it discourages low-income patients from getting adequate care. Finally, some argue that cost sharing can discourage low-cost preventive or primary care, necessitating more expensive care later once medical conditions get out of hand.

A significant, and currently growing, body of expert opinion in the United States and elsewhere regards moral hazard as the central problem in health care finance policy. This concern is largely founded on economic theory. If one believes that economics completely explains human behavior, the existence of excess demand in the face of full insurance is as inescapable as the fact that apples fall when dropped. Concern about moral hazard, moreover, also finds support in empirical evidence. Most notably, the RAND health insurance experiment in the early 1970s — the most ambitious controlled trial ever conducted of health care finance — is generally interpreted as supporting the notion that full insurance leads to wasteful consumption of health care services. Further, the experience of other countries, particularly Singapore and South Africa, with medical savings accounts is cited as further evidence that increased cost sharing is very effective in controlling health care costs. The theory and empirical evidence behind the consumer-driven movement will be discussed in chapters 7 and 8.

Each of these four issues — skewed costs, affordability, supply-side organization and payment, and moral hazard — must be acknowledged by any nation designing a health care finance system. The kind of system with which a country ends up will depend to a considerable extent on which issue it decides is most important. CDHC advocates are clear about what they see as central: the problem of moral hazard. They begin with the problem of moral hazard and the need for consumer cost sharing. They recognize the problem of skewed costs and therefore accept the need for catastrophic insurance. Some CDHC advocates, in particular Regina Herzlinger, are very much concerned about the supply side. Much of Herzlinger's writing is concerned with how to organize and provide information about providers to make a consumer-driven system work. But most consumer-driven health care advocates are concerned primarily with getting the demand side incentives right and believe that the supply side will largely take care of itself. Finally, most consumer-driven advocates recognize that some kind of government program is needed to assure access for those who cannot afford insurance, though many believe this to be a fairly insignificant problem.

Most health care systems of the world begin with the first issue listed above, recognizing the need for insurance to counter the skewed nature of health care costs. They continue, however, quickly and decisively to the second issue: the need to make health care affordable for all. They recognize that public insurance is necessary to solve this problem for many people. Every country has a different approach toward how to provide public insurance and how to supplement it with private insurance or out-of-pocket payments. But all countries other than the United States make sure that everyone is covered for at least basic medical services, and most do so through programs that are not limited to the poor. Each country reaches its own resolution of the problem of how to organize and deliver health care products and services, and finally, each addresses to some extent the problem of moral hazard. Most countries impose some user fees for some services, and almost all rely on private payment for the services most at risk of moral hazard, such as cosmetic surgery and nonessential dental work. Many also attempt to remedy the problem of provider-induced demand, either through payment incentives or some form of utilization review. But in most countries moral hazard is viewed as a secondary issue. There is greater concern with the barriers that user fees pose to access to health care than with the costs that they deter.

I will disclose at the outset that I also begin with the problem of health care affordability. I believe that all people should have access to basic health care products and services regardless of their ability to pay. I arrive at this position because of the teachings of my faith — I am a Christian — but many religious faiths and philosophies also support the notion of equality of opportunity and generosity to the poor. I take all four problems seriously, however. None, including the problem of moral hazard, is trivial. This book is an exploration, therefore, of how to understand the problems facing our own American health care system and how the incredible complexity of each of the four issues outlined above should be confronted in solving those problems.

I begin in the next chapter by describing the problems that plague the American health care system. Chapter 2 presents the CDHC solution to this problem, while chapter 3 explores the beliefs and stories on which the CDHC approach is based. Chapters 4, 5, and 6 are historical, describing first America's earlier experiences with CDHC, then how and why we ended up with an employment-based health insurance system (which CDHC advocates by and large reject), and finally, the history of the CDHC movement. Chapters 7 and 8 examine and critique first the economic theory and then the empirical evidence on which CDHC is based. Chapter 9 explores the legal and ethical ramifications of CDHC. Chapter 10 considers how other countries organize their health care systems, exploring alternatives to CDHP. Finally, chapter 11 concludes with a proposal for reorganizing our American health care system, incorporating CDHC but recognizing its limitations.

I would like to thank all of those who helped me write this book: Timothy Diette, Peter Hammer, and John Nyman, who read parts of earlier drafts; James Knight, John Goodman, Haavi Morreim, Mark Hall, Caleb Alexander, Ted Marmor, Evan Malhado, and Pat Butler, who contributed helpful ideas; Lindsay Swift, my research assistant, who spent endless hours editing and formatting; Vera Mencer, my omnicompetent secretary; Linda Newell, who found every source I requested, no matter how obscure; and John Doyle, who helped find references. I thank Fred Kameny of Duke University Press for excellent editing. I thank the Frances Lewis Law Center and the Robert L. Willett family for financial support. I gratefully acknowledge permission from the *Wake Forest Law Review* to use material from "Our Broken Health Care System and How to Fix It: An Essay on Health Law and Policy," which included an earlier version of chapters 1 and 11. Finally, I thank Ruth, Jacob, Micah, and David, who put up with me through a year when, frankly, I was pretty grouchy much of the time.

CHAPTER 1

Our Broken American Health Care System

Criteria to Judge a Health Care System

The consumer-driven movement has been able to gain purchase as a policy initiative because of a widespread consensus that our health care system is in desperate straits and in need of a radical change. This chapter examines the problems plaguing our health care system to which the consumer-driven movement offers a solution. Chapter 2 lays out the consumer-driven solution, and later chapters examine the appropriateness of that solution to our problems. I will revisit the problems examined here in chapter 10, which compares the performance of the American health care system with the systems of other countries. When placed in a comparative light, the performance of the American system is even more distressing. Recognizing that there will be some overlap between these chapters, I begin by considering our own system in isolation.

Most health care policy experts identify three touchstones by which the health care systems of countries should be evaluated: access, cost, and quality (European Economic and Social Committee 2004). First, do all those within the system have access to health care when they need it? Second, is health care available at reasonable cost given the resources of a nation, and are increases in the cost of health care from year to year kept to reasonable levels? Third, is the health care of acceptable quality? Does it achieve the best possible outcomes, and are avoidable errors kept to a minimum?

Judged by each of these standards, the health care system of the United States fails dramatically. First, by one recent count nearly forty-seven million Americans lack health insurance, and the number is growing (DeNavas-Walt, Proctor, and Lee 2006, 20). Of course not all of the uninsured lack access to all necessary health care, but many face severe access limitations. Even many who do have insurance still experience serious difficulties in affording needed health care products and services. Second, the cost of our health care system is now approaching $2 trillion, or 16 percent of our gross domestic product, and is growing at unsustainable rates (Catlin, Cowan, Heffler, Washington, and National Health Accounts Team 2007, 143). Finally, the quality of American health care is seriously deficient. One example is the conclusion by the Institute of Medicine that from 44,000 to 98,000 Americans die every year from medical errors (Institute of Medicine 2001b, 1). In sum, the American health care system is in trouble.

There are other criteria by which a health care system can be judged. One of these, given particular emphasis by CDHC advocates, is freedom of choice. Another criterion might be whether patients are treated with respect; whether, for example, they are allowed to make decisions with respect to their own health care and whether their medical information is kept private. Yet another criterion is whether the system encourages innovative research regarding medical problems, their causes and cures, and whether it stimulates the creation of new medical products and procedures. Judged by some of these criteria the American health care system does reasonably well; judged by others, it scores rather poorly.

This chapter examines the performance of the American health care system with respect to each of these criteria, focusing first on the central concerns of access, cost, and quality. Readers already familiar with the problems of the American health care system may wish to skip this chapter. But because CDHC advocates minimize the seriousness of the problem of access to health care, which they do not convincingly address, and because they only partially address other problems that plague the American health care system, it is necessary to fully explore the seriousness of these problems before moving on to the CDHC prescriptions.

Access: The Forty-six Million Uninsured

In 2005, according to estimates by the Census Bureau, 46.6 million Americans lacked health insurance at some point (DeNavas-Walt, Proctor, and Lee 2006, 20).[1] This number has grown significantly over the past half-decade, as employer-sponsored coverage has declined dramatically and public coverage has not expanded quickly enough to fill the void (Holahan and Cook 2005, W5-499–W5-502).[2] The number of the uninsured is likely to grow to 56 million by 2013 (Gilmer and Kronick 2005, W5-148). This is the most serious problem facing the American health care system, and a problem that CDHC largely ignores.

To get an accurate perspective on the problem of health insurance in the United States, however, one needs a movie, not a snapshot. If one examines the phenomenon of un-insurance over time, one sees that many more people — almost 82 million, or one-third of all non-elderly Americans — were uninsured at some point during 2002 and 2003 (Families USA 2004, 3).[3] One also sees a very dynamic picture — people moving from private to public insurance, from public to private insurance, or among private insurers; people lacking insurance for long periods, perhaps the entire two years; and people uninsured for a single short period, or for repeated short periods (Short and Graefe 2003, 247–49). Most of those uninsured at any one time have been uninsured for a year or more (over 80 percent according to one survey), and many of those currently insured were uninsured during the previous year — sixteen million according to one survey (Collins, Davis, Doty, Kriss, and Holmgren 2006, 4–5).

Although health policy discussions commonly draw a bright line between the insured and the uninsured, the ultimate issue is access to health care, not insurance. The degree of difficulty experienced in gaining access to health care varies tremendously among both the insured and the uninsured. Just because a person is uninsured does not mean that he has no access to health care. But neither does the mere fact that one is insured mean that one can gain access to health care without difficulty or undue expense. It is necessary, therefore, to examine in greater detail the experience of both the uninsured and the privately and publicly insured.

About 80 percent of uninsured Americans are either employed or in the household of someone who is employed (Glied 2001, 91).[4] Most American employers offer health insurance, although many, particularly small businesses, do not (Kaiser Family Foundation / Health Research and Educational

Trust 2006, sec. 2, p. 1). But most of the employed uninsured do not have health insurance available from their place of employment. Many are low-wage, part-time, or seasonal employees or work for very small businesses (Institute of Medicine 2001a, 60–62, 67–70; Fronstin 2006b).[5] Other uninsured people are in fact eligible for health benefits at their place of employment, but decline the offer rather than pay the employee's share of premiums.[6]

Many uninsured Americans are otherwise disadvantaged. The uninsured tend disproportionately to be drawn from minority groups — especially Hispanics.[7] Uninsured adults are also more likely than the insured to report fair or poor health (Graves and Long 2006, 3). Most uninsured persons have very low incomes: 25 percent are from households with incomes below the poverty level, and 54 percent from households with incomes below 200 percent of the poverty level (Cover the Uninsured Week 2006).

The picture is complicated, however. For example, 17 percent of America's uninsured are from households that earn $75,000 a year or more (Cover the Uninsured Week 2006). As an increasing number of Americans have become independent contractors, consultants, contingent or temporary employees, and "1099 workers," and as whole industries have moved away from a traditional full-time employment model, many of the uninsured are middle- or upper-class Americans who simply do not have access to traditional employment-related insurance (Schwartz 2004, 18–28). Yet others are reasonably well off but temporarily between jobs.[8] Very few, however, choose to be uninsured because they believe insurance to be unimportant. In one recent survey, 1 percent of non-elderly adults reported having "no need for insurance," while most others polled reported primarily the high cost of insurance (54 percent) or job-related reasons, such as loss of employment (41 percent), for being uninsured (Graves and Long 2006, 4).

Many of the uninsured are young people who have not yet entered the employment market or who are working at low-wage jobs. During the period from 1996 to 2000, two-thirds of young adults aged nineteen to twenty-three went without insurance coverage at some point, and almost a quarter were uninsured for more than two years. (Collins, Schoen, Kriss, Doty, and Mahato 2006, 4). Young adults are often healthy, but many are not. Three and a half million women aged nineteen to twenty-nine become pregnant every year, one-third of HIV diagnoses are made among young adults, and traumatic injuries requiring emergency room visits are much more common among young adults than among children or older adults. When offered health insurance, nearly three-quarters of employed young adults take it up (Collins, Schoen, Kriss, Doty, and Mahato 2006, 5–7).

A significant proportion of older Americans are also uninsured. More than half of adults aged fifty to sixty-four in households earning less than $25,000 have been uninsured at some time since turning fifty. More than one-third of older adults in working households either have had a problem with a medical bill in the past twelve months or are paying off accrued medical debt (Zeldin and Rukavina 2007; Collins, Davis, Schoen, Doty, and Kriss 2006, viii).

Many of the uninsured (particularly children) are eligible for Medicaid or for their state's SCHIP program, but are not enrolled. Bureaucratic barriers, including burdensome application procedures, frequent and onerous redeterminations, and lack of enrollment education efforts on the part of the states, discourage enrollment (Mann and Westmoreland 2004, 416, 419). Some potentially eligible people would rather not identify themselves to the government. The onerous proof-of-citizenship requirements recently adopted in the Deficit Reduction Act of 2005 are likely to increase further the rolls of the uninsured. In some states, moreover, certain categories of persons potentially eligible for Medicaid are not covered unless they are desperately poor (Kaiser Family Foundation 2005b).

The experience of being uninsured varies. Healthy middle-aged executives who are temporarily between jobs may also get by without any ill effects. But even higher-income uninsured Americans suffer. They are significantly less likely than insured Americans to receive recommended medical services (Ross, Bradley, and Busch 2006, 2032–33). They often run into financial trouble because of medical costs. One recent study of uninsured persons found that problems with medical bills and debt were most frequent among those with higher incomes. Almost half of working-age adults with incomes of $40,000 or more who had been uninsured at some time in the previous year reported problems with medical debt or bills (Collins, Davis, Schoen, Doty, and Kriss 2006, ix).

The "insured," on the other hand, are also far from monolithic. At the one extreme, employees of large employers still covered by collective bargaining agreements may have first-dollar medical coverage through a preferred provider organization (PPO) with a comprehensive network and no requirements for utilization review, supplemented by pharmaceutical, dental, and vision coverage with minimal cost sharing, as well as a flexible spending account (FSA) or health reimbursement account (HRA) to cover any costs not otherwise covered. At the other extreme, individuals and families insured in the nongroup (individual) market may have deductibles as high as $10,000, co-insurance as high as 50 percent, co-payments of $200 a day for hospital coverage, exclusions for preexisting conditions, and no coverage for mental health, maternity, or prenatal care (America's Health Insurance Plans 2005b, 11, 13, 17, 26). Adults in the nongroup market are at much higher risk for high financial burden than those with group coverage or public insurance (Shen and McFeeters 2006, 207–8). The Tonik "thrill-seeker" plan offered by Blue Cross of California covers four physician visits a year, has a deductible of $5,000 and an emergency room co-payment of $100, and covers only generic drugs. An uninsured person in an area with a good safety-net system may in fact have better access to health care than an "insured" person with this level of exposure.[9] The access difficulties experienced by low-income, privately insured persons are quite similar to those experienced by Medicaid recipients (Coughlin, Long, and Shen 2005, 1081–82).

In between these extremes are many people insured through HMOs or PPOs with limited networks of available providers, significant gaps in coverage, and high cost-sharing obligations. Deductibles and co-payments have increased dramatically in recent years, and additional forms of cost sharing, such as separate deductibles for hospital care, are becoming common (Kaiser Family Foundation / Health Research and Educational Trust 2006, sec. 7, pp. 1–2). Recent research has demonstrated that a significant number of Americans experience serious financial problems because of health care expenses, and that most of them are insured. Nearly two-fifths of Americans report serious problems paying for their own or their family's medical care, including half of Americans earning less than $50,000 a year (Schoen, How, Weinbaum, Craig, and Davis 2006, 6, 7). One-third of working-age adults are either paying off accrued medical debt or have had medical bill problems in the previous year, and three-fifths of these were insured (Collins, Davis, Schoen, Doty, and Kriss 2006, viii). Nearly three in ten adults report that there was a time in the preceding year when they did not have enough money to pay for medical care; 62 percent of these were insured (USA Today / Kaiser Family Foundation / Harvard School of Public Health 2005). Many Americans have credit card debt attributable to medical expenses (Zeldin and Rukavina 2007). Some lose their homes when they cannot pay off home equity loans they have taken out to cover their medical debt, or find themselves unable to rent apartments because their credit rating has been ruined by medical debt. About half of all bankruptcies have some medical cause (Himmelstein, Warren, Thorne, and Woolhandler 2005). Most bankrupts with medical debts are insured.

Disparities in the extent of insurance coverage would not matter so much if third-party health care financing were not so necessary for getting health care in the United States. In general the uninsured get less health care than the insured, and get it later, when it is often less effective (Wolman and Miller 2004, 399–400). Because of the Emergency Medical Treatment and Active Labor Act (EMTALA), it is possible for even the uninsured to gain access to emergency care in the United States without health insurance (Furrow, Greaney, Johnson, Jost, and Schwartz 2000, 512–23). Care provided under EMTALA is not free, however, and some choose to forgo it rather than incur further medical debt. It is much more difficult, moreover, to gain access to preventive or primary care or care for chronic conditions than it is to get emergency care. Over one quarter of uninsured adults with chronic medical conditions reported no visits to health professionals in the twelve months preceding a recent survey (Urban Institute / University of Maryland 2005, 4). One-quarter of Americans with below-average incomes have to wait six days or more to see a doctor when sick, compared to only 13 percent of Americans with above-average incomes (Huynh, Schoen, Osborn, and Holmgren 2006, 7). Among uninsured Americans of working age, 60 percent report not filling a prescription, not seeing a specialist when needed, skipping a medical test or treatment, or not seeing a doctor for medical problems because of lack of insurance (Collins, Davis, Schoen, Doty, and Kriss 2006, 9). Americans with medical debt are also much less likely to get needed medical care than those who do not have problems with medical debt (Doty, Edwards, and Holmgren 2005).

Not surprisingly, the uninsured suffer higher morbidity and mortality. An estimated eighteen thousand adults die prematurely every year from lack of insurance (Institute of Medicine 2004, 8). Even those who are insured for part of the year receive much worse care than those continuously insured in terms of delayed care, unmet medical needs, and unfilled prescriptions (Olson, Tang, and Newacheck 2005). It is also clear that the uninsured get less health care not by choice, and not because they fail to perceive the need for care—the uninsured understand that they need care to the same extent as the insured do, but they are half as likely to get it (Hadley and Cunningham 2005, 1–2).

Not only individuals suffer from lack of insurance: families and communities suffer as well (Institute of Medicine 2002b; Institute of Medicine 2003b). The financial problems of the uninsured are even worse than those of the population generally as described above. More than half of those adults who have been uninsured at any time in the preceding year report medical debt problems, and 40 percent of those currently uninsured with medical debt problems have difficulty paying for basic necessities because of medical bill problems. Half have used up all their savings, 11 percent have taken out a mortgage or loan to pay for medical debt, and almost a quarter have taken on credit card medical debt (Collins, Davis, Schoen, Doty, and Kriss 2006, 7; Seifert and Rukavina 2006). Hospitals in communities with high rates of non-insurance offer fewer services to vulnerable populations and have worse financial margins (Wolman and Miller 2004, 401–2). Even higher-income residents of areas with high levels of noninsurance suffer — from overcrowded emergency rooms or deterioration of the health care infrastructure (Institute of Medicine 2003b, 82–119). Indeed, the entire country loses because of the diminished productivity of those whose diseases and disabilities go untreated for lack of health insurance.[10]

As bad as our disparities are, they seem to be getting worse. The number of the uninsured is growing much more rapidly among the poor than among those relatively well off (Holahan and Cook 2005, W5-500–W5-501). High-end, private health insurance plans continue to improve access and service for their members, emphasizing specialized and technical care, improved quality, and consumer service, while at the same time Medicaid coverage and safety-net services are deteriorating, particularly with respect to coverage for mental illness and pharmaceuticals (Hurley, Pham, and Claxton 2005). Health care is local, and disparities in some localities are worse than in others. But across the entire United States lack of access is a very serious health policy problem, and it is getting worse.

Cost: The Two-Trillion-Dollar Health Care Bill

In 2005, the last year for which cost data are more or less complete, we spent $2 trillion on health care. This amounts to $6,697 per person (Catlin, Dowan, Heffler, Washington, and National Health Accounts Team 2007, 143). We spend more on health care than we do on anything else — more than we spend on food, more than we spend on housing, more than we spend on transportation (Blue Cross Blue Shield Association 2006, 7). As is examined further in chapter 10, we also spend far more on health care than any other country. Moreover, the cost of health care is steadily increasing. From 2000 to 2004 the cost of health care increased at an average annual rate of about 7.9 percent, causing the proportion of GDP attributable to health care to grow from 13.8 percent in 2000 to 16 percent in 2005 (Catlin, Cowan, Heffler, Washington, and National Health Accounts Team 2007, 143). Under current projections, the cost of health care will grow by 2013 to $3.36 trillion, or 18.4 percent of GDP (Heffler, Smith, Keehan, Clemens, Zezza, and Truffer 2004, W4-80). Why do we pay so much for health care? This question is best answered by comparing our experience with those of other countries, a topic that will be taken up in chapter 10.

Is the high and growing cost of health care a problem? Although we spend more of our GDP on health care than other countries do, other countries spend more on housing and food than we do, yet we do not necessarily perceive those countries as having food or housing crises. Just as we spend more of our GDP on health care than we did twenty years ago, we spend more on computers than we did twenty years ago, but we do not believe that we are facing a computer crisis.

And although health care is expensive, it is also very valuable. In *Your Money or Your Life* (2004), David Cutler argues convincingly that the benefits of our improved ability to alleviate cardiovascular problems and to preserve the lives of low–birth weight babies dramatically outweigh the cost of the interventions. Improvements in our ability to treat mental illness and to replace worn-out hip and knee joints have significantly increased the quality of life for many Americans. The high prices that we pay for health care encourage investment in new technologies (Garber, Jones, and Romer 2006), which have dramatically expanded the length and quality of life for many people. Our health care system is very costly, but arguably its benefits greatly exceed its costs.[11]

Nonetheless, the high and rapidly growing cost of American health care is troubling. First, the rapid growth in health care costs is one of the primary causes of the increasing lack of access to health care. Historically, most Americans have received health insurance through their place of employment. Economists agree that because the cost of insurance is passed along to employees in the form of lower wages, in effect it is the employees rather than the employers who pay for health insurance, at least in the long run (Pauly 1997). But the amount that the employer pays for health benefits, when added to the cost of other employment benefits and of wages, cannot in the long run exceed the value of the employee's labor. As health care costs have increased, therefore, some employers have eliminated health insurance coverage as an employee benefit. In 2005 only 60 percent of employers offered health benefits to their employers, down from 69 percent in 2000, with most of the loss among small employers (Fronstin 2006b, 3). Three-quarters of the employers who do not offer health insurance cite the high cost of health insurance as the reason for their failure to do so (Kaiser Family Foundation / Health Research and Educational Trust 2006, sec. 2, p. 9).

Many employers, moreover, have increased the amount that employees must pay for health insurance premiums and the amount of cost sharing that employees must bear, making insurance policies both more expensive and less valuable to their employees. This trend has led to an ever-increasing share of employees who decline insurance coverage offered by their employers. Those who lose employment-based coverage usually become uninsured altogether.

The cost of health insurance has also led to a decline in the number of employers offering retirement benefits.[12] In 1988 66 percent of all large firms offered retiree benefits; today only 33 percent do (Kaiser Family Foundation 2005b). This in turn has led to higher levels of noninsurance among retirees who are not yet eligible for Medicare, and to higher out-of-pocket expenditures for Medicare beneficiaries.

Second, high and rising health care costs also put public programs under stress. Over 45 percent of health care in the United States is now paid for by public programs (Catlin, Cowan, Heffler, Washington, and National Health Accounts Team 2007, 146). Even though public insurance (Medicare and, for those with low incomes, Medicaid) covers the elderly and the disabled in the United States — a much more expensive population to insure than the working-age population — public insurance payments have grown at about the same rate as private insurance premiums. Medicare spending, for example, increased at an average annual rate of 8.9 percent from 1970 to 2004, while private health insurance premiums increased at a rate of 9.9 percent (Kaiser Family Foundation 2005b). But as our population continues to age, the public contribution to health care costs is likely to increase. We will thus have to come up with more public money to fund the programs, or dramatically cut them.

Yet the financial sources that we rely on for our public programs are problematic. Medicare Part A (institutional care insurance) is financed on a pay-as-you-go basis through payroll taxes. Over the next few decades, as baby boomers retire, the share of the population that is in the labor force and paying those taxes is likely to decrease relative to the population that is receiving benefits, increasing the burden on workers subject to payroll taxes (Board of Trustees 2006). Part of the cost of Medicaid (our program for the poor), on the other hand, is covered by state taxes. Medicaid is a counter-cyclical program—its enrollment and thus its costs increase when the economy worsens, just as state tax revenues are in decline. Periodic Medicaid cost crises are thus almost certain.

Medicare Parts B (which funds professional services) and D (the drug program) and the federal Medicaid share are largely financed through the federal income tax. Though Americans of all political persuasions are pleased to receive money from the federal government, they have never been sold on Justice Holmes's aphorism that taxation is the price we pay for a civilized society, and identify more strongly with the libertarian assertion that taxation is theft. It is very difficult, therefore, to raise tax revenues to keep up with medical cost increases. The fundamental problem with publicly funded health care in the United States is that even if one accepts the assertion by Cutler (2004) that the value of health care exceeds its cost, the people receiving the value are not necessarily the same as those paying the cost. Those paying the cost are becoming increasingly restive.

Third, Americans pay for a great deal of health care out of pocket, and these expenses represent an increasing burden. Though only about 20 percent of medical expenses are paid out of pocket, because of the skewed nature of medical costs, most of the costs covered by insurance are attributable to high-cost individuals. The average American, who is not receiving high-cost health care, pays for 35 percent of medical costs out-of-pocket (Kaiser Family Foundation 2006b).[13] For 18 percent of Americans, health care is their second-largest expense after rent or mortgage payments (USA Today / Kaiser Family Foundation / Harvard School of Public Health 2005). If CDHC advocates get their way, this amount will increase dramatically. But Americans, insured as well as uninsured, are already experiencing serious problems because of medical debt and medical bills, as noted earlier. The high and growing cost of health care is therefore a real problem.

Quality: The 44,000 to 98,000 Deaths

The third leg of the health policy triangle is quality. While we have long known that Americans have worse access to health financing and pay more for health care than the residents of other countries do, we have still prided ourselves on having "the best health care system in the world."[14] Those who make this claim seem to be saying that we have the smartest doctors; the latest drugs, devices, and procedures; and the best-equipped and shiniest hospitals.

In fact, however, a series of studies over the past decade and a half, beginning with the Harvard study of hospitals in New York and culminating in the Institute of Medicine's reports *To Err Is Human* and *Crossing the Quality Chasm*, have revealed that the quality of our health care system is seriously deficient (Brennan, Leape, Laird, Hebert, Localio, Lawthers, et al. 1991; Leape, Brennan, Laird, Lawthers, Localio, Barnes, et al. 1991; Institute of Medicine 2000; Institute of Medicine 2001b). *To Err Is Human* reached the startling conclusion that from 44,000 to 98,000 Americans die every year from medical errors, more than die of breast cancer, AIDS, or automobile accidents (Institute of Medicine 2001b, 1). This report, and many others like it, amply document the failures of communication, coordination, and knowledge, and sometimes the sheer incompetence, that plague our health care system.

There is considerable evidence that health care products and services in the United States are overused, underused, and misused. There is tremendous variation in the use of medical procedures (Baicker, Chandra, Skinner, and Wennberg 2004). Specific procedures or drugs are used in situations where they have no demonstrated value (Merenstein, Daumit, and Powe 2006, 521–27; Fisher and Welch 1999). Demonstrably effective procedures, on the other hand, are not being used in situations where they clearly would be of value (Maciosek, Coffield, Edwards, Flottemesch, Goodman, and Solberg 2006). There is some evidence that we are making progress in improving the quality of health care, but progress is slow and much remains to be done (Agency for Healthcare Research and Quality 2005).

It is more difficult to identify a fundamental cause of our quality failures than it is to describe why we have problems with access and cost. Many analyses of the problem, however, including the Institute of Medicine reports, point to system and coordination deficiencies (Institute of Medicine 2001b, 4–9, 61–89). These coordination failures often occur within institutions, resulting, for example, in preventable medication errors that harm 1.5 million Americans a year and cost at least $3.5 billion for hospital medication errors alone (Institute of Medicine 2006, 2). Coordination failures also exist within the larger health care system, for example when a patient with a chronic disease is passed from one physician to another because the patient's employer has changed insurers and thus provider networks, or because the patient has changed employers and thus has to find a new physician in the new employer's physician network (Tai-Seale 2004, 508). The United States is lagging far behind other developed nations in implementing electronic health information technology that would facilitate better coordination among providers (Anderson, Frogner, Johns, and Reinhardt 2006, 822–29).

Incentives for improving the quality of care in the United States are rather weak. The system provides few incentives for taking a long-term approach to problems because it is based on short-term relationships — insurance contracts are written year to year. Thus there is little reason for an insurer to take steps that cost more now but might save money (or health) down the road, when the patient will in all likelihood no longer be its responsibility (Herzlinger ed. 2004, 31–32). In most parts of the United States it is difficult for consumers to find information that would allow them to identify the providers offering the highest quality of care (Federal Trade Commission / Department of Justice 2004, 25–27). Neither public nor private insurance programs do much to reward superior providers or punish inferior ones by "paying for performance" (Federal Trade Commission / Department of Justice 2004, 25–28).[15] We do have licensure, certification, and accreditation programs in place to ensure that professionals have the basic knowledge and providers the basic structural capacity to offer care of adequate quality (Jost 1988, 542–53, 582–87). These programs have not, however, been successful in assuring a high quality of care, nor are they designed to do so.[16] Clearly, if we do have the "best health care system in the world" (and no one knows whether this is true), it is not because the quality of our health care is particularly admirable, but rather because other nations are also struggling to get a handle on how to identify and to achieve a high quality of health care and how to avoid medical errors.

Choice, Respect, and Innovation: A Mixed Record

The American health care system offers a great deal of choice to some participants and much less choice to others. Medicare beneficiaries (elderly and disabled Americans) arguably have the greatest freedom of choice. Virtually all hospitals and the vast majority of doctors participate in the Medicare program (Medicare Payment Advisory Commission 2006, 80; Cunningham, Staiti, and Ginsburg 2006). Most Medicare beneficiaries have the choice of at least one Medicare Advantage managed care plan and two Part D prescription drug plans.

The most common form of private insurance coverage currently is the PPO, and while PPOs by definition encourage their members to use restricted provider networks, many PPOs have quite comprehensive networks, offering their members access to most hospitals, pharmacies, and physicians in their coverage area.[17] Health maintenance organizations (HMOs) and point of service (POS) plans offer more restricted networks and are also more likely to limit members' choice through pre-admission or pre-procedure screening or other utilization review requirements, but they too have become less restrictive over the past decade. Many larger employers also offer a choice of two or more employee benefit health plans, which broadens the menu of choices for insureds (Kaiser Family Foundation / Health Research and Educational Trust 2005, sec. 4, p. 2). This is much less common among small employers.

Because of low provider payment rates, many physicians do not participate in Medicaid, our federal and state health care program for the poor. In some states, Medicaid recipients must use emergency rooms for routine care because of the difficulty of otherwise getting access to medical care.[18] Poor persons who are uninsured are often very restricted as well in their choice of provider, limited to public facilities, to physicians or institutions that offer charity care, or to emergency rooms, which must accept all comers who are in fact experiencing a medical emergency.[19]

According to one recent survey, 81 percent of non-elderly adults with employer-sponsored insurance reported having at least "a fair amount" of choice of provider, compared to 70 percent of those with individual insurance, 64 percent of those with "public insurance" (primarily Medicaid), and 47 percent of the uninsured (Lambrew 2005, 2). Only 14 percent of the uninsured reported having "a great deal" of choice, compared to 35 percent of those with employer-sponsored insurance. Choice of provider correlates with both income and health status, with higher-income Americans and those in good health having more choice of provider than lower-income Americans or those in fair or poor health (Lambrew 2005, 2–3). Higher-income Americans are also more likely to have a choice of health plans, with almost 59 percent of Americans with annual incomes of $60,000 or more offered a choice of employer-sponsored insurance plans and only 37 percent of those with incomes of less than $20,000 reporting a choice of plans. A quarter of those who have little or no choice of provider report being dissatisfied with their health care, compared to only 4 percent of those with a great deal of choice (Lambrew 2005, 3).

Other factors limit choice of provider as well. Residents of rural areas have fewer provider choices than those who live in urban or suburban areas. On nights and weekends, most Americans have only the choice of the emergency department if they need to see a physician and cannot wait until morning (or Monday).[20] One quarter of adults with health problems report visiting the emergency department for treatment that could have been provided by a regular doctor had the doctor been available (Davis, Schoen, Schoenbaum, Audet, Doty, Holmgren, et al. 2006, 20). In fact, most adults who are frequent users of emergency departments are insured and have a usual source of care, but are in poor health (Hunt, Weber, Showstack, Colby, and Callaham 2006). On the whole, however, choice is uneven in the United States, and often related to economic status.

It is difficult to evaluate comprehensively how our health care system responds to patients. We have arguably made progress over the past half-century in involving patients in their own treatment through "informed consent," protecting the privacy and confidentiality of patient information, and allowing patients access to their own information. Patients and their families are much more closely involved in making end-of-life decisions, and medical professionals are more concerned about pain experienced by their patients.

On the other hand, survey data show that we have far to go. According to one recent survey, a quarter of patients left a doctor's appointment at some point in the two preceding years without getting important questions answered; half of patients reported that their regular doctor "rarely," "never," or only "sometimes" told them about their care and treatment options and asked for their opinions; over one-quarter reported that their regular doctor "rarely," "never," or only "sometimes" clarified specific goals for care and treatment, or gave clear instructions about their symptoms and about when to seek further care; a quarter reported that their doctor "rarely," "never," or only "sometimes" spent enough time with them; and three-quarters reported that they wanted but did not have access to their medical records (Davis, Schoen, Schoenbaum, Audet, Doty, Holmgren, et al. 2006, 18). Of the six nations included in the survey, the United States ranked last in patient-centeredness rankings.

The one criterion on which the United States scores the highest is in encouraging creativity and innovation. The United States has in recent years been the world leader in pharmaceutical innovation (Grabowski and Wang 2006). Our health-related research and development is fueled by massive federal investments, $27.6 billion in 2003.[21] Americans tend to be very supportive of medical research and optimistic about its possibilities, and have significantly greater confidence in science and research than Europeans do (National Science Board 2004, 7-22–7-29). New medical technology is not only created disproportionately in the United States, it is also adopted more quickly and pervasively in the United States than in most other countries (Anderson, Frogner, Johns, and Reinhardt 2006, 822). Lack of price controls, generous coverage policies, and vast public funding for basic research and for training of research scientists place the United States in the lead for innovation.

On the other hand, there is real controversy as to whether the high prices paid for pharmaceuticals and medical services are really necessary to encourage innovation. An enormous amount is spent by American pharmaceutical companies on marketing of debatable value.[22] And not all innovation is really progress, as recent experience with Vioxx and other highly advertised drugs makes clear (Spitz and Abramson 2005, 331–34). A great deal of money is wasted on new technologies and medicines of questionable effectiveness, and on the excessive and inappropriate use of new medical technologies (Deyo and Patrick 2005). In sum, while our health care system scores high on innovation, this may not be as much of an advantage as some advocates claim, and it does not justify our system's other serious deficiencies.

If one accepts that our health care system denies access to health care to too many Americans, costs too much, and is of uneven and often inadequate quality, and that its performance with respect to other values does not make up for these deficiencies, what is to be done? The CDHC movement has an answer, to which we turn next.

CHAPTER ⌈ 2 ⌋

The Consumer-Driven Prescription

The Diagnosis

CDHC has become to the middle of the first decade of the twenty-first century what managed care was to the 1980s and 1990s and health planning to the 1970s: the latest panacea that will solve the problems of the American health care system. The fundamental idea of CDHC is that patients can be turned into health care consumers if they can be compelled to pay a larger share of the costs of health care that they consume. This can be done by raising health insurance cost sharing, and in particular by raising deductibles to a high enough level that health insurance does not cover routine health care costs. If patients have to purchase health care with their own money, making the same trade-offs between cost and quality that they make in purchasing other products and services, they will only purchase health care if it is as valuable to them as other products and services. This will bring down the cost of health care while increasing consumer choice and improving health care quality.

CDHC advocates form a subgroup of a larger movement for greater market competition in health care, which has traditionally emphasized three strategies for strengthening markets in health care. The history of the movement is discussed in greater detail in chapter 5, and the strategies advocated by it will only be introduced briefly here.

One of the earliest contributions of the pro-market movement was to describe the suppression of competition in health care by providers and provider associations, aided and abetted by government regulation. The strategy called for by one group of advocates, therefore, is based on enforcement of the antitrust laws and deregulation to stimulate market competition (Friedman 1962; Kessel 1958; Kessel 1970; Havighurst and Goodman 1980).

The second market-based strategy is "managed competition." Advocates of managed competition call for organized competition among managed care plans to create a structured, competitive market for health insurance, which in turn, they contend, will bring down the cost and improve the quality of health care. Managed competition advocates argue that individuals can act most effectively as rational consumers when they are not in the throes of a health crisis, but rather can thoughtfully and at their leisure compare the cost and quality of care offered by competing alternative health plans offering sufficiently similar products to make comparison shopping possible. Forced to offer competitive packages and premiums, health plans will in turn control the practice of affiliated providers to hold down the cost and improve the quality of medical care. The managed competition strategy has been used successfully in the Federal Employees Health Benefits Program and was at the heart of the ill-fated Clinton Health Security Act, as well as of several largely unsuccessful efforts to introduce market competition into the Medicare program, the most recent of which is the Medicare Advantage program.

CDHC market advocates, by contrast, contend that the most effective point to introduce market competition into health care is at the moment when consumers decide whether to purchase particular health care items and services. Most of these advocates reject managed competition (some quite vehemently) as inefficient because it depends on government regulation for structuring markets and on managed care organizations rather than consumers for making purchasing decisions (Cannon and Tanner 2005, 38–40; Goodman, Musgrave, and Herrick 2004, 201–12; Herzlinger ed. 2004, 96–97). Indeed, some CDHC advocates reject managed care itself, claiming that it imposes private bureaucratic rationing in place of public rationing (Herzlinger 1997, 117–27).

CDHC is firmly rooted in a belief that moral hazard is the key problem in health policy, and more specifically that excess insurance is the primary driver of increasing health care costs (Pauly and Goodman 1995, 129). In this view, if we can simply strip away insurance, leaving the consumer to purchase health care out of his or her own pocket, competition for consumer dollars will control health care costs. People must make health care purchasing decisions just as they make purchasing decisions for everything else. Indeed, they must be prepared to trade off their preferences for health care against their preferences for all other consumer goods and services. If consumers are forced to make these decisions, providers and professionals, forced to compete seriously for the consumer dollar, will lower their prices and improve the quality of their services.[1] Physicians will become more conscious of the price of the services that they recommend and will discuss prices with consumers. Consumers, on the other hand, will buy only the number and intensity of products and services that they really need (or want, or can afford) and bargain for lower prices, thus bringing down health care utilization to the correct level (Goodman and Musgrave 1992, 29–31).

The ultimate solution to the problem of moral hazard — simply outlawing health insurance — is not embraced by even those most convinced that over-insurance is the heart of the health care cost problem. They understand the problem of catastrophic costs — of the skewed nature of health care costs that accounts for health insurance in the first place. Few people can afford to pay out of pocket for a heart transplant or for the services required to respond to the major traumatic injuries caused by a car accident.[2] Many of those afflicted with expensive chronic diseases would soon find themselves unable to afford further health care without health insurance (Druss, Marcus, Olfson, and Pincus 2002). Since many of these conditions are caused or aggravated by genetic or environmental factors, it is not fair to hold these persons solely responsible for their suffering, no matter how one may feel about individual as opposed to societal responsibility in other contexts. Bankruptcy solves the problems of some of those faced with enormous expenses and no insurance, but it deals with costs already incurred and does not assure ongoing care to the chronically ill. Bankruptcy, moreover, only shifts the costs of care to providers, who themselves may be financially unable to absorb the loss.[3]

Acknowledging the problems that would attend the elimination of health insurance, CDHC advocates rather call for limiting insurance to truly catastrophic cases through the imposition of high deductibles that would encourage consumers to make better purchasing decisions at the margin. Many also advocate coupling health savings accounts (HSAs) with high-deductible health insurance policies. They call for tax subsidies to cover contributions to the HSAs (whether they come from employers or employees), as well as payments for high-deductible health plans (Goodman and Musgrave 1994, 88–92).

They contend that HSAs will introduce point-of-purchase competition into health care and save the cost of claims processing, thus reducing total health care costs. At the same time, HSAs will assure that consumers have funds available to purchase health care, thus improving access, and encourage consumers to shop for better products and services, thus improving quality (Goodman and Musgrave 1992, 231–61).

The Program

Medical savings accounts were introduced onto the national health policy stage by the Health Insurance Portability and Accountability Act of 1996 (HIPAA), which granted tax subsidies to MSAs on a limited and experimental basis to determine whether they could live up to the promises of their supporters.[4] MSAs were also introduced on an experimental basis into Medicare by the Balanced Budget Act of 1997.[5] Even though both experiments were failures — no insurer has yet signed up for a Medicare MSA and few people signed up for the HIPAA MSAs[6] — Congress extended tax benefits to a much larger category of MSAs (rechristened "Health Savings Accounts," or HSAs) through the Medicare Modernization Act (MMA) in 2003.[7]

The MMA offers a tax exclusion to employers and a deduction to employees for funds contributed by an employer or employee to an HSA.[8] The HSA must, however, be coupled with a high-deductible health insurance plan (HDHP), and this plan must, as of 2007, have a deductible of at least $1,100 a year for a single individual or $2,200 a year for a family.[9] The catastrophic policies that accompany an HSA must also have caps on out-of-pocket expenditures, which cannot exceed $5,500 for an individual and $11,000 for a family (in 2007).[10] The tax subsidies for contributions to the HSA are limited to a fixed amount, adjusted annually for inflation, which for 2007 was $2,850 for individual coverage and $5,650 for family coverage.[11]

Money contributed to an HSA can be spent for "qualified medical expenses" without being subject to income tax,[12] but it is subject to both income tax and a 10 percent excise tax if spent for other purposes.[13] "Qualified medical expenses" are broadly defined, however, to include many things not covered by traditional health insurance, such as nonprescription drugs and transportation or lodging while away from home to receive medical care.[14] HSA expenditures are controlled only by very infrequent audits from the Internal Revenue Service, whose auditors have no particular health care expertise (U.S. Department of the Treasury 2005). It is likely, therefore, that HSA expenditures will be limited only by the imagination and good faith of their owners. If HSA funds are not spent for health care, they can be withdrawn for any purpose once the account holder dies, becomes disabled, or reaches the age of sixty-five.[15] HSA funds may continue to be withdrawn after the age of sixty-five for qualified medical expenses, including Medicare premiums, free from taxation.[16] If they are used for other purposes, withdrawals are taxed as income, but no penalties are attached. At the death of the HSA account holder, funds may be passed on to the owner's spouse, but others who inherit them must pay income tax on the funds received.[17]

The HSA has been joined by another new health savings device, the health reimbursement account, or HRA. The HRA was created not by a statute but rather by the Internal Revenue Service, which in, 2002 determined that existing legislation authorized the offer of tax subsidies for employer contributions to health savings vehicles fully funded by employers.[18] The HRA has proved attractive to employers because the accounts can be held as notional accounts and need not be fully funded, and because the funds in them also need not go with the employee if he or she leaves employment. The use of HSAs grew rapidly after enactment of the MMA. Whereas roughly 438,000 individuals were covered by HSAs in 2004, by early 2006 the number stood at over 3.2 million (America's Health Insurance Plans 2006, 2–3). In 2006, however, growth leveled off considerably, with relatively few employees choosing consumer-driven plans when offered other options (Gabel, Pickreign, and Whitmore 2006, 1–2; Fronstin and Collins 2006, 1).

Efforts are also under way to introduce consumer-driven models into state Medicaid programs. The Deficit Reduction Act of 2006 authorized ten state demonstration projects permitting states to offer Medicaid HSAs coupled with HDHPs (Milligan, Woodcock, and Burton 2006, 2). Several states, including Florida and West Virginia, have already begun to experiment with health accounts for Medicaid recipients under the waivers authorized by the Department of Health and Human Services under its 1115 demonstration project waiver authority (Milligan, Woodcock, and Burton 2006, 1–2). The Bush administration has also attempted to revive the moribund Medicare HSA program through a demonstration project (CMS Office of Public Affairs 2006).

The Politics

The HSA concept grew out of the CDHC movement and is vigorously supported by pro-market advocacy groups. (These groups, their academic supporters, the assumptions they make, and the stories they tell are analyzed at greater length in chapter 3.) HSAs have also received strong support from the Bush administration and from the Republican Party leadership. They also offer significant opportunities for specific interest groups, which have thrown their support behind HSAs as well.

First, HSAs are very attractive as tax-sheltered investment vehicles for higher-income Americans. Many of the early purchasers of HSAs (and of MSAs) were professionals or ranchers who have relatively high incomes but lack ready access to a group health plan since they are self-employed (Bilyk 2006). According to one scenario, a family that invests the maximum amount in an HSA over a forty year period, paying for their medical expenses out of pocket rather than from the HSA, could accumulate $1.5 million in tax-free savings that could be withdrawn at retirement.[19] If the family instead used the account to cover $1,000 in medical expenses each year and encountered a significant medical event requiring the payment of the full deductible once every decade, the family would still end up with $1.25 million after forty years. HSAs are not subject to the income limits that apply to Roth IRAs and traditional IRAs, and are thus very attractive to those earning above those limits. Contributions may be made to HSAs, moreover, even if their owners have contributed the maximum possible to IRAs and 401(k) plans. After the age of sixty-five, HSA funds can be withdrawn without penalty. In addition, HSA funds may continue to be withdrawn after the age of sixty-five without tax liability for qualified medical expenses, including Medicare premiums and long-term care insurance premiums.

HSAs are potentially very valuable to banks. They represent a massive transfer in capital from the insurance to the banking industry.[20] Banks have been starved for capital in recent years, as consumer demand for home purchases and refinancings has been high while the interest on bank accounts has been low compared to potential returns on other investments. Though it is likely that the large accumulations held in HSAs over time will eventually end up in more lucrative investment vehicles, in the short run HSA funds are likely to be deposited in banks. Indeed, much of the money invested in HSAs is likely to remain in banks over the long term, readily available for medical expenses. One expert estimates that up to $300 billion a year may eventually be held in HSA deposits, representing "the largest legislated opportunity for asset capture in the United States" (Knight 2005). Most banks charge $50 to $75 for establishing an HSA, and collect about $40 or more a year in maintenance and service fees (Dash 2006). One source states: "Financial institutions have the potential to capture $3.5 billion in revenues driven by account and asset management fees" (Diamond Cluster International 2006). It is not surprising, therefore, that the American Bankers Association and the American Bankers Insurance Association have formed the HSA Council to promote HSAs ("Bankers Form Health Savings Account Council" 2005).

Much of the money now being deposited in HSAs would formerly have gone to insurance companies in premiums (and to insurance agents in commissions) to pay for first-dollar insurance coverage. Insurance companies and brokers stand to be the losers as money that was formerly paid in low-deductible insurance premiums is moved to HSAs. A number of insurance companies have tried to protect their income by buying or partnering with banks. United has opened Exante Bank (and acquired two smaller insurance companies that had specialized in HSAs), and Aetna is partnering with J. P. Morgan. The Blue Cross Blue Shield Association has announced that it will open its own Blue Healthcare Bank in 2007. Insurance companies are also permitted by the federal law to administer HSAs. This would be a new and unfamiliar line of business for insurance companies, however, which is one reason why in the short run HSA money seems to be ending up in banks.

HSAs are also popular with some physicians, who are tired of struggling with managed care companies. Physicians have had to offer deep discounts to HMOs and PPOs, and have had to endure managed care utilization reviewers second-guessing their treatment decisions. Simply handing a bill to a patient for whatever amount the physician chooses, and swiping the patient's debit card (to withdraw funds from the HSA) or credit card (if the patient's HSA is exhausted), seems like a very attractive alternative (White 2006). Further, most physicians are small businessmen with high incomes. This is exactly the group to which HSAs are most attractive as a means of sheltering income for retirement.

Of course, CDHC is not an unmixed blessing for providers. Managed care organizations commonly require that when billing HDHP plan members with HSAs, providers who participate in their managed care plans must offer discounts that they have negotiated with the plans, even while the members are still under the deductible limit. Managed care organizations also often require that providers and plan members comply with utilization review requirements in incurring expenses that will be set off against the deductible (Jost and Hall, 2005, 408; Hall and Havighurst 2005, 1497–98). Moreover, if providers really do start publishing their fees online and competing with each other for consumer business, there is the possibility that their fees will be pushed down.

It is also likely that some providers will be stuck with bad debt as they themselves provide services on credit to consumers still under the deductible limit (White 2006).

CDHC could also prove a boon to employers. Though economists almost unanimously agree that in the end it is employees rather than employers who pay for employment-related health insurance (as discussed in chapter 1), employers (and employees) generally do not seem to believe it (Pauly 1997). At least some employers — those with a large number of minimum-wage employees or with rigid collective bargaining agreements — do absorb much of the cost of increased health insurance premiums, at least in the short run. In recent years these increases have consistently been much higher than inflation generally (Fronstin 2006b, 2).

CDHC advocates believe that HSAs coupled with high-deductible health plans will bring down health insurance premiums. Catastrophic policies clearly cost less than full coverage policies, and it is possible that together the catastrophic premium and the employer's HSA contribution might amount to less than the cost of a full coverage policy of equivalent value. It is also hoped that the cost of health insurance premiums will grow more slowly once consumers are spending money out of their own HSAs, using fewer health care services, and looking for bargains when they purchase health care. The experience of early adopters seems to bear out this possibility. Their experience, as well as the question of whether this will be the general experience of all adopters, is discussed in chapter 8.

But even if inflation in the cost of employment-related health insurance coverage is not significantly retarded, many employers may prefer HSAs. With HSAs, employers will be able to decide how much they want to contribute to employee HSAs in addition to deciding how much they want to pay for health insurance premiums. They will thus be better able to control how much they contribute in total toward the cost of health care coverage for their employees. Currently 35 percent of employers are holding onto some of the savings from reduced HDHP premiums rather than contributing the full amount to employee HSAs (National Association of Health Underwriters 2006). Many employers, therefore, and particularly small employers, are likely to support consumer-driven care. It is also likely that some employers will also see increased tax subsidies for individually purchased HSAs as a reason for eliminating their own health plans, thus increasing the number of persons who do not have employment-related insurance.

On the other hand, employment-related insurance is offered as a fringe benefit to attract and hold employees, and if employees are not sold on HSAS and HDHPs, it will be difficult for many employers to move to them. At this point, many employers are holding off on adopting HSAS or are offering them only as one option in a menu of plans (National Association of Health Underwriters 2006).

Finally, CDHC is a boon for the consumer credit industry. When HSAS are exhausted but deductibles have not been met, American consumers are likely to turn to credit cards to pay for health care, as they do for everything else (Zeldin and Rukavina 2007).[21] They may also ultimately turn to home equity loans. Because health care costs are often unexpected and significant in size, many consumers will carry credit card balances, possibly large balances, for some time. There is a great deal of money to be made here in interest charges and fees.

There will, of course, be losers from CDHC as well. Unions and government employees have opposed CDHC, which they see as shifting more costs to workers and undermining employment-related insurance (Yeager 2006; Regopoulos, Christianson, Claxton, and Trude 2006, 769). They believe that HSAS will encourage employers to drop health insurance, just as IRAS and 401(k) plans have allowed employers to abandon traditional pensions (Schor 2006). As already noted, insurance brokers and insurance companies that cannot diversify to market HSAS will lose premium business. Low-income consumers who have had HMOs or PPOS through their employment and whose employers have covered most of the premium cost of that insurance will suffer if their employers move them to high-deductible plans without significantly lowering the employee's premium contributions. Consumers whose income is low enough that they are not required to pay income tax will gain nothing from the tax deductions offered for HSA contributions. Indeed, if their employers drop or decrease insurance coverage, reasoning that their employees can now get coverage through nongroup HDHPs, low-income employees will come out behind since they do not have to pay payroll taxes (their only real tax liability) on employer health insurance contributions.[22] Medicaid recipients in particular stand to be big losers from CDHC, as they have virtually no disposable income with which to cover higher cost-sharing obligations (Park and Solomon 2005).

Consumers with chronic health problems who previously had HMO coverage with low cost-sharing through their employers, but who now will have to move to a high-deductible policy without significant HSA employer contributions, may end up paying a lot more for health care, though for these consumers, a great deal depends on how the plan is designed.[23] Brand-name pharmaceutical companies may lose if consumers switch to generics or simply stop taking prescribed drugs when face with higher cost sharing, but even brand-name pharmaceutical companies may be winners if they are able to charge higher prices or reach bigger markets once freed from the negotiated discounts or formulary arrangements that they currently have with pharmaceutical benefit management companies. Hospitals will be winners if they can figure out how to collect directly from consumers without having to extend credit, but will be losers if they end up with more bad debt (Wilensky 2006).

At this point the winners from CDHC are easier to identify — and much easier to organize — than the losers. Most of the opposition to CDHC seems to come from politicians and political advocacy groups that see CDHC as a step in the wrong direction. In particular, the Democratic leadership in Congress is concerned that additional tax subsidies for HSAs may encourage employers to drop employee coverage altogether (Bohan 2006).

The bottom line, however, is that there are well organized, well funded, politically powerful groups that stand to gain financially from CDHC. Its political future, therefore, is bright.

CHAPTER 3

Consumer-Driven Health Care Advocates: Who They Are and What They Believe

Who Are They?

The CDHC movement is formidable. It is well funded and organized and has a clear and articulate message, which it hammers home at every opportunity. CDHC advocates include academics, political advocacy groups, political entrepreneurs, and industry interest groups. They have been extraordinarily effective.

A number of pro-market advocacy groups have adopted the cause of CDHC, including the Heritage Foundation, the National Center for Policy Analysis, the Cato Institute, the Galen Institute, the American Enterprise Institute, and the Progressive Policy Institute. Most of these groups identify themselves as conservative or libertarian and generally support Republicans, though the Progressive Policy Institute bills itself as a moderate group that supports moderate Democrats, thus bringing a bipartisan flavor to the issue. Regional market advocacy organizations such as the Heartland Institute, Pacific Research Institute, and the Buckeye Institute, as well as advocacy organizations from other countries including the Fraser Institute in Canada and the Institute of Economic Affairs in the UK, also call for consumer empowerment in health care markets.

Though all these organizations support market-based approaches to health policy, they differ to some extent in their policy recommendations. For example, *Healthy, Wealthy, and Wise: Five Steps to a Better Health Care System* (2005), by John Cogan, R. Glenn Hubbard, and Daniel Kessler, the most recent health policy book sponsored by the American Enterprise Institute and the Hoover Institution, calls for tax deductibility for all health care expenditures. On the other hand, Robert Moffit, Stuart Butler, and Nina Owcharenko of the Heritage Foundation, among the most active advocates of market-based health policy, publish a steady flow of briefing papers calling for replacing tax deductions and exclusions with tax credits for health insurance, as well as for the deregulation of the health care, insurance, and pharmaceutical industries and for limiting remedies available to malpractice victims. Michael Cannon and Michael Tanner of the Cato Institute promote the same agenda in their recent book, *Healthy Competition: What's Holding Back Health Care and How to Free It* (2005), although their solutions appear somewhat more radical. Though both Heritage and Cato support HSAs, they see them as part of a larger deregulatory strategy.

HSAs are the primary focus of the National Center for Policy Analysis and the Galen Institute. John Goodman, the long-time president of NCPA, has played a key role in developing CDHC theory and continues to produce a great volume of reports, studies, and books supporting consumer-based strategies for reorganizing health care. Also affiliated with the NCPA is Devon Herrick, who also writes extensively about CDHC. Galen's health policy point person is Grace-Marie Arnett Turner, who has also produced a number of books and articles on CDHC.

These advocacy organizations are generously funded. The budget for the Heritage Foundation in 2004 was over $36 million, while the Cato Institute's annual budget runs at about $17 million (Source Watch). Some of their funding comes from health care industry groups that stand to benefit from their deregulatory agenda. The NCPA, for example, has received funding from the Eli Lilly and Company Foundation, the Lilly Endowment, and the Procter and Gamble Fund, while the Heritage Foundation has received funding from Johnson and Johnson, GlaxoSmithKline, America's Health Insurance Plans, Pfizer, the Bristol-Myers Squibb Foundation, and PhRMA (Source Watch). But industry support makes up a relatively small part of their total funding, most of which comes from right-wing foundations, including the Castle Rock Foundation, Earhart Foundation, Roe Foundation, Koch Family Foundations,

Scaife Foundations, Lynde and Harry Bradley Foundations, and until recently the John M. Olin Foundation.

A number of prominent academics have provided intellectual support for the CDHC movement. One of the most prolific, creative, and open-minded has been Mark Pauly of the University of Pennsylvania, who has long advocated the creation of a consumer-driven national health care system based on tax credits. Though Pauly has been a primary intellectual force behind the consumer-driven movement, he has rejected tax subsidies for HSAs as inconsistent with the need to reduce tax subsidies for health care, and he seems unconvinced that HSAs would make a major contribution to controlling health care costs (Pauly 1994). Martin Feldstein of Harvard played a key early role in describing the incentives created by tax subsidies in American health care finance, and he continues to publish regularly on health economics topics. The works of other health economists, including Gail Jensen, Jonathan Gruber, Frank Lichtenberg, Richard Zeckhauser, Michael Morrisey, Joseph Newhouse, and Mark Duggan, are frequently cited in CDHC literature, though not all identify fully with the CDHC agenda.

With two thick books on CDHC and frequent public appearances, Regina Herzlinger of the Harvard Business School is one of the most conspicuous academic supporters of the consumer-driven health care movement. While most consumer-driven health care advocates focus on the demand side, Herzlinger focuses much more on the supply side. The primary concerns of her work seem to be how best to configure providers to compete for the business of health care consumers and how to provide information to consumers to promote competition among providers (Herzlinger ed. 2004, 102–21). Herzlinger also favors competition for the sale of insurance as well as for the sale of health care. At times she questions whether high-deductible insurance policies will be attractive to consumers, valuable to them, and effective in holding down health care costs (Herzlinger ed. 2004, 102–3). She even advocates limiting out-of-pocket maximums to amounts that people can really afford given their income (Herzlinger 1997, 258). Herzlinger's concern with the nature of supply-side competition is also shared by other business school academics, such as Michael Porter of Harvard and Elizabeth Teisberg of the University of Virginia, who have recently published a book, *Redefining Health Care*, advocating "value-based" competition but offering only qualified support for consumer cost-sharing as a strategy to encourage competition (Porter and Teisberg 2006, 90–94, 496–97).

Several legal academics have also supported market-driven health care, although not the full CDHC agenda. Clark Havighurst (sometimes writing in conjunction with James Blumstein) provided significant early support for increasing the role of markets in health care, although Havighurst's writings on contract-based competition in health care have focused more on competition at the level of purchase of health insurance coverage than at the level of purchase of goods and services. Havighurst's most recent writings contend that managed care and medical savings accounts could be complementary strategies to bring down health care costs (Hall and Havighurst 2005).

Richard Epstein, another law professor, holds down the libertarian fringe position on health policy in his book *Mortal Peril* (1997).[1] Epstein's favored position of abolishing all public support of health care for the poor, leaving indigents to rely on charity, finds little explicit support among other CDHC advocates, most of whom, like Goodman, recognize the need for a residual public program to support those who truly cannot help themselves, and some of whom, like Pauly, recognize the need for a quite extensive public program (tax credit–based) to assist those priced out of the health insurance market. Epstein also regards tax-subsidized MSAs as at most a second-best solution to the moral hazard problem (Epstein 1997, 181–82).

Of all legal scholars, Haavi Morreim has been the most consistent supporter of HSAs. Her recent scholarship (discussed in chapter 9) thoughtfully explores the legal ramifications of CDHC for the relationship between patients and health care providers (Morreim 2006). Marshall Kapp also advocates CDHC (Kapp 2006). Other legal scholars, including Richard Kaplan, John Jacobi, Wendy Mariner, and Mark Hall, have explored CDHC, but from the standpoint of neutral or skeptical scholars rather than as enthusiastic advocates.

Finally, a number of political entrepreneurs support CDHC. Newt Gingrich, in his new incarnation as a public intellectual, has probably written the most about CDHC, focusing on both the supply and the demand sides. A broad coalition of politicians ranging from conservative Republicans to moderate Democrats have supported CDHC initiatives in Congress and in the states.

The CDHC literature, both academic and advocacy, presses a number of themes. On some issues the authors diverge sharply. But one also finds a striking uniformity of assumptions, stories, and messages. Most CDHC advocates start from the same underlying assumptions about how the world operates. Most also tell the same stories about the history and nature of the American health care system and the health care systems of other countries. Most preach the same message of salvation for the American health care system.

What They Believe

What then are these underlying assumptions? First, and ultimately most important, CDHC advocates believe that economics, and more particularly the microeconomics of the Chicago school, provides the most reliable and accurate explanation of human behavior, and indeed a comprehensive tool for understanding human behavior. This underlying assumption is rarely articulated expressly, but it seems always to be there.[2] This belief in the necessity and sufficiency of economic explanations for human behaviors — to the exclusion of alternatives such as history, sociology, psychology, philosophy, theology, or political science — pervades the CDHC literature. Economics tells us that if we just let self-interest do its work, everything will be fine (Goodman and Musgrave 1994, 33–37).

Second, CDHC advocates believe in the vital importance of individual freedom of choice in health care transactions (Goodman and Musgrave 1994, 117, 120). As noted in chapter 1, health policy experts from other traditions usually describe the ideal health care system as possessing three attributes: accessible to all, reasonable in cost, and high in quality. The European Commission and Council, for example, articulate the three long-term objectives of European health care systems as "accessibility of care for all, based on fairness and solidarity," "high-quality care for the population," and "long-term financial sustainability of this care [delivered in a system] as efficient as possible."[3] *Healthy Competition*, the Cato Institute's latest book on CDHC, articulates a different trio of values: "quality, affordability, and choice" (Cannon and Tanner 2005, 2). Choice appears to be the most important value of the three, because "individual choice actually promotes lower prices and higher quality" (Cannon and Tanner 2005, 5). Any constraint on individual freedom of choice, be it imposed by the government through regulation or by private arrangements such as managed care, impedes the achievement of economic efficiency. Freedom of choice is not just freedom to choose a particular provider or insurer, moreover, but also the freedom to choose the method of treatment or no treatment at all.

Individual freedom to exercise control over resources is not just an economic issue to most advocates; it is a moral and political value as well. Some advocates believe that recognizing this right requires rejecting a positive right to health care, with which it is in irreconcilable conflict. Accepting a positive right of access to health care for all on any basis other than ability to pay would mean, in the words of one group of authors, "imposing an obligation on Jones to provide health care for Smith," thus limiting the right of Jones to choose how to direct his own resources (Cannon and Tanner 2005, 35).

Third, health care market advocates believe that the best way to express, and conversely to gauge, individual preferences is through the expenditure of money (Epstein 1997, 32, 34–35). People should spend their own money (and not be allowed to spend other people's money) on health care services. Only when consumers can "vote with their dollars" can an industry be run efficiently (Herzlingler 1997, 15). Only by requiring consumers to spend their own money on health care services can we be sure that they truly value health care goods and services more than other goods and services.

In sum, CDHC advocates believe that health care products and services are in fact pretty much like all other goods and services, subject to the same laws of supply and demand, or at least capable of being rationally traded off for other goods and services (Goodman, Musgrave and Herrick 2004, 7; Epstein 1997, 164–65). Consumers can — and should — decide rationally whether to spend $50,000 on a new high-end car, a child's college education, or a bone marrow transplant; whether to spend $100 on food for the next week or on hypertension medication. Health care enjoys no special status as a consumer good (Epstein 1997, 112).

Fourth, advocates believe that health care professionals and providers, just like consumers, are primarily motivated by economic considerations (Herzlingler 1997, 28). Correspondingly, the best way to get health care providers to offer better or less expensive care, as well as to encourage innovation, is to get the financial incentives right by creating competitive markets (Goodman and Musgrave 1992, 129–31). Thus Herzlinger argues that providers ought to be able to set their own terms for selling their services; to charge higher prices, for example, if they think that they can get them in competitive markets (Herzlinger ed. 2004, 77, 80). If producers are freed from the price constraints currently imposed by managed care plans and government programs, they will configure themselves so as to maximize productivity and quality, which in Herzlinger's vision will lead to the creation of focused health care factories — production units that focus on treating particular diseases in high volumes (Herzlinger ed. 2004, 105–10; Herzlinger 1997, 157–99). Further, if patients (rather than insurers or providers) pay providers directly, providers will respond to the needs of consumers (Herzlinger 1997, 84). If competition can be introduced into health care, prices will fall, just as they have fallen for cars, clothes, computers, and other products traded in functioning markets

(Herzlinger ed. 2004, 128). As proof of this hypothesis, advocates point to the markets for cosmetic surgery, eyeglasses, and over-the-counter drugs, in which patients do pay directly and prices have come down dramatically in recent years (Cannon and Tanner 2005, 6–7; Herzlinger 1997, 31).

Fifth, CDHC advocates tend to reject the notion of a "need" for health care. CDHC advocates believe that health care services have value only insofar as they are valued by individuals. Consistency, therefore, would require that they reject the notion of a "need" for medical services independent of demand for medical services. This indeed seems to be the position of some advocates at least some of the time. They may seem quite skeptical of the value of health care services (Cogan, Hubbard, and Kessler 2005, 15; Epstein 1997, 156–57).[4] Or they may criticize the "wasteful proliferation of technology" driven by third-party payment (Herzlinger 1997, 226, 233), or claim that much of the money spent on preventive care is wasted (Goodman and Musgrave 1992, 87–92). They are particularly critical of the wastefulness of government health care programs (Cannon and Tanner 2005, 80–81).

But CDHC advocates are ambivalent on the value of health care. While they at times seem to reject the concept of "need" for health care, they can also wax eloquent about the wonders of modern medicine. This is particularly true when they compare health care in the United States to that found in other countries (Cannon and Tanner 2005, 17–23; Herzlinger 1997, 101–2). In this mode, they emphasize the innovativeness and creativity of American health care research (Cogan, Hubbard, and Kessler 2005, 8–13; Cannon and Tanner 2005, 17–18).[5] Other countries with publicly funded health care systems, they suggest, discourage innovation and depend on the United States to move medicine forward (Cannon and Tanner 2005, 17–18). Advocates point out that other countries ration health care, by which they mean that other countries deny "needed" health care products or services (Goodman, Musgrave, and Herrick 2004, 17–22).

CDHC advocates not only question the "need" for health care, they also question its role in promoting or protecting health. Some advocates assert that individual lifestyle choices are at least as important as medical care in determining the health status of individuals or populations (Herzlinger 1997, 48–49, 210; Goodman and Musgrave 1992, 86, 92–94). If people, would stop smoking, drinking, using drugs, overeating, and having illicit sex, they contend, these behavioral changes would have a much greater impact on health than additional medical services would. If people in other developed countries have longer life expectancies and lower infant mortality rates, it is because they behave better, not because they have universal access to health care (Goodman and Musgrave 1992, 86, 93).

Some advocates go so far as to assert that people engage in risky and unhealthy behaviors partly because they have too much health insurance, or at least because the prices they pay for health insurance do not reflect their risky lifestyle choices (Herzlinger 1997, 64–69). If people had to pay for their own health care out of pocket, they would live healthier lives (Goodman and Musgrave 1992, 94). Some go even further and claim that if people choose to live unhealthy lives, it is wrong for society to bail them out by providing health insurance (Epstein 1997, 54–58). This is particularly true for the poor, who are encouraged by government programs, in this view, to behave in ways that increase the cost of those programs (Cannon and Tanner 2005, 91; Herzlinger 1997, 280). As usual, Epstein (who, to be fair, is not a mainstream CDHC advocate) takes the most extreme position on this, arguing that the provisions of the Emergency Medical Treatment and Active Labor Act guaranteeing all access to emergency care encourages risky behavior, because those who engage in such behavior know they will get emergency care when they suffer its consequences (Epstein 1997, 102). But the underlying theme that too ready access to medical care can result in worse health is found in the work of other authors as well.

Sixth, CDHC advocates believe that there are no inherent limits to the demand for health care (Goodman and Musgrave 1992, 75–80). If consumers are not required to pay the full cost of medical products and services, their demand for services will be limited only by the opportunity cost of the time that it takes them to acquire the services or by whatever bureaucratic barriers a health care system places in their way to ration care (Goodman and Musgrave 1992, 111; Goodman, Musgrave, and Herrick 2004, 3, 4). Again, moral hazard is seen as the central problem of health policy.

Some consumer-directed advocates really seem to believe that if we do not do something soon to make patients pay the full cost of health care, we will be spending our entire GDP on health care (Goodman, Musgrave, and Herrick 2004, 1–2). Goodman projects that we will reach this point in 2062 (Goodman and Musgrave 1992, 76). Advocates are particularly concerned with new diagnostic tests, such as full body scans, that allow even the healthy to spend large amounts of money on searching for possible diseases; with the potential of personalized genetic medicine that will be very effective but very expensive;

and with the limitless demand for cosmetic surgery (Goodman, Musgrave, and Herrick 2004, 2). If health services are not rationed by price and by ability to pay, there is no other limit to demand for them.

A common trope in the consumer-driven literature is to liken first-dollar health insurance coverage to first-dollar coverage for car maintenance, housing costs, or restaurant dining, which, they argue, would lead to wanton abuses (Herzlinger 1997, 251).[6] This analogy ignores, of course, the fact that health care is usually time-consuming, inconvenient, unpleasant, uncomfortable, and sometimes just plain painful. A few people do pathologically pursue health care services, but most of us have better things to do. Designer prescription sunglasses, evoked by some advocates to epitomize health care consumption, are in fact not typical of health care products and services.

Problems and Solutions

From these philosophical and political assumptions grows a particular understanding of how health care systems function. To some extent this understanding is based on observations of reality, that is to say that it is empirical in nature. But it also follows deductively from the assumptions outlined above. Their observation of the world, that is to say, confirms that which CDHC advocates already know.

First, CDHC advocates believe that insurance as it now exists in the United States (and indeed throughout the world) is the problem, not the solution. We do not have too little health insurance in the United States but rather far too much. The uninsured are not the problem; the overinsured are. Insurance reduces the cost of health care to less than its full cost, which encourages unnecessary spending (Cogan, Hubbard, and Kessler 2005, 16; Cannon and Tanner 2005, 46; Goodman, Herrick, and Musgrave 2004, 4). Indeed, consumers are forced by our current system to buy insurance that they do not even want. Overinsurance results in overutilization and waste. It also results in care of poor quality, since it discourages patients from shopping for high-quality care (Cannon and Tanner 2005, 52–54). Insurance misaligns incentives for providers, requiring providers to cater to the demands of insurers (or to deceive insurers) rather than to serve the needs of their patients (Cannon and Tanner 2005, 48–51). It thus undermines the doctor-patient relationship (Cannon and Tanner 2005, 57–58).

CDHC advocates, as noted earlier, do not reject insurance altogether. They acknowledge the skewed nature of health care costs and realize that insurance plays an essential role in medical catastrophes. Most believe, however, that insurance should be available only for high-cost, low-frequency events, as other forms of insurance are (Goodman, Herrick, and Musgrave 2004, 238–40). Some argue, moreover, that insurers should make lump sum payments to patients when insured conditions occur (as with other forms of insurance), and then allow patients to choose and pay their providers directly, perhaps even to decide how to spend the insurance payments (Goodman, Musgrave, and Herrick 2004, 5, 244–46). Other CDHC advocates would not limit health insurance to catastrophic coverage. They would allow consumers to choose any insurance policy they preferred — including high-benefit policies with low deductibles and co-payments — as long as consumers paid the full actuarial cost of whatever policies they chose (Herzlinger ed. 2004, 75). Indeed, Herzlinger seems to see consumer choice taking place primarily among insurance plans, though without the structure of managed competition (Herzlinger ed. 2004, 156).

CDHC advocates believe that health insurance should be sold in competitive markets just like any other product. Whatever resources individuals choose to spend on insurance is the right amount, and whatever risks individuals choose to cover with insurance is correct. Neither the government nor employers should second-guess these decisions. Moreover, insurers should risk-adjust their rates so that persons purchasing insurance pay the actuarially fair rate for the risks that they bring to the insurance pool (Goodman, Musgrave, and Herrick 2004, 237; Herzlinger 1997, 255). Insurance should cover capricious risk, but only among people who have the same risk profile to begin with. The purpose of health insurance is not to achieve social solidarity — to pool and share risk across a population — but rather to smooth health insurance expenditures for individuals from period to period and to absorb unexpected health shocks (Epstein 1997, 52–54). Community rating and guaranteed issue requirements thus distort insurance markets, and are in any event futile since they will be evaded by insurers (Goodman, Musgrave, and Herrick 2004, 204–7). Indeed, community-rated premiums result in ex ante moral hazard, i.e. they encourage unhealthy behavior, such as smoking, inactivity, and overeating (Epstein 1997, 125). Not all CDHC advocates, however, oppose all forms of insurance regulation. Some call for guaranteed renewable insurance to facilitate the smoothing function of insurance (Herzlinger ed. 2004, 75; Goodman and Musgrave 1992, 126).

Second, CDHC advocates generally reject any significant role for government in regulating or financing health care. This opposition is in large part driven by their general belief that governments are markets carried on by other means (and less efficiently than real markets) (Epstein 1997, 15).[7] Laws, including those that govern health care, are the means through which organized groups with political power further their own interests, which often means protecting themselves against real market competition (Cannon and Tanner 2005, 35). In particular, the concentrated interests of providers tend to triumph over the more diffuse interests of consumers (Goodman, Musgrave, and Herrick 2004, 196).

Though CDHC advocates accept market failure as a theoretical possibility that might justify regulation, they believe that market failures rarely occur in real life. Restraint of trade by monopolies or cartels is an infrequent problem that can be solved through antitrust enforcement (Epstein 1997, 19). Even when markets fail in some significant respect, government intervention is rarely the best "second-best" solution. Some advocates see a marginal role for government in providing information to consumers or in prosecuting fraud (Herzlinger ed. 2004, 182, 183). But the role of government is quite limited.

Real markets are grounded in the interests of all individuals as those individuals themselves perceive those interests, and thus better represent the public interest than government does. Government regulation inevitably distorts markets, introducing waste and inefficiency. Insurance benefit mandates, for example, dramatically increase the cost of health insurance without providing real value to insureds (Cogan, Hubbard, and Kessler 2005, 16–17, 44–45; Herzlinger 1997, 45; Goodman and Musgrave 1992, 47–49). Insurance rating regulation, which limits the range of insurance premiums or the ability of insurance companies to underwrite risk, results in higher premiums and decreased coverage (Cogan, Hubbard, and Kessler 2005, 50). Government regulation of pharmaceuticals, health professionals, and institutions also increases costs without corresponding benefits (Cannon and Tanner 2005, 116–24, 130–38; Epstein 1997, 86–87).[8] In total, one advocacy group asserts, government regulation of health care costs $169.1 billion annually, rendering 7.5 million Americans uninsured and causing 22,200 deaths a year (Cannon and Tanner 2005, 111–12).[9]

Similarly, government programs that provide benefits are the means through which powerful political interests take wealth away from the less powerful (Epstein 1997, 15). Like regulatory programs, benefit programs are inherently inefficient and distort health care markets (Cannon and Tanner 2005, 35–38).

Government benefit programs encourage inadequate care and restrict beneficiaries' choice of providers and services, while administered pricing formulas distort competition.[10]

Health care programs for the poor also impose perverse incentives on their recipients, discouraging work and savings and crowding out private insurance (Cannon and Tanner 2005, 96–97). They impose high administrative costs and are inevitably attended by government corruption (Epstein 1997, 49–50). Though government programs often aspire to providing only a "decent minimum" of care, it is impossible to define what this means, and the programs usually end up providing far more services and products than are necessary (Epstein 1997, 51). Finally, regardless of their intent or structure, government-funded health benefit programs are unavoidably inefficient because they depend on taxation for funding, and taxation is inherently distortive and inefficient (Cannon and Tanner 2005, 34; Epstein 1997, 2, 176).

Advocates are uniformly critical of public health insurance programs in other countries as well (Goodman, Musgrave, and Herrick 2004). Other countries, CDHC advocates assert, provide high cost; low quality of care, rationed through interminable waiting lists; obstacles to innovation and the use of new technologies; intolerable administrative burdens; and policies that discriminate against the elderly, minorities, the poor, and people who live in rural areas (Goodman, Musgrave, and Herrick 2004, 147–65; Goodman and Musgrave 1992, 112).

CDHC advocates also reject tax expenditure programs. Indeed, opposition to the federal tax subsidies for employment-related health benefits is a defining characteristic of the CDHC movement. Pro-market health care advocates have for decades argued that the employment tax subsidy encourages the purchase of excessive health insurance, which in turn leads to the purchase of excessive and wasteful health care (Cogan, Hubbard, and Kessler 2005, 15–16, 27–33; Cannon and Tanner 2005, 48–49, 61–73; Goodman and Musgrave 1992, 50–51). Cannon and Tanner assert that these subsidies have "restricted consumer choice and competition, reduced patients' control over their health care decisions, increased the cost of health insurance and medical care, caused many to go without health insurance for extended periods (and many more for brief spells), discouraged saving, lowered wages, eliminated jobs, reduced consumers' health insurance choices, discriminated against those who cannot obtain employer-sponsored coverage, and left Americans poorer" (Cannon and Tanner 2005, 62). By subsidizing overinsurance, the tax subsidy "encourages riskier behaviors (smoking, overeating, inactivity) [and] discourages prudent behaviors (saving for future medical expenses, exercise, preventive care)" (Cannon and Tanner 2005, 64). It also decreases productivity and entrepreneurship, by locking workers into their jobs (Cannon and Tanner 2005, 64). One CDHC advocate argues that eliminating the subsidy would lower the costs of health insurance to the point that it would be affordable by the uninsured (Herzlinger 1997, 279).

CDHC advocates see tax subsidies (along with the wage and price controls imposed during the Second World War) as the key culprits in causing our "accidental health care system." They believe that the employment-based American health insurance system exists not because Americans want it, but rather because perverse government tax and regulatory policy brought it into being. This central claim is the subject of chapter 5.

Market advocates part company, however, when they try to delimit the proper role of government in meeting the health care needs of the poor. Epstein, ever at the fringe, claims that we need to just say no to medically needy persons (Epstein 1997, 181). Most CDHC advocates, however, agree that some form of government program is necessary to provide medical care for the poor. In general, advocates favor shifting government programs from a defined-benefit to a defined-contribution basis, providing beneficiaries with funds to purchase health insurance (Cannon and Tanner 2005, 86). Some favor tax credits to support the purchase of health insurance, at least for those otherwise unable to afford it (Cogan, Hubbard, and Kessler 2005, 38–39). Cogan, Hubbard, and Kessler favor expanding the availability of tax preferences to cover noninsured health care expenses, thereby at least eliminating the distortion caused by tax preferences that apply only to insurance (Cogan, Hubbard, and Kessler 2005, 33–35).[11] Herzlinger is troubled by the current tax subsidies (Herzlinger 1997, 250–52) but unsure whether tax credits for insurance or for MSAs are the best substitute for them (Herzlinger 1997, 256–57). Goodman, who would favor government-funded MSAs for at least some of the poor (Goodman and Musgrave 1992, 60), also suggests giving Medicaid funds to local communities along with the power to decide how to spend them, effectively returning us to the early twentieth century when welfare was a local function (Goodman and Musgrave 1992, 67).[12]

Third, CDHC advocates are in general skeptical about the seriousness of the problem of the uninsured. They believe that most people who do not purchase health insurance or health care are simply choosing to spend their money on other things that are of more value to them (Goodman, Musgrave, and Herrick 2004, 218–20). Only a small group of the poor and chronically ill have difficulty obtaining individual health insurance coverage (Cogan, Hubbard, and Kessler 2005, 50). Many of the uninsured are well-to-do young people who simply choose to self-insure, and many more are already eligible for public programs (Goodman, Musgrave, and Herrick 2004, 35). Some proportion of the uninsured (Goodman estimates one-quarter) chooses not to purchase insurance "because of the price-increasing effects of state regulation" (Goodman and Musgrave 1992, 100). And most of the uninsured are without coverage only for short periods (Goodman, Musgrave, and Herrick 2004, 35).

Advocates believe that insurance in the nongroup market is affordable to almost all the uninsured.[13] Many of the uninsured are also eligible for a Medicaid or another government program but have chosen not to participate in it, preferring uninsured status to Medicaid.[14] And many of the uninsured have access to free medical care or Medicaid whenever they need it (Goodman, Musgrave, and Herrick 2004, 36–37, 221–22). In any event, the problem of access for the poor is best solved by the transfer of money to poor people to allow them to decide how much to spend on health care. Alternatively, tax credits could be made available to support the purchase of catastrophic insurance policies (Cogan, Hubbard, and Kessler 2005, 38–39). Poor persons who refuse to insure, even with tax credits, can borrow money for health care and go bankrupt if necessary (Goodman and Musgrave 1992, 103). Advocates also claim that CDHC will make health insurance more affordable for the poor, while it will also develop special products better fitted to their needs (Herzlinger ed. 2004, 161–62; Goodman and Musgrave 1994, 101).

CDHC advocates are skeptical of the claim that the paucity of consumer information is a major barrier to having consumers take charge of their health care.[15] To the extent that it exists, market failure in health care caused by lack of information can be solved by private entrepreneurs (Cogan, Hubbard, and Kessler 2005, 52).[16] Indeed, if we had real competition in health care, providers themselves would give consumers the information they need to make appropriate health care purchases (Cannon and Tanner 2005, 58–59).

Relevant information can also be produced as needed to support competition in insurance markets. CDHC advocates reject the position of managed competition supporters that standardized insurance policies are necessary to facilitate choice. They argue that standardization simply denies choice (Herzlinger 1997, 260–62). If standardization makes sense, the market will standardize without government intervention (Herzlinger 1997, 263). The primary reason why we do not have the information needed to make markets work is that "bureaucrats" want to keep it from us (Goodman and Musgrave 1992, 34). Insurers can be trusted to figure out which choices are most valuable to consumers and to focus the information that they provide to consumers on those choices (Herzlinger ed. 2004, 97–98).[17] The problem of lack of information will be easily solved if health care markets are unleashed.

CDHC advocates have a great deal of faith in the capacity of the internet to solve information deficiencies. Health care consumers can already find web sites that allow them to figure out what medical care they need, and will soon be able to shop for health care providers on the internet, comparing quality and price from their own homes. Advocates argue that shopping for health care is no more complicated than shopping for investments. Developments in the financial industry over the past two decades prove that anyone can master complex decisions and that private entrepreneurs will step forward to provide any information that consumers need to make wise decisions (Herzlinger ed. 2004, 3–23).

Advocates also believe that favorable selection, or "cherry picking," by insurers or providers is not a major problem in health care markets. To the extent that problems of risk selection do exist, they can be solved through risk adjustment (Herzlinger ed. 2004, 77, 79, 80–83, 170–75). Some advocates propose that employer payments for employment-related health benefits be risk-adjusted to assure access to health insurance (Herzlinger ed. 2004, 77, 79, 80–83, 159). This risk adjustment would, they argue, distort markets less than required community rating would. Government payments should also be risk-adjusted, allowing insurers to charge each insured the actuarially fair rate. Other advocates are skeptical about the potential of risk adjustment, which they see as being at best a poor second-best to just letting markets function without intervention (Goodman, Musgrave, and Herrick 2004, 208–9).[18]

These are among the key beliefs and claims of consumer-directed health care advocates. The chapters that follow examine and evaluate the extent to which these beliefs and claims mirror reality. I begin by examining the historical evidence in the next three chapters. The chapters that follow will explore in turn the theoretical, empirical, and comparative beliefs and claims of CDHC advocates.

CHAPTER 4

Consumer-Driven Health Care the First Time Around

The Consumer as King: The Late Nineteenth
Century and Early Twentieth

One fact seldom mentioned by CDHC advocates is that we have tried CDHC before. From the beginning (and indeed until the middle of the twentieth century) there was only consumer-directed health care in the United States. Health insurance has been a significant factor in American health care finance only since the 1930s. Before that time most Americans paid for their own health care out of pocket (Cathell 1922, 272–73). Doctors did sometimes provide care without charge to their poorest patients, while dispensaries provided basic medical services in poor neighborhoods and most hospitals offered charity care.[1] State and local governments were responsible for providing health care to indigents, and special state institutions existed for the mentally ill and, to a lesser degree, victims of tuberculosis (Committee on the Costs of Medical Care 1932, 4–5).[2] But most patients paid out of pocket for medical services, and they paid it directly to the service provider. In this first incarnation, unregulated, consumer-driven health care was not the Eden that its current supporters envision.

In general, the markets of health care products and services in the nineteenth century and early twentieth were active and competitive. This was certainly true of the patent medicine market (Shryock 1947, 249–51). The turn of the century was the golden age of patent medicine, when fortunes were made selling nostrums over the counter for cash (Starr 1982, 127–34). Patent medicines were usually ineffective, sometimes addictive, and occasionally deadly (Shryock 1947, 249–55, 270). But the patent medicine market was vigorously competitive, with heavy direct-to-consumer advertising (Mann and Plummer 1991, 50–51). Not only did patented medicines compete with each other, but they also faced vigorous competition in the form of counterfeits and parallel imports from countries in which the products lacked patent protection (Mann and Plummer 1991, 32–36).

Competition among doctors was fierce and fired by professional animosities (Starr 1982, 93–94). Doctors were poorly trained, largely ineffective, sometimes dangerous (Starr 1982, 37–59). Throughout the nineteenth century and into the twentieth, medical schools were generally of poor quality, with limited and inadequate training facilities. Not surprisingly, Americans had little respect for doctors (Starr 1982, 31).

Doctors competed in particular for wealthy and socially prominent patients (Starr 1982, 88–89). They generally practiced price discrimination, charging high prices to their wealthier patients and much lower prices to their working-class patients (Rosen 1946, 2, 58; Davis 1941, 52–54). It was essential, therefore, that they attract wealthy patients to remain in business. Doctors depended on lay referrals for business, and were very conscious of their image (Starr 1982, 41, 86–87). Daniel Webster Cathell, whose medical practice management manual went through multiple editions in the late nineteenth century and early twentieth century, advised doctors to dress well, observe personal hygiene, keep up appearances of wealth, and when possible maintain their dignity by insisting that patients see them in their offices rather than making home visits (Cathell 1922, 74, 108–9, 304).

Patients saw themselves as consumers purchasing services in an active market. Some believed that they were better able than their doctors to diagnose and treat their own conditions, and argued with their doctors over prescribed treatments (Cathell 1922, 199). Patients changed doctors frequently, either to avoid paying doctors to whom they owed money or to try out new doctors recommended by others, and thus there was little continuity or coordination of care (Cathell 1922, 176–77, 179; Shryock 1947, 383). In times of illness they sought help not only from physicians but also from clinics, hospitals, patent medicines, home remedies, and other resources (Cathell 1922, 176–77). One study found that "[c]ost or the fear of cost is a pervasive element, commonly influencing choice, often causing delay in securing care, and frequently impelling change from one medical resource to another" (Davis 1941, 27).

Commentators also expressed concern about the effects on the physician-patient relationship of out-of-pocket payment, then a nearly universal practice: "A financial relation between doctor and patient necessarily becomes part of their personal relation, and generally embarrasses it, or worse. Paying fees to doctors does not contribute toward intimate personal relationships with them but rather–especially when uncertain, variable, and possibly large fees are involved–is an obstacle to intimate and continuous relationships. Fine personal relations between physicians and patients exist despite the fee system, not because of it" (Davis 1941, 42).

Billing and collecting from patients were a constant source of worry and frustration for doctors (Cathell 1922, 305). Even deciding what to bill patients was problematic. Although doctors' bills were in principle based on the wealth of their patients, this was often very difficult for doctors to gauge (Davis and Rorem 1932, 50). Doctors struggled continually with the travails of collecting debts from patients who failed to value medical services and refused to pay, or simply could not pay (Cathell 1922, 269–312; Thompson 1954, 333, 401). Many patients expected doctors to provide services on credit, and were then reluctant to pay once their health improved (Thompson 1954, 400–401). Other patients with serious medical problems went deeply into debt to finance their care and then could not pay the debt (Thompson 1954, 538). Doctors sometimes had to accept payment in kind (Thompson 1954, 576). They were repeatedly warned to do business on a cash basis only, but often were too embarrassed to collect their fees at the time services were delivered (Cathell 1922, 285, 29). Doctors did, however, freely decline patients from whom they expected problems with compliance or payment (Cathell 1922, 164, 299). Many patients therefore lacked access to medical care. Because doctors were often unable to collect bills from patients, and because they had to keep their fees low to avoid losing patients, the incomes of physicians were very low throughout the late nineteenth century and into the twentieth. Many supplemented their income by farming or by operating other businesses, such as drugstores (Starr 1982, 65). Some also provided unnecessary care to increase their income (Thompson 1954, 374–75). Capable people were discouraged from going into medical practice (Rosen 1946, 7–8, 89; Shryock 1947, 265–66).

The turn of the century also saw the rise of the modern hospital. Throughout much of the nineteenth century, patients who could afford it were generally treated at home, even having surgery in their homes.[3] Hospitals were simply too dangerous. As antisepsis became better understood and anesthesia improved, hospitals became less dangerous and more comfortable (Stevens 1989, 30; Shryock 1947, 347). Doctors, moreover, increasingly preferred to treat their private patients in the hospital, where nursing staff and state-of-the-art facilities were available.

By the 1920s hospitalization became common, especially for children. Tonsillectomies, adenoidectomies, and appendectomies became the most frequent surgeries, indeed childhood rites of passage (Stevens 1989, 106–7).[4] Many were undoubtedly unnecessary. Expectant mothers were also increasingly hospitalized to deliver babies (Stevens 1989, 106–7).

Although most nonprofit hospitals had begun as charitable institutions for the care of sick and disabled indigents, by the end of the nineteenth century almost all had begun to compete for private pay patients as well. Hospitals often sought to segment the market, offering private rooms to their wealthiest patients, semiprivate rooms to middle-class patients, and ward facilities for the poor, who were increasingly seen as a nuisance rather than a mission (Stevens 1989, 47–48). Some hospitals accommodated private patients in separate buildings, with food cooked in separate kitchens, and with longer visiting hours (Stevens 1989, 10). Hospital facilities mimicked hotels, as if to convince patients of their value by their costliness (Stevens 1989, 36–37, 108–9). Some hospitals even advertised, one describing its private rooms as appealing to "those of the most cultivated tastes" (Stevens 1989, 36, 109–10). Hospitals also competed for the doctors by offering the latest technology, as the doctors had the authority to admit private pay patients (Stevens 1989, 33–35).

In parts of the country where community hospitals were scarce, for-profit hospitals, often owned by the doctors who practiced within them, became common. These were wholly dependent on attracting private pay patients for their continued existence and sought them actively (Stevens 1989, 20).

As hospitals became more safe and comfortable, they also became dramatically more expensive (Stevens 1989, 134; Starr 1982, 160). The itemized hospital bill, with multitudinous and incomprehensible charges for technical services, supplemented by separate charges for the services of physicians and surgeons, became common in the 1920s (Stevens 1989, 134). Hospitals expected their bills to be paid first, before physicians were paid, leading to increasing friction between hospitals and doctors (Stevens 1989, 135). Though many hospitals still offered charity care, hospitalization increasingly became a real burden to those ineligible for charity.

Organized Medicine Rejects Market Competition

Though a competition-based health care system imposed burdens on many consumers, it was simply not tolerable for the competitors. During the last quarter of the nineteenth century and the first quarter of the twentieth, allopathic physicians achieved considerable success in eliminating competition from other sources of healing and in regularizing competition among themselves. The wide-open market that characterized the middle of the nineteenth century for the services of persons who claimed to be healers changed dramatically as the century drew to a close. The medical licensure laws that the states adopted beginning about 1870 drove unlicensed lay healers, herbalists, and bonesetters out of business (Starr 1982, 102–12). Though these laws generally permitted members of competing schools such as homeopaths and eclectics to continue their practice, these practitioners were marginalized by the growing power and authority of allopathic medicine and eventually lost their market. Organized medicine was also successful in closing down substandard proprietary medical schools, and thus limiting entry into the profession (Starr 1982, 112–23, 218–20).

Organized medicine also attacked patent medicines. The American Medical Association mounted an active effort to investigate and report on quack medicines (Shryock 1947, 355). Working closely with journalists, the AMA exposed and discredited ineffective proprietary medicines (Starr 1982, 128–131). In 1905, the AMA established its Council on Pharmacy and Chemistry to set standards for drugs and evaluate them (Starr 1982, 131). By the early twentieth century, advocacy by the American Medical Association had succeeded in creating a new category of "ethical" medicines sold only by prescription, giving doctors new control over drugs and thus over patients (Starr 1982, 134). By the end of the first quarter of the twentieth century, allopathic medicine had consolidated its grip over the practice of medicine in the United States, and the prices of medical care were on their way up.

As the twentieth century unfolded, active competition, never encouraged, was increasingly frowned on by organized medicine (Cathell 1922, 279). "Stealing patients" from other doctors was strongly discouraged (Shryock 1947, 267). Advertising to attract business was condemned as unethical, as was denigrating another doctor (Cathell 1922, 122–23).[5] Underbidding another doctor to get business was reprehensible, as was criticizing the fees charged by another doctor (Cathell 1922, 295). Doctors were counseled to bill adequately for their services, to be diligent in collecting their fees, and to be careful to impress upon their patients the value of their services (Rosen 1946). Doctors were encouraged to bill on a fee-for-service basis and to avoid "contracts for annual attendance," under which they would agree to attend to all of an individual's or family's medical needs for a year for a set fee, a common practice in the early nineteenth century that was now seen as encouraging abuse (Rosen 1946). Doctors were also discouraged from the apparently common practice of billing annually or semiannually (Cathell 1922, 273–73). Local medical associations tried harder to get their members to conform to agreed-upon fee schedules, though enforcing conformity was a source of ongoing frustration (Starr 1982, 63).

It is tempting to understand these developments as cartelization. Organized medicine gained control of the power of the state through the medical licensure boards, and then used this power to eliminate rival schools of healing, to limit entry to the profession by closing down medical schools, and to subjugate other health care professions such as nursing.[6] It also suppressed effective competition from the proprietary medicine business through private and then public regulation and brought pharmaceuticals under its control through the prescribing power.

Paul Starr argued convincingly in his *Social Transformation of American Medicine* that this is not the whole story. As the twentieth century progressed, consumers themselves came to believe the claims of allopathic physicians to special knowledge and skills that made their services worth paying for (Starr 1982, 134–44). Surgery was safer and more effective. Diagnoses were becoming more scientific and accurate. Medicines emerged that were effective in treating disease if used properly. Infectious diseases that formerly killed many children were becoming treatable (Shryock 1947, 304–335). Death in childbirth, also once distressingly common, was becoming rarer. Doctors and hospitals were making a real difference in the lives of consumers, and consumers were willing to pay for their care and services. There is little evidence that consumers resisted organized medicine's efforts to escape market competition.

The Failure of Consumer-Driven Health Care and the Search for Alternatives

Eventually consumers did become concerned about how much health care cost. As hospitalization became more and more common for the middle class, it also became more expensive. Doctor's fees also increased rather dramatically, particularly during times when doctors were in short supply like during the First World War. The main problem was not so much the cost of routine medical care, or even the proportion of the national economy devoted to medical care, but rather the costs imposed on particular individuals and families at the time of medical crises.

Then as now, a small fraction of the population was responsible for the vast majority of medical costs, and for these people the cost of health care was often crippling (Committee on the Costs of Medical Care 1932, 16–19). Then as now, the problem was how these catastrophic medical costs could be managed. One approach that today seems obvious is insurance. Although a few commercial insurers offered health insurance as an adjunct to life or disability insurance in the nineteenth century, most commercial insurers believed that health was uninsurable (Starr 1982, 241–42, 298), the problem of adverse selection insurmountable (Simons and Sinai 1932, 176). Few commercial insurers offered health coverage before the First World War (Somers and Somers 1961, 262).

Some patients belonged to "consumer clubs," often ethnically based, that pooled their resources to provide health care and disability or burial benefits (Starr 1982, 206–7). But this form of payment for care never became really widespread.[7] Some patients also worked for employers that offered the services of a company doctor (Starr 1982, 200–202). This was particularly true in remote and inaccessible areas where health care might not otherwise have been available. Mining and timber companies were particularly likely to offer access to a company doctor, more often in the West than in the settled East (Davis and Rorem 1932, 202). But these arrangements were opposed by organized medicine and remained rare in most of the country.

The truly indigent could turn to the government (usually local government) for care or receive charitable services. Publicly funded care was indeed quite common, but only for the "worthy" needy, and the process of establishing eligibility was intrusive and humiliating.[8] Private charitable care was also available through charitable hospitals, dispensaries, and private doctors who provided free care to indigents (Cathell 1922, 296–97). Charitable care was available only to the neediest, however, and often in crowded and unpleasant hospital wards or in dispensaries.

Physicians constantly complained about abuse of the dispensaries by patients who could afford to pay for services, and made certain that dispensaries remained unpleasant enough to discourage patients who had resources. Patients who used dispensaries might have to spend the whole day waiting in close quarters with others who had contagious diseases, only to be seen for a few minutes by an overworked and harried doctor rushing on to the next patient. Even those who clearly qualified for charity often tried to avoid these conditions by scraping together enough to be seen by a private physician (Starr 1982, 182–83).

In the absence of insurance, people paid for health care from their current income where possible, or from their savings where it was not. Some hospitals set up programs to help people save for anticipated medical expenses, such as the birth of a child. An article in the *Bulletin of the American Hospital Association* in 1928 presciently referred to these savings accounts as "health savings accounts" (Bacon 1928, 69). It advised: "Economic preparedness of the individual in connection with the use of the modern hospital is largely a matter of public education and training . . . Practicable and easy plans might well be formulated to encourage use of the item 'sickness' in the family budget as actively as the items 'insurance' and even 'clothes' are budgeted" (Bacon 1928, 68). The Farmer Security Administration in the 1930s also attempted to set up an account-based medical savings program for its borrowers, though it later abandoned the program in favor of a group prepayment program (Williams 1939, 585–86).

In the end it appears that budgeting for major medical care expenses proved impractical. Patients found it difficult to know ahead of time how much care would cost. Doctors' fees varied dramatically and were difficult to determine before a service was rendered. Proposals were considered to reduce uncertainty by disclosing the total costs of hospitalization at the time of admission, but this did not address the problem of skewed medical costs, for which an insurance model was needed (Davis and Rorem 1932, 90–99, 184–89, 198–99, 200–201). Medical costs were a "serious and often staggering financial burden for those who suffer them. Even budgets well above the poverty line, large enough to care for ordinary current expenses on a reasonable standard of living and including a certain amount of regular medical services, are shattered and the family driven to the wall financially when these high-cost-illnesses befall" (Davis and Rorem 1932, 51–52).

When their pockets were empty, patients had to borrow the money to pay for health care services. Usually the lender would be the doctor or hospital that provided the care. As earlier noted, doctors commonly billed for their services after the services were rendered, and when bills were not promptly paid they became debts carried by the doctor (Starr 1982, 63; Davis 1941, 54–55). For a period in the 1920s and early 1930s loans to cover medical costs were common, sometimes offered by hospitals and at other times by commercial lenders (Stevens 1989, 146). Some medical societies organized "medical service bureaus" to provide installment loans to pay for medical services. The Cleveland Hospital Council in 1933 set up a hospital finance corporation to determine the creditworthiness of patients and to make individual loans to them (Stevens 1989, 146). One small-loan company reported that 30 percent of all its loans were for medical payments (Davis 1941, 54). The interest and expenses attributable to these loans substantially increased medical costs (Davis 1941, 54–55).

But borrowing to purchase health care is obviously quite different from borrowing to start a business or buy a home or farm, both from the standpoint of the debtor and from that of the creditor. Major purchases and investments are planned for, and can be put off until earning capacity is sufficient to carry the debt. High-cost episodes of medical care are usually unanticipated and often interfere with earning capacity. Lenders often see debtors with serious medical problems as poor credit risks. Finally, a surgery, unlike a new appliance, cannot be repossessed if payments are not made.[9] Debt financing for medical costs, therefore, was never commonly used before the growth in the popularity of credit cards (which made unsecured loans with little attention to credit-worthiness widespread).

While the cost of medical care, and in particular hospital care, stretched the means of many consumers and threatened the financial stability of doctors and hospitals under the best of circumstances, these problems became devastating during the depressions that periodically swept the country. The precipitating cause of the change in the American system of health care finance was the Great Depression of the 1930s, during which not only isolated high-cost patients suffered ruin but the financial life of the nation's hospital system itself was seriously threatened (Starr 1982, 270–71).

The Depression brought on dramatic decreases in both occupancy and payment for the nation's hospitals. Occupancy rates in the hospitals in Cook County, Illinois, dropped by 50.5 percent during 1932 (Davis and Rorem 1932, 4–5). Occupancy rates in government hospitals grew, but occupancy fell in voluntary hospitals (Davis and Rorem 1932, 24–25). Two out of five hospitals owned by individuals or partnerships, and one out of six hospitals owned by nonprofit or for-profit corporations, closed between 1928 and 1936 (Stevens 1989, 147).

The Depression, moreover, came at a time of continually increasing medical costs. Though costs had been increasing throughout the nineteenth century, they rose especially rapidly during the 1920s (Rosen 1946, 46, 89; Starr 1982, 258–59). This increase in costs was accompanied by an even more troubling increase in the variability of costs. The cost of high-cost cases, that is to say, climbed even faster than the cost of average cases (Starr 1982, 260). When this rise in costs collided with the fall in incomes brought on by the Depression, it precipitated the first major health care cost crisis in American history.

An immediate effect was the convening of the Committee on the Costs of Medical Care, whose final report, *Medical Care for the American People*, was published in 1932. The committee, formed in the late 1920s, consisted of a distinguished group of economists, physicians, and public health specialists, led by Ray Lyman Wilbur, a physician who was a past president of the AMA and current president of Stanford University, and who later became the secretary of the interior (Starr 1982, 261). Despite what its name might suggest, the committee did not find that expenditures on health care were excessive (Committee on the Costs of Medical Care 1932, 13–15). The primary concern of the committee was that the amount of medical care provided in the United States fell far short of the services actually "needed," that is, of the "standards for good medical care published by the Committee" (Committee on the Costs of Medical Care 1932, 7). The report concluded that medical services received were less than those needed for all income groups, including wealthy Americans, but particularly for the poor and for African Americans (Committee on the Costs of Medical Care 1932, 7–10).[10] "The Committee report on the need for medical care set out the position that: The real need for medical care is a medical, not an economic, concept. It can be defined only in terms of the physical conditions of the people and the capacities of the science and art of medicine to deal with them. Thus, it is not always a conscious need, still less an active desire backed by willingness to pay. The ordinary layman lacks the knowledge to define his own medical needs and can rely only on the expert opinion of medical practitioners and public health authorities" (Lee and Jones 1933, 12).[11] The committee described needed medical care in some detail and identified the personnel and facilities needed to meet that need.

One reason why provision fell short of need, in the eyes of the committee, was the skewed distribution of medical costs (Committee on the Costs of

Medical Care 1932, 48). "No one fact is more clearly demonstrated by the Committee studies than this one: That costs of medical care in any one year now fall very unevenly upon different families in the same income and population groups" (Committee on the Costs of Medical Care 1932, 18). Because of this skewed burden the committee concluded that budgeting for medical costs was impracticable: "it is impossible for 99 per cent of the families to set aside any reasonable sum of money with positive assurance that that sum will purchase all needed medical care" (Committee on the Costs of Medical Care 1932, 19).

Out-of-pocket payment for medical care on a fee-for-service basis caused problems not only for patients but also for physicians and other providers. Incomes of physicians dependent on out-of-pocket payment varied widely, while fee-for-service medicine resulted, the report asserted, in unnecessary care and "fee-splitting," or kickbacks from specialists to general practitioners for referrals (Committee on the Costs of Medical Care 1932, 22, 24).

In short, the committee concluded that consumer-driven health care had failed. The solution to the problems facing Americans was some form of sharing of risk. "Inevitably the Committee has been led to the conclusion that the cost of medical care should be distributed over groups of people and over period of time" (Committee on the Costs of Medical Care 1932, 48). This kind of risk pooling, the committee concluded, was only possible through taxation or insurance. The committee was skeptical of the potential of commercial insurance to achieve cost sharing, believing that insurers would remove incentives for efficiency and economy and threaten the quality of care by forgoing "professional participation in the formulation of policies" (Committee on the Costs of Medical Care 1932, 51). The committee also rejected the notion of a program aimed only at poor people, which would have to offer services more limited in scope or lower in quality than that received by the population as a whole (Committee on the Costs of Medical Care 1932, 128).

Rather, the majority of the committee supported group health insurance, financed by regular premium payments from individuals and families at a level that they could pay "without undue hardship," supplemented where necessary by local taxes, especially to cover the costs of the poor (Committee on the Costs of Medical Care 1932, 68). In communities where incomes were too low for local taxes to cover medical care, the local taxes could be supplemented by state or even federal tax funds (Committee on the Costs of Medical Care 1932, 68, 122). The majority of the committee favored maintaining a voluntary insurance system, at least until sufficient experience was gained to support a compulsory insurance system (Committee on the Costs of Medical Care 1932, 127). The committee recognized, however, that families with low or irregular incomes, as well as the self-employed and small businessmen, were unlikely to purchase insurance voluntarily (Committee on the Costs of Medical Care 1932, 127). A minority report endorsed a compulsory insurance system, contending that voluntary insurance could never cover "the unorganized, low-paid working group who are not indigent but live on a minimum subsistence income" (Committee on the Costs of Medical Care 1932, 131).

The recommendations of the majority report were met with a strongly dissenting minority report. This dissenting minority was composed primarily of the physician members, and their main concern was for preserving the economic perquisites of physicians, particularly-fee-for-service practice (Committee on the Costs of Medical Care 1932, 151). They strongly opposed the expansion of insurance, but in paradoxical contrast to today's critics of insurance, they challenged insurance as promoting competition among providers, which they viewed as destructive (Committee on the Costs of Medical Care 1932, 165). Voluntary insurance, they claimed, had everywhere failed (Committee on the Costs of Medical Care 1932, 163). "Wherever [voluntary insurance plans] are established there is solicitation of patients, destructive competition among professional groups, inferior medical service, loss of personal relationship of patient and physician, and demoralization of the professions" (Committee on the Costs of Medical Care 1932, 164). The minority recognized the problem that medical cost imposed on the chronically ill, but suggested that physicians themselves, or perhaps medical plans sponsored by county medical societies, bear the risk, and that the government help to finance care for the indigent (Committee on the Costs of Medical Care 1932, 168–81).

In the end, however, the majority of the committee realized that in its first incarnation, consumer-directed health care had failed. Even though medical costs were much lower than they are now, saving and borrowing were not adequate to the task of paying for health care, at least for those with the most serious problems. The solution to which the country turned was health insurance. That solution is the subject of the next chapter.

CHAPTER 5

The Nonaccidental System

The Origins of American Health Insurance

A primary message of the CDHC movement is that we have too much health insurance. Economics teaches us, however, that consumers do not purchase "too much" of a product in a properly functioning market—whatever amount consumers demand is the right amount. To sustain their claim of "overinsurance," therefore, CDHC advocates must establish that the market for health insurance in the United States is distorted in some way. In fact, this is what they do claim: that the market for health insurance in the United States is distorted because insurance is purchased by employers rather than insureds, and employers purchase too much insurance because of the incentives offered by perverse federal government policy.

Central to the message of the CDHC, therefore, is the belief that our health insurance system is an "accident" of bad public policy, not the result of consumer demand (Cannon and Tanner 2005, 61; Cogan, Hubbard, and Kessler 2005, 2; Gabel 1999). Repeatedly throughout CDHC literature one finds reference to "the accidental health insurance system." The story told by CDHC advocates is that employment-related health insurance began in the United States during the Second World War because the National War Labor Board (NWLB), acting under the

Stabilization Act of 1942, put a cap on wage increases but allowed employers to increase fringe benefits, including health insurance, instead. Employment-related health benefits continued to grow after the war, the story continues, because an Internal Revenue Ruling issued during the war held that insurance benefits could be offered to employees free from taxation to both employer and employee, a position confirmed by the Internal Revenue Code of 1954.

In fact there is some truth in both claims. The NWLB did exempt health insurance benefits from wage controls under some circumstances during the latter part of the war, resulting in some expansion of health insurance benefits. Tax exemption for employee benefits also was a factor in the expansion of employee benefits in the second half of the twentieth century, particularly after the middle of the 1950s once the tax code clarified the tax status of health insurance. The primary reason why we have employment-related health insurance in the United States, however, is the same reason why many developed countries historically began their health care financing systems with employment-related health insurance and why many countries still have employment-related insurance today. Health insurance is a product that consumers want, and one of the most efficient ways to provide it is through places of employment, which meliorates the problem of adverse selection and reduces marketing and underwriting costs (Glied 2005; Hyman and Hall 2001). Health insurance came into existence in the United States in the 1930s, not during the Second World War, and it came into existence because the CDHC system described in chapter 4 had failed. Employment-related insurance expanded dramatically throughout the 1940s and 1950s in both the number of employees and the extent of services covered, and it did so even though throughout this period most employees paid for health insurance with their own, after-tax income. Health insurance coverage expansion during the 1940s and 1950s was largely driven by collective bargaining, as unions fought to provide employer-funded insurance coverage for their members, and as other employers attempted to resist unionization by unilaterally offering richer health insurance benefits to their employees.

Employment-related insurance continued to expand, covering more employees and becoming more comprehensive throughout the 1970s and 1980s, in part because of the tax subsidy, but also because employees valued insurance as a means of responding to rapidly increasing health care costs and because employers understood the value of health insurance to their employees.

Contrary to the claims of some CDHC advocates, employee cost sharing continued to be significant from the 1950s until the coming of managed care in the late 1980s and early 1990s. Despite this, health care cost inflation grew at historically high levels throughout this period, only to be reined in by managed care in the 1990s, even though, paradoxically, employee cost sharing decreased markedly under managed care. The true story of America's nonaccidental health care system, in sum, is quite different from the version presented by CDHC advocates. This chapter tells that story.

Prepayment for Health Care: Blue Cross

One route that the United States could have taken to address the increasingly prominent problem of medical costs discussed in chapter 4 would have been to establish a public health insurance program. Germany had been the first country to establish a social insurance program for workers in 1883, and other countries in Europe soon followed, including the United Kingdom in 1911 (Jost 2003, 71–72, 205–6). The first major drive for a national health social insurance program in the United States took place in the second decade of the twentieth century. Though for a time an impressive coalition of business, labor, and even medical interests supported this legislation, it ran into stubborn political resistance and ultimately came up short (Starr 1982, 243–57). Subsequent efforts in the 1930s and 1940s met with more determined opposition from organized medicine and business interests, and also failed.

What arose in the place of either a public national social insurance program or a private system for financing medical debt was voluntary insurance through private nonprofit prepayment plans, Blue Cross and later Blue Shield. The first "hospital service plan" was started by Baylor Hospital in Dallas in 1932. Baylor entered into a contract under which white public school teachers paid fifty cents a month into a prepaid hospital services plan with the assurance that they would receive up to twenty-one days of hospital care if they needed hospitalization, and a one-third discount on the next 344 days (Stevens 1989, 137; Payton and Powsner 1980, 216).

Hospital service plans filled an obvious need and spread quickly during the 1930s. Although other service plans based on a single hospital were established, like that of Baylor, state and regional hospital plans quickly became much more common. In 1936 the American Hospital Association established the Commission on Hospital Services, which ultimately became the Blue Cross Association (Dickerson 1963, 152). This commission encouraged and supported the spread of state and regional Blue Cross plans. Blue Cross plans were heavily advertised, and found a responsive audience (Stevens 1989, 185). By

1937 twenty-six plans had 600,000 members, and by 1940 seventy-one plans had 4.4 million members (Stevens 1989, 182).

Blue Cross plan members paid a fixed sum every month for the assurance that their needs would be covered if they had to be hospitalized. Blue Cross plans were available on a community-rated basis to employment-related groups, professional and community associations, and in some cases individuals. The plans negotiated "service benefit" contracts with the hospitals, under which the plans would cover up to a fixed number of days of hospitalization for a per diem fee established in the contract. Initially plans covered an average of twenty-one days, but by 1949 most members were covered for thirty-one days, and by 1956 seventy days of hospital coverage seemed most common, with some plans covering six months or more (Somers and Somers 1961, 278). Blue Cross plans also provided either service benefit or indemnity coverage for "extras" such as emergency and operating room charges, or laboratory tests (U.S. Senate 1951, 38).[1] Blue Cross plans did not initially impose deductibles or require coinsurance payments for hospital services, rather providing "first-dollar" coverage for the full cost of hospitalization up to the maximum number of days.[2] The Blue Cross strategy proved remarkably successful for the hospitals. Blue Cross plans were also very popular with consumers and spread rapidly.

As it became increasingly clear that there was a substantial market for hospital benefits, private commercial insurers began also to market health insurance products. Initially most entrants into the market were life insurers, who were experienced in underwriting based on health conditions (Somers and Somers 1961, 263). Commercial insurance policies were very different from the Blue Cross products. Like Blue Cross, they covered hospital care, but many also covered surgical care as well (Stevens 1989, 188). In the late 1930s and early 1940s they even began to cover medical costs (nonsurgical physician's services). By the late 1950s home and office visits also began to be covered, especially under individual policies (Somers and Somers 1961, 281, 334).

Commercial health insurance was sold on an indemnity basis. Insureds would pay medical providers in cash for services and then file a claim with the insurer for an indemnity payment. These payments would be for fixed sums per service, which were set forth beforehand in the insurance contract. Some commercial policies included deductibles, which became more common over time (Somers and Somers 1961, 282).[3] The fixed level of indemnity payments was the insurer's strongest protection against excessive use by insureds. Insureds had to pay for the difference between the indemnity payment and the doctor or hospital charge out of their own pocket, which encouraged them to search for and purchase lower-cost care and to avoid overuse (Frech and Ginsburg 1978, 27–29).[4]

One of the major problems that the Blue Cross plans faced in competing with the commercial insurers was their lack of coverage for medical and surgical benefits. The success of the hospitals in offering prepaid benefits was soon noticed by physicians. In 1939 the first of the medical benefits plans that came to be known as Blue Shield plans became available (Somers and Somers 1961, 318). Blue Shield plans initially covered surgical benefits in hospital, later expanding to cover medical benefits in hospital and eventually medical benefits out of hospital.

Blue Shield plans combined the Blue Cross and commercial insurance approaches to providing benefits. Though some plans offered only service benefits or only indemnity coverage, most plans offered both (Reed 1947, 205–15). Members whose incomes fell below a fixed income level (an average of $2,050 for a single individual and $3,500 for a family in 1949) received service benefits (U.S. Senate 1951, 41). Doctors agreed to accept negotiated payments from the plans as payment in full for these patients (Reed 1947, 212–14). Members with incomes above these levels, on the other hand, received indemnity payments and had to pay the difference between whatever the doctor chose to charge them and the indemnity amount (U.S. Senate 1951, 41). In 1949 about one-quarter to one-third of Blue Shield members had service benefit plans, the remainder indemnity plans (U.S. Senate 1951, 41). Blue Shield plans were initially community-rated, but over time they moved to experience rating to compete with the commercial insurers (Ehrenreich and Ehrenreich 1970, 151–54). Over time Blue Shield plans also began to impose deductibles and coinsurance payments.

During the 1930s and 1940s other models of health care coverage arose based on comprehensive prepayment for health care (Somers and Somers 1961, 341–63). These plans were generally known as the "independent" plans. Some of these, such as the Kaiser plan, were initially industry sponsored; others, like the Ross-Loos plans, were sponsored by physicians; while yet others, like the Washington Group Health Insurance Plan, grew out of the old consumer-sponsored plans. These plans generally did not impose cost sharing, because they were better able to control costs directly through their control over doctors (Starr 1982, 292–93). The independent plans, precursors of our modern staff-model HMOs, were vigorously opposed by organized medicine, particularly those that were not sponsored by physicians. Organized medicine preferred cash-and-carry medicine (as it does today), but was willing to tolerate prepayment and indemnity insurance as long as insurance did not subject doctors to lay control. Lay control of medical practice was unacceptable, and health plans that employed doctors were fought tooth and claw by the AMA through much of the twentieth century, resulting in the 1940s in a criminal conviction of the AMA for antitrust violations.[5] These efforts by the AMA succeeded in keeping prepaid medical practice marginal through much of the twentieth century.

Employment-Related Insurance: A Choice, Not an Accident

Blue Cross plans, and later commercial and Blue Shield plans, were sold primarily to groups. It was much less expensive to market health insurance to groups than to individuals, and marketing to employment-related groups in particular also went far toward solving the perennial problem of adverse selection (Reed 1947, 59–60; Glied 2005, 40–41). Blue Cross plans sold insurance to groups of various types, including professional associations. Primarily, however, they contracted with employment-related groups. Persons healthy enough to work were reasonably good risks for health insurance, and employers could deduct the premium from the employee's paycheck, assuring that premiums would be paid.[6]

While most group plans were employment-related, they were not initially paid for by employers. Employers permitted the sale of group policies to their employees, facilitated the formation of groups, and often deducted the premiums from pay checks through a payroll check-off system. But few employers financed the plans themselves. Indeed most government employers were legally prohibited from contributing, or even from providing payroll check-offs (U.S. Senate 1951, 9, 66).

The limited role of employers in these plans began to change in the 1940s. Insurance coverage also grew dramatically during the war. One reason was wartime wage stabilization and tax policies. Labor was scarce during the war, and excess profit taxes were very high, up to 85 percent (Brown 1997–98, 651). The Stabilization Act of 1942 allowed the NWLB to exclude a "reasonable amount" of insurance benefits from wage controls,[7] and board rulings exempted some health insurance benefits from the board's general policy of limiting wage increases to increases in the cost of living (Klein 2003, 179–80). An IRS ruling of 1943 also allowed businesses to deduct payments to health and welfare funds as business expenses, and provided that these benefits would not be taxable to employees.[8]

Yet there are several reasons to be skeptical of the claim that wage policy was the primary reason for the expansion of health insurance coverage during the war. First and foremost, as just noted, health insurance as an employee benefit was already well established and growing rapidly before the war began. Second, the NWLB did not uniformly exempt health insurance benefits from price controls. Although it did in 1943 adopt a general policy of allowing employers and unions to agree to new employee benefit plans costing up to 5 percent of payroll, in individual contested cases it refused to require benefit increases (Klein 2004, 40–42; Klein 2003, 177–83). The board's primary goal was to preserve labor peace while keeping inflation in check. It thus kept employers from cutting back on fringe benefits, but it did not require them to expand benefits. Indeed, in at least one case it refused to make an employer provide an insurance plan wholly funded by employees, opining that the mere provision of a payroll check-off would be too much of a burden for the employer (Klein 2003, 180).

Third, most of the growth in wartime employment and health insurance coverage took place before the NWLB policies came into effect. The NWLB wage freeze went into effect in 1942. Both the Revenue Act of 1942, which imposed excess profit taxes, and the NWLB fringe benefit exemptions went into effect in 1943. American industry had in fact been gearing up for the looming war since 1939, and while employment increased 49 percent between 1939 and 1943, it only increased another 4 percent between 1943 and 1945 (Dobbin 1992, 1437). More importantly, while the number of American employees carrying employment-related commercial group health insurance increased from 3.5 million in 1939 to 6.5 million in 1943, it only increased another half a million between 1943 and 1946 (Ilse 1953, 189). Employment-related insurance coverage also continued to increase rapidly after wage price stabilization controls expired in 1946, suggesting again that expansion was not driven primarily by wage stabilization policy. The wage stabilization policy was in any event routinely circumvented, as it allowed wage increases in conjunction with promotions, and "in-job promotions" quickly became common (Dobbin 1992, 1438).

Finally, throughout the war employment-related insurance continued almost always to be paid for by employees rather than employers, and thus wage controls were largely irrelevant. By the end of the war only 7.6 percent of Blue Cross enrollees were participants in groups to which employers contributed (U.S. Senate 1951, 67). Under contracts negotiated during the war, employers often simply contributed a percentage of payroll (2–3 percent) for fringe benefits generally, and much of this went to life or accidental-death policies (U.S. Department of Labor 1947, 2).

The Evolution of Employment-Related Health Insurance

In fact, the most explosive growth in health insurance coverage came after the war. The number of workers covered by health insurance under collective bargaining agreements (which usually provided the most generous benefits) grew from half a million in 1945 to 3 million in mid-1948, over 7.5 million in early 1950, and finally 11.3 million — 70 percent of all workers under collective bargaining agreements — by 1954 (Rowe 1955, 1). By 1950 75 million Americans, or half the population, had some form of private health insurance, up from 6 million in total in 1939 (U.S. Senate 1951, 1–2).[9] By 1965, the year Medicare and Medicaid were adopted, private hospital insurance covered 156 million Americans,[10] or about 80 percent of the population (Health Insurance Institute 1966, 5, 10–13).[11]

Not only did the number of employees covered grow after the war, but coverage became more comprehensive as well. The most important of the new forms of coverage to emerge in the 1950s was major medical coverage, through which commercial insurers (who by the 1950s had caught up with and in some parts of the country surpassed the Blues in covered lives) provided catastrophic coverage for hospital and medical care. Major medical policies usually supplemented basic hospital and surgical-medical coverage. Comprehensive coverage, which arrived soon after major medical, bundled basic and major medical coverage to provide the most complete coverage available (Somers and Somers 1961, 383).[12] During the 1940s and 1950s Blue Cross and Blue Shield plans began to combine forces to offer similarly comprehensive coverage, as well as coverage that was convertible nationwide among Blue plans (Somers and Somers 1961, 299–300, 324–25). Finally, during the 1960s and 1970s insurance coverage began to expand to cover dental care and pharmaceuticals, with improved coverage for maternity care, mental health, and some preventive services within basic coverage. By 1977, 87 percent of employees were covered for pharmaceutical benefits, as were 75 percent for outpatient mental health benefits (Gabel 1999, 68).[13]

Another important trend after the war was increased employer responsibility for employee health benefits. During the late 1940s and early 1950s employer contributions to collectively bargained plans increased exponentially. Employers generally turned to commercial insurers for health insurance coverage, and commercial insurers offered employers generous premium rebates that sharply reduced the cost to the employer of coverage (Klein 2003, 225–26). A survey of collectively bargained plans in 1950 found that employers paid half the initial gross premium cost for their employees' insurance coverage, but only 37.5 percent of the net premium cost after taking into account rebates received from insurers (U.S. Senate 1951, 66).[14] By comparison, employers had only paid 25 percent of gross and 10 percent of net cost for collectively bargained plans in 1945. By 1959 employers paid the entire premium for hospital insurance for virtually all unionized employees in multi-employer plans and for 37 percent of employees subject to collective bargaining agreements in single-employer plans (U.S. Department of Labor 1960a, 6–7).[15]

Employer contributions to premiums in non-unionized places of employment increased more slowly. As recently as 1950 only 12.2 percent of Blue Cross participants were enrolled in groups to which employers contributed (U.S. Senate 1951, 67). By 1964, however, about 48 percent of employees had the total cost of their health insurance covered by their employer, and only 2.4 percent paid the entire cost themselves (Health Insurance Institute 1966, 28). Employer contributions to health insurance expanded even further during the 1970s and 1980s. By 1980 large employers paid for over 90 percent of health insurance premiums, while medium-sized firms paid two-thirds of individual coverage and half of family coverage (U.S. House of Representatives 1984, 101). By 1988 employers covered in total 90 percent of the cost of individual coverage and 75 percent of the cost of family coverage (Gabel, DiCarlo, Fink, and de Lissovoy 1989, 120).

Why Employment-Related Group Insurance?

There are several reasons for these impressive expansions in the number of workers covered, the benefits provided, and the level of employer contributions in the third quarter of the twentieth century. One was certainly pressure from the labor unions. Unions provided health benefits to their members as early as the 1880s, although they vacillated between the desire to provide welfare benefits for their members and the need to focus solely on compensation (Munts 1967, 3–12). Unions were at the peak of their strength in the mid-twentieth century. At the close of the war over 30 percent of the nonfarm labor force was unionized; union membership had increased by six million between 1939 and 1945 (Brown 1997–98, 659). In the late 1940s unions pushed hard for increased compensation, and particularly for fringe benefits. One insurance company executive was quoted at the time as saying: "Unions are the direct initiating influence in 75 percent of the group health policies now being written, and may be the most important influence in the other 25%" (Baker and Dahl 1945, 10).

The Inland Steel case in 1949 clarified that employee benefits were included within the "terms of conditions of employment" subject to collective bargaining under the National Labor Relations Act, giving new impetus to union demands for health benefits.[16] The unions saw their ability to provide health insurance as important to securing the allegiance of workers, particularly where benefit plans were union-administered (Brown 1997–98, 657–66). Unions were also, moreover, genuinely interested in the health needs of their members (Baker and Dahl 1945, 19).

Although some of the major unions, notably the United Mine Workers, insisted on union-run health plans, employment-related plans on the whole remained under the control of employers (Klein 2004, 44–52).[17] Unions tended to favor Blue Cross and Blue Shield contracts, which offered more comprehensive coverage,[18] but large employers favored commercial insurers, who offered them more flexibility in the design of plans as well as the rebates already mentioned (U.S. Senate 1951, 88; Klein 2004, 51). Employers with healthy workforces also favored commercial insurers because they used experience rating and thus could offer lower rates (Stevens 1989, 260).

The unions' push for benefits affected even firms that were not unionized. Employers realized that fringe benefits were a potent bargaining tool of the unions and offered liberal fringe benefits to forestall unionization (Brown 1997–98, 666). Employers also saw health insurance as a means to stabilize employment (by making it more difficult for employees to leave), to keep workers healthy and productive, and to ward off a national social health insurance program (Baker and Dahl 1945, 25).[19]

Another factor underlying the growth of employment-related insurance was the continuing increase in health care costs. The proportion of the gross domestic product spent on health care grew from 3.9 percent in 1930 to 5.1 percent in 1950. At the same time, changes in medical technology were making medical care much more effective, and thus more valuable (Thomasson 2002, 236). While patients valued medical care more and more, they found it less and less affordable, especially if they had high-cost conditions. One study in 1952–53 found that 15 percent of American families were in debt for medical care, and this only included debt to health care providers, not debt to financial institutions for loans incurred to cover medical care (Dickerson 1963, 33–34). The growing burden of health care costs led in turn to an increased desire to pass costs on to insurers, and ultimately to employers.

A third factor was the enactment of the Employee Retirement Income Security Act (ERISA) in 1974, which encouraged employers to self-insure. Self-insurance seems to have caught on quickly, as it gave employers increased power to control health care costs and the right to receive interest on reserves, as well as the opportunity to avoid state health insurance premium taxes, health insurance mandates (which became common in the early 1980s), capital and reserve requirements, and state risk pool contribution requirements (Gabel, Jajick-Toth, de Lissovoy, Rice, and Cohen 1988, 59). By the end of the 1980s self-insurance had become common for big employers. Whereas only 5 percent of group health claims were paid by self-insured plans in 1975, an estimated 60 percent of employees were in self-insured plans by 1987 (Gabel, Jajick-Toth, de Lissovoy, Rice, and Cohen 1988, 58).[20] Self-insurance meant, however, that the employer took on a significant share of the cost of the insurance rather than simply passing it on to the employee.

Finally, tax policy certainly played a role. The IRS ruling of 1943 provided support for the argument that employment-related group health insurance premium contributions were deductible business expenses for employers and not taxable income for employees, although the question remained unsettled.[21] The Internal Revenue Code (1954) explicitly recognized the nontaxability of employment-related benefits, and as more and more Americans began to pay income tax, the tax benefits of health insurance became more important (Thomasson 2003).[22] Employers and unions were aware that health benefits were exempt from taxation, and thus more valuable than cash wages (Munts 1967, 87). In particular, tax policy played a role in increasing employer contributions to employment-related health insurance (Munts 1967, 87). But tax policy was only one factor, and perhaps not the most important, in the expansion of health coverage. Other fringe benefits, such as life insurance and disability benefits, were also tax exempt, but did not become as widespread. In the end it was primarily consumer demand as mediated through the unions and recognized by employers — not unwise government policy — that drove the expansion of health insurance.

The True Story of Cost Sharing

While health insurance coverage expanded and employers took on responsibility for an ever growing share of insurance premiums during the second half of the twentieth century, insureds continued to bear much of the cost of health care itself. Six forms of cost sharing have played an important role in the history of health insurance in the United States. Three of these are the standard forms of cost sharing used by contemporary health insurance plans: deductibles, coinsurance, and co-payments. The fourth form is the balance-billing that results when indemnity insurance fails to cover a provider's entire bill. The fifth form is the costs that an insured incurs when medical bills exceed maximum coverage. The final form is payments that are made out of pocket for health care services not covered by insurance.

From the beginning, Blue Cross and Blue Shield generally offered first-dollar coverage. This did not mean that the Blues covered the full cost of care for their members. Initially they had rather conservative coverage limits. Twenty-one-day maximums for hospital coverage, for example, were standard with the earliest plans, and thus insureds faced the possibility of considerable costs once coverage limits were exceeded. Many plans also had fixed dollar limits on ancillary cost coverage (U.S. Senate 1951, 39). Second, Blue Shield coverage for insureds whose income was above a threshold level took the form of indemnity coverage, and therefore insureds had to pay providers extra where they balance-billed (U.S. Senate 1951, 39). In addition, Blue Shield medical payments often began only after a certain number of days of hospitalization (two to six days), which was a form of deductible (U.S. Senate 1951, 39).

Commercial insurance was built on an indemnity model and thus offered limited coverage. Members of commercial plans routinely faced balance-billing from individual providers as well as the possibility of exceeding their coverage and being exposed to further costs. Indeed, indemnity payments were often intentionally set below expected fees to assure that the insured bore part of the cost of care (U.S. Senate 1951, 55). In 1950, for example, commercial insurers covered 45–55 percent of their enrollees' hospital costs and 29 percent of physician services, in contrast to to comparable coverage rates of 70–80 percent for Blue Cross and 45 percent for Blue Shield (U.S. Senate 1951, 4–5). Commercial plans also began imposing deductibles and coinsurance obligations quite early.

The development of the major medical plan in the 1950s brought significant changes in coverage. The major medical plan usually supplemented existing basic coverage, imposing a "corridor" deductible between the basic coverage and the major medical umbrella. The corridor deductible on a major medical plan was usually $100 to $150 (the equivalent of $700 to $1,050 today). Major medical plans also routinely imposed coinsurance obligations of 20 to 25 percent (Department of Labor 1961). The primary selling point of major medical plans was that they offered broad and catastrophic coverage, much like today's high-deductible plans,[23] with coverage limits set at much higher levels than those common in the 1930s and 1940s. By 1959 major medical maximum coverage amounts were usually between $5,000 and $10,000, compared to maximums of around $2,000 for traditional hospital coverage.

The late 1950s, 1960s, and 1970s witnessed contradictory trends in cost sharing. One the one hand, comprehensive plans which emerged in the late 1950s boasted high coverage limits and comprehensive coverage like major medical plans, but much lower deductibles ($25 to $50) and more limited coinsurance obligations (U.S. Department of Labor 1961, 9). Independent prepaid plans had long offered coverage essentially without cost sharing, and now the comprehensive plans also offered the same protection to those with conventional coverage. Coverage under commercial plans also seems to have become more protective as indemnity plans (or at least major medical plans) began to cover "reasonable and customary" charges rather than fixed dollar amounts for indemnity (U.S. Department of Labor 1961, 6–7). Blue Cross and Blue Shield plans also started offering "extended benefit" contracts in competition with commercial comprehensive policies (U.S. House of Representatives 1976, 221).

On the other hand, deductibles and coinsurance continued to be common through the 1970s and into the 1980s, and indeed spread to Blue Cross and Blue Shield plans. The most common deductible amount in 1982 was $100, though 15 percent of employment-related plans had no deductible (U.S. House of Representatives 1984, 289). The most common coinsurance level was 20 percent. Specific deductibles for hospital care became more common in the mid-1980s, as the traditional Blue Cross service benefit finally yielded to the major medical model (Short 1988, 188). In fact cost sharing for hospital care seems to have increased in the mid-1980s, even as cost sharing for other services was decreasing (Short 1988, 88).

It was only with the coming of managed care in the 1980s that cost sharing diminished dramatically. Prepaid independent plans had long existed, antedating both the Blues and commercial insurance, but they had been limited to a few markets (notably California) and a few major plans (notably Kaiser). The Nixon administration, however, decided to base its national health policy on the expansion of prepaid health care — rechristened health maintenance organizations (HMOs), by Paul Ellwood — and in 1973 Congress adopted legislation to encourage the growth of HMOs. HMO coverage grew slowly but steadily through the 1970s (from 6 million members in 1976 to 8.3 million in 1979), but after 1983 enrollment exploded, rising from 12.5 million members in that year to 29.3 million by the end of 1987 and 34 million by 1990 (Gruber, Shadle, and Polich 1988, 198; Health Insurance Association of America 1991, 17). The mid-1980s also brought on the emergence of new forms of managed care: the preferred provider organization, or PPO, and the fee-for-service plan with utilization review, which spread rapidly after 1984 (Gabel, Jajick-Toth, de Lissovoy, Rice, and Cohen 1988, 51). By 1990 one source claimed that 38 million Americans had PPO coverage (Health Insurance Association of America 1991, 21).

HMOs had traditionally imposed only minimal cost-sharing obligations both to encourage preventive care and because they used other strategies for controlling costs.[24] As HMOs spread in the early 1980s, they usually had no or low deductibles. They also commonly relied on co-payments instead of coinsurance. PPOs retained deductibles and coinsurance, but primarily for out-of-plan providers. In the mid-1980s PPOs typically charged 20 percent coinsurance rates for out-of-network care, 5 percent to 10 percent for in-network care (Rice, de Lissovoy, Gabel, and Ermann 1985, 37). By the 1990s indemnity insurance practically disappeared, and with it cost sharing in the form of balance-billing. This development seems to have been of particular benefit to higher-income insureds, who saw out-of-pocket medical expenditures for health care drop from $732 to $452 in constant 1990 dollars from 1990 to 1997 (Gabel, Ginsburg, Pickreign, and Reschovsky 2001, 51). For employees generally, out-of-pocket expenditures dropped from $504 to $404 from 1990 to 1997 in constant 1990 dollars (Gabel, Ginsburg, Pickreign, and Reschovsky 2001, 51). These trends toward lower cost sharing are also apparent in the national health care accounts. Only in 1979 did the amount that private health insurance paid for health care begin to exceed the amount paid out of pocket, but once the gap was opened it continued to widen at an increasing rate through the 1980s and 1990s (Health Insurance Association of America 1990, 59).

When CDHC emerged in the 1990s, therefore, it encountered a situation atypical historically in terms of the proportion of health care costs borne by consumers. In fact, high-deductible policies are not a new discovery; they simply return us to the situation that existed a quarter century earlier.

Although cost-sharing obligations remained substantial until the coming of managed care, however, health care cost inflation remained high throughout most of the second half of the twentieth century. Personal health expenditures grew at a rate of 12.7 percent a year between 1965 and 1970, 12.3 percent between 1970 and 1975, and 13.7 percent between 1975 and 1980 (National Center for Health Statistics 2005, 362). The share of the GDP spent on health care grew from 5.1 percent in 1960 to 12 percent in 1990. There were many factors behind the growth in health care costs during this period, most significantly the creation of the Medicare and Medicaid programs in 1965 and the subsequent large-scale expansion of coverage to many who had not been covered by private insurance. It remains a fact, however, that the coming of managed care in the 1990s brought about a radical diminution in both cost sharing and health care cost inflation. Health care costs increased only 7.3 percent between 1990 and 1995 and 5.6 percent between 1995 and 2000, while the proportion of the GDP devoted to health care actually decreased, from 13.4 percent in 1995 to 13.3 percent in 2000. This happened even though the share of health care costs covered by out-of-pocket expenditures dropped from 27.1 percent in 1980 to 25.5 percent in 1990 to 17 percent in 2000.

Lessons to Be Learned

What can we learn from the history of American private health insurance? First, that our health insurance system is not accidental. We have employment-related group health insurance because employees wanted it, so much so that until the late 1950s they paid for it primarily themselves, without assistance from employers or tax subsidies. Even today, when employees are asked whether they prefer employment-related health insurance that costs a specified amount or the same amount in taxable wages, 80 percent prefer the insurance when the price is set at $6,700, as do 66 percent when it is set at at $10,000. Only 17 percent of current workers are extremely or very confident that they could purchase health insurance on their own if their employer ceased offering coverage and gave them an equivalent amount of cash, and lower-income workers are much less confident of this than higher-income workers (Fronstin 2006a, 10). When asked how much additional taxable income they would need to give up their health coverage, the median amount cited by covered employees is $11,000 (Helman, Mathew Greenwald & Associates, and Fronstin 2006, 2). Tax subsidies undoubtedly encouraged the expansion of health insurance, but they were only one of several factors that did so.

Finally, first-dollar insurance coverage has not been the norm in American history: it is largely a result of the spread of managed care in the 1980s and 1990s. And first-dollar coverage is not the cause of the rise in health care costs over the past half-century. Paradoxically, the spread of first-dollar coverage accompanied a decrease, not an increase, in health care cost inflation. In sum, CDHC advocates present a rather distorted view of the history of American health insurance.

The CDHC movement also has its own history, to which we now turn.

CHAPTER 6

The Origins of Consumer-Driven Health Care:
A Short History of American Health Economics

The Discovery of Moral Hazard

The consumer-driven health care movement not only has its own version of history; it has its own history. Understanding this history can assist us in better understanding the movement. The history of CDHC is largely the history of moral hazard.

From the earliest beginnings of health insurance in the United States observers were concerned about the possible effects of moral hazard.[1] This concern was based in part on the perceived experience of European social insurance systems. Richard Shryock, writing in the 1940s about the German and English systems, saw excessive demand growing out of malingering, craving for medicine, and neurotic patients (Shryock 1947, 388). Shryock also viewed with alarm the early American experience with health insurance. "Quality of medical services was poor, . . . the personal relationship was lost, and . . . malingering or a desire to 'get something back' was encouraged" (Shryock 1947, 410).

A. M. Simons and Nathan Sinai, writing in the early 1930s, also recognized the significant impact of moral hazard. They observed: "Insurance patients, like private ones, are subject to the suggestive power of skillful advertising and ask for the 'latest thing' in highly touted remedies" (Simons and Sinai

1932, 94). "The person who has made regular payments to an insurance fund and sees himself required to pay these indefinitely in the future comes to look upon himself as 'owning' the sum thus accumulated. As this sum grows, there also grows a mental accumulation of desires and excuses to obtain possession of it" (Simons and Sinai 1932, 158). But Simons and Sinai were not wholly sold on the economic model of demand under insurance, concluding: "Such reasoning rests on the discarded, and never accurate, idea that consumers reason out the expenditure of their income instead of buying what is most effectively sold to them" (Simons and Sinai 1932, 171).

In the end Simons and Sinai concluded, like most health policy observers of their generation, that the benefits of health insurance outweighed its costs (Simons and Sinai 1932, 162–63, 206–9). Several million people in the United States were without insurance, incapable of affording medical care without sacrificing other things still more essential for health (Simons and Sinai 1932, 171, 173). Even those who might be able to save for medical care would have problems doing so, because "saving for such emergencies is a hard thing to market against the much more effective salesmanship used for other goods" (Simons and Sinai 1932, 171). Americans needed insurance.

But as health insurance became more prevalent, with it came a growing awareness of the effect of health insurance on health care costs, and in particular on the cost of health insurance itself (LaDou and Kikens 1977, 94–96, 98–99, 101). The cost of health insurance grew rapidly during the 1950s. Part of the increase in insurance cost was attributed to the "well-known" fact that doctors increase charges when caring for insured persons (Harris 1964, 66; U.S. Senate 1951, 88; Starr 1982, 319). Another factor was physician-induced demand (Dickerson 1963, 272). Yet another was the high overhead costs of insurance: 47 percent for private companies (although only 11 percent for Blue Cross) (Harris 1964, 243). But the most important cause of increased health care costs was increased utilization, in particular of hospitals (Harris 1964, 66; Somers and Somers 1961, 523). Seymour Harris reported in 1964 that during a recent nine-year period, premiums for Blue Cross had risen 112 percent and for Blue Shield Surgical by 50 percent, while hospital prices had risen by only 80 percent and the price of surgery by 20 percent. The excess in costs was generally attributed to increased utilization (Harris 1964, 23).

One reason why use of hospitals increased was that throughout the 1950s and 1960s, hospitalization was covered by insurance, while other services were not (Harris 1964, 239).[2] Expanded health insurance coverage increased utilization by making hospital care free at the point of service. One study found one-third of insured hospital admissions "faulty" (excessive or unnecessary), as opposed to 14 percent of noninsured admissions (Harris 1964, 242). But insurance also made health care more widely available to persons with lower incomes, bringing their level of use up to that of higher-income groups (Harris 1964, 24, 240–41). And increased use of hospitals was also due to factors other than insurance, including higher incomes, greater educational attainment, and the shift toward childbirth in hospitals rather than at home. Some also believed that the rapid spread of health insurance might have simply released "pent-up demand" (Somers and Somers 1961, 406).[3]

A remarkable feature of the literature of this period was the extent to which "moral hazard" was viewed as a truly moral issue. O. D. Dickerson, writing in 1959 about "The Problem of Overutilization in Health Insurance," identifies several causes, including the hypochondriac who "forms a 'crush' on the physician . . . and finds in continued medical treatment the attention or affection missing in daily life," psychosomatic illnesses and accident-proneness, and deliberate malingering "to get rest in the comparative luxury of a hospital bed, a free baby-sitter, or to build up a substantial liability claim against a third party" (Dickerson 1959, 65–66). Dickerson also faulted physicians, who would charge patients more and "order 'the works'" when the patient had health insurance, as well as hospital administrators who would "look upon health insurance primarily as a device to keep their hospitals filled to capacity with paying patients" (Dickerson 1959, 66–67). Finally, Dickerson faulted insurers, who overpaid for procedures and encouraged unnecessary hospitalizations by extending coverage to hospital care alone, and then passed on ever-increasing costs to subscribers (Dickerson 1959, 67).

The introduction of Medicare and Medicaid further fueled the rapid escalation of health care costs. Medicaid, which was initially projected to be a low-cost program, far outran its cost estimates (Starr 1982, 384). This was in part because costs were poorly controlled under the initial legislation, but also because physicians and hospitals began to charge for services that they had previously provided as charity (Stevens and Stevens 1970, 385). Health care costs reached 7 percent of GDP in 1970 and 8.8 percent in 1980. The use of cost-based reimbursement by Medicare also seems to have been a major factor driving up cost (Lave and Lave 1970; Worthington 1978, 248).

Some observers recommended greater cost sharing to control moral hazard, even limiting insurance to catastrophic coverage (U.S. Senate 1951, 10–12;

Dickerson 1963, 99, 277–29; Dickerson 1959, 71). Indeed, the position of the AMA at mid-century was that insurance should be limited to catastrophic care: "Minor illnesses should be left as a responsibility of the individual, since, from this view, their costs ordinarily would not represent a serious financial problem" (U.S. Senate 1951, 40). But there was also some hesitation about imposing cost sharing. Herbert Klarman, one of the most prominent health economists of the period, noted, "There is reason to believe . . . that coinsurance may be an ineffective deterrent to extravagant spending by the well-to-do, while imposing excessive burdens on the average family" (Klarman 1957, 37).

Alternative Approaches to Cost Control

Cost sharing was only one alternative proposed for controlling demand. Another was increased utilization review (Harris 1964, 243; Somers and Somers 1961, 235; Starr 1982, 319). American commentators viewed favorably attempts by Canada to control utilization through administrative review of physicians' services (Sinai, Hall, and Homes 1939). Other commentators called for more peer pressure within insured groups to handle overusers (Dickerson 1963, 283; Dickerson 1959, 70).

The primary strategy pursued for controlling costs at mid-century, however, was planning to control excess capacity. Health planning seems to have originated primarily as a solution to the problem of poor distribution and local undersupply of health care resources. In the 1930s the Committee on the Costs of Medical Care, drawing on British sources, had recommended planned, coordinated systems of health care delivery, organized regionally (Melhado 1988, 15, 27). The Hill-Burton hospital construction program of 1949, the most important federal health care initiative until the Medicare and Medicaid programs, required states to plan for hospitals regionally, with a goal of creating a "scientifically planned" hospital system, as a condition of receiving Hill-Burton funds (Stevens 1989, 220).

Over time, however, the rationale of health planning focused increasingly on cost control. The economic justification for planning came to be articulated in Roemer's law, "if a hospital bed is built it will be used,"[4] suggesting that the best way to control hospital costs would be to control hospital construction (Payton and Powsner 1980, 269; Starr 1982, 364; Somers and Somers 1961, 175, 138). New York in 1964 became the first state to regulate capital expenditures of hospitals and nursing homes (Melhado 1988, 33; Starr 1982, 398; Stevens 1989, 307). By 1972, in the wake of the explosive growth in health care costs that followed on the adoption of the Medicare and Medicaid programs, twenty-three states required health care institutions to obtain state approval for major construction projects and capital investments (Stevens 1989, 307). In that year Congress created the Section 1122 health planning program, which authorized the Department of Health, Education and Welfare to deny Medicare capital cost reimbursement for hospitals and nursing homes that had not received approval from state health planning agencies (Melhado 1988, 33). Finally, in 1974 Public Law 93-641 created a new comprehensive federal health planning program, replacing the health planning agencies developed by the states with a national system of regional health agencies that would finally control capital investment in health care institutions, and thus health care costs (Starr 1982, 401–2).

The planning strategy aimed to achieve cost control through supply-side limitations. It was a strategy that reflected the high social value placed on technically advanced medical care, and a continuing belief that it was possible to identify an objective standard for the need for care (Melhado 1988, 31). At least at the beginning, however, planning largely ignored the importance of demand in driving, and limiting, health care costs.

The Birth of Health Economics and Demand Theory

By the 1960s economists became increasingly interested in the application of mainstream economics, including the concept of demand, to health care. Although several prominent economists had written about health issues early in the twentieth century, often as advocates for national health insurance, mainstream economists paid little attention to health care from the 1920s through the Second World War (Fox 1979, 302–14). In part this neglect may have been due to the general belief at the time that medical care was not subject to the normal laws of supply and demand, because need for medical care was based on objective scientific judgment and because consumers had "no basis for critical judgment" in making purchasing decisions (Fox 1979, 311). Milton Friedman's doctoral dissertation, criticizing restrictions on entry into the medical profession, forcefully argued that medical care was subject to economic analysis, but although written in 1937, it was not published until 1945 (Fox 1979, 314–15). The seminal breakthrough in the application of economic thought to health care was Kenneth Arrow's paper "Uncertainty and the Welfare Economics of Medical Care" (Arrow 1963).

Arrow had been commissioned by the Ford Foundation to bring to the field of health care the insights of a theoretical economist who had not previously worked in the field (Hammer, Haas-Wilson, and Sage 2001, 838). Arrow focused on the problem of risk and uncertainty as the central problem in medical care markets, a focus captured in the title of his article. He accepted a conventional view of insurance as a means of pooling risk in the face of uncertainty and affirmed its role in medical care markets (Arrow 1963, 959–60). To Arrow the pooling of medical risk through insurance potentially resulted in a "net social gain which may be of quite substantial magnitude" (Arrow 1963, 960). He also argued that the value of medical care might exceed its cost, because recovery from an illness could mean return to productivity and relief from "dissatisfactions" (Arrow 1963, 960–61).[5] Where insurance financed this care it would be welfare enhancing, because it would facilitate access to medical care that a person might otherwise have forgone because of its cost. Arrow concluded therefore that "[t]he welfare case for insurance policies of all sorts is overwhelming" (Arrow 1963, 961). And, he argued, "It follows that government should undertake insurance in those cases where [the market for insurance], for whatever reason, has failed to emerge" (Arrow 1963, 961). Arrow recognized the problem of moral hazard but suggested several ways of dealing with it, including coinsurance and "third party control" (Arrow 1963, 961–962). He did not see moral hazard as an insurmountable problem that negated the welfare-enhancing character of insurance for medical care.

In 1968 Mark Pauly published a brief response to Arrow's article, arguing that moral hazard was a much more serious problem than Arrow had recognized. Pauly noted that the practical effect of insurance without cost sharing is to reduce the price of medical care to zero, and thus to increase the amount of medical care consumed (unless the demand for medical care is wholly inelastic) (Pauly 1968, 532–33). In the presence of insurance, each individual faces a prisoner's dilemma, recognizing that it is in his individual interest to consume more medical care, even though doing so will inevitably raise premiums for the entire insured group, including himself (Pauly 1968, 534). Significantly, Pauly recognized that there was nothing immoral about "moral hazard" — it was not necessarily the result of "malingering" or "hypochondria" as earlier writers had claimed — but simply a rational response to a price reduction (Pauly 1968, 535). Yet because of moral hazard, medical care insurance could, at least for some persons, result in a welfare loss rather than gain, contrary to the opinion of Arrow (Pauly 1968, 534). The ramifications of this conclusion, in Pauly's view, were that (1) different kinds of insurance should be made available to meet the demands of different people, (2) medical insurance should focus on events which were most likely to be random and as to which there would be the least elasticity of demand, such as medical catastrophes, and (3) coinsurance was needed to reduce moral hazard (Pauly 1968, 536–37).[6]

Pauly rejected the basic belief that "need" for health care existed independently of demand, a belief which had grounded much of health policy for the preceding half-century — including health planning (Melhado 1988, 228). Health care was subject to the same economic laws as any other product. Consumer preferences, not expert planners, should therefore determine the utilization of health care. Consumer demand, moreover, was elastic, and insurance, particularly in the absence of cost sharing, encouraged excessive demand.

Pauly was joined in this belief by other economists, notably Martin Feldstein. Feldstein did his doctoral work at Oxford in the 1960s, studying the economics of the British National Health Service (Melhado 1998, 223). By the 1970s Feldstein had reached the same conclusions as Pauly: need for medical care did not exist independently of consumer demand, and consumer demand was driven by the presence of health insurance. Feldstein further concluded that the increased demand for medical care created by insurance increased the price of medical care, which in turn increased the demand for insurance, creating an endless cycle of price inflation (Melhado 1998, 241). He also pointed out that the demand for insurance was artificially inflated by federal income tax subsidies, which encouraged employers to provide generous first-dollar insurance policies that contributed to inflation (Melhado 1998, 241). While Pauly had identified the possibility that health insurance might result in welfare loss, Feldstein saw the scope of the welfare loss as much greater, particularly given the tendency of tax subsidies to encourage the already present bias toward "overinsurance."

Other economists also picked up these themes. An article by Judith and Lester Lave in a symposium of *Law and Contemporary Problems* in 1970 begins with a parable about "prepaid dining clubs" that reads very much like Regina Herzlinger's chapter on breakfast insurance three decades later (Lave and Lave 1970). The Laves described the problem of excessive consumption of medical services where insurance reduced the cost of care to zero, the issue of physician-induced demand, and the relatively small improvement in health effected by increased medical care as opposed to, for example, measures to alleviate poor nutrition or substandard housing (Lave and Lave 1970, 253, 263, 254–55). Older themes, however, persisted at this time alongside the newer ones. Another article in the same symposium, by Milton Roemer, focused almost solely on health care regulation and planning as the primary vehicle for assuring the quality and controlling the cost of medical care (Roemer 1970, 284–304).

While the theoretical work of Pauly, Feldstein, and others was important in laying the intellectual foundations of CDHC, the work of Joseph Newhouse, Charles Phelps, and their collaborators in the Rand Health Insurance Experiment (HIE) was vital in placing the theory of insurance-induced demand on a solid empirical footing. The HIE remains the most ambitious controlled experiment ever undertaken examining health care finance. The experiment involved 3,200 families, lasted five years (for some of the participants), and cost $32 million in 1973 dollars (Newhouse 1974, 5–24). The HIE was funded initially by the Office of Economic Opportunity to examine how financing health care for the poor under the Medicaid program could be improved, but was taken over by the Department of Health, Education and Welfare and broadened to consider generally "the demand for medical services under any particular insurance plan" (Newhouse 1974, 6; Melhado 1998, 245). The experiment focused primarily on examining the effects of different levels of deductibles and coinsurance on demand for health services, but a subsidiary goal was to determine the utility of health care service: to see whether insurance improved the health of the poor or simply led to the purchase of ineffective or unnecessary health services (Melhado, 1998, 246; Newhouse and Insurance Experiment Group 1993).

The results of the HIE were clear and powerful. They are discussed in detail in chapter 8, but the basic conclusion of the study was that cost sharing has a significant effect on the utilization of health care. Health care consumers do respond to price, and thus insurance results in moral hazard, which can be controlled by cost sharing. The experiment thus powerfully supported the assertion of economists like Pauly and Feldstein that "need" for medical services had no meaning independent of demand, or consumer preference. Moral hazard was in fact a serious problem.

The Varieties of Market Theory

By the early 1970s the notion that health care was largely subject to normal rules of supply and demand and thus was best governed through markets like other products and services was firmly established. Yet at the same time, the different market approaches introduced in chapter 2 began to diverge. One strand embraced competition among integrated health plans as the best approach. Paul Ellwood, working through his think tank InterStudy, promoted the use of prepaid group medical practices as the building blocks of a consumer-based, competitive health care system (Oliver 2004, 706). Ellwood coined the term "health maintenance organization," or HMO, to leave behind the political baggage carried by traditional prepaid group practice (Oliver 2004, 706). HMOs formed the basis of President Nixon's "rear-guard" action against continuing Great Society proposals for national health insurance (Starr 1982, 394–97). They were embraced as federal policy in the HMO Act of 1973.

HMOs became part of a larger strategy of managed competition with the work of Alain Enthoven. Enthoven published a series of articles in the *New England Journal of Medicine* in 1978,[7] which subsequently were incorporated into his book *Health Plan: The Only Practical Solution to the Soaring Cost of Medical Care* (1980). Like other economists, Enthoven concluded that exploding health care costs were due to the absence of competitive markets in health care. But he rejected a key role for cost sharing in controlling health care costs, arguing that cost sharing was already common yet had not stopped inflation, that deductibles would have no effect once their limits were exceeded, that insufficient information about the prices and benefits of treatment was available to make point-of-service competition work, that patients were not in the best position to make purchasing decisions when they urgently needed medical care, and that the cost-sharing strategy ignored the supply side of the medical care market (Enthoven 1980, 32–36). Enthoven believed that structured competition should rather take place among integrated, well-managed health plans, with competition among plans bringing down the cost of health care coverage, and health plans bringing down the cost of health care itself. The managed competition market approach became the basis for President Clinton's proposed Health Security Act. It was incompletely realized by managed care plans that began to dominate health care financing in the late 1980s and have continued through the present time.

The second approach emphasized the need to overcome the anticompetitive aspects of the existing organization of medical care, and in particular of self-regulation. As we have seen, the AMA had been criminally prosecuted for antitrust violations in the 1940s; Reuben Kessel had been writing about the anticompetitive nature of the regulation of physicians since the 1950s, and of course Milton Friedman's doctoral thesis had attacked the anticompetitive nature of professional regulation (Kessel 1958; Kessel 1970). The leading thinker in this line of inquiry was Clark Havighurst, who as the editor of *Law and Contemporary Problems* and in his own scholarly work contended that many aspects of professional regulation and self-regulation were better understood as attempts to suppress competition than as reflections of special characteristics of the medical profession (Havighurst 1973). The Supreme Court's decision in Goldfarb v. Virginia State Bar Association,[8] holding that professionals were engaged in commerce and thus subject to the antitrust laws, led to a flurry of antitrust enforcement, turning back some of the most egregious forms of anticompetitive conduct. The scholarship of Havighurst and others who saw health planning as a forum for carrying on anticompetitive activities also contributed to the erosion of support for federal health planning efforts, which led in turn to the repeal of the federal health planning laws in 1986.

Advocates of the third competitive approach envisioned competition at the point of purchase of service, with consumer choice driven by cost sharing. Pauly and Feldstein each developed consumer-oriented proposals for national health insurance (which in the early 1970s still seemed almost inevitable). Feldstein's proposal, called Major Risk Insurance, was based on high deductibles and cost sharing, subject to an income-related cap (Feldstein 1971). Pauly's Variable Subsidy Insurance was similar: catastrophic insurance available to all, with graduated deductibles, coinsurance, and premiums based on income (Pauly 1971).[9]

The "overinsurance" thesis also continued to be developed through the 1970s and 1980s (Pauly 1980, 201). But since market advocates in general believed in consumer sovereignty, they faced a paradox: If insurance was inefficient, why did consumers continue to demand it? Market advocates increasingly homed in on tax subsidies for insurance as the cause of this problem. Throughout the 1980s and indeed until the present, market advocates criticized tax subsidies for employment-based insurance as the key cause of overinsurance and of the distortions that it introduces into the health care system (Vogel 1980, 220; Taylor and Wilensky 1983, 163).

The Origins of Medical Savings Accounts

Yet high levels of cost sharing also posed a problem. How would consumers pay for health care with the high deductibles envisioned by the proposals put forth by cost-sharing advocates? One possibility would have been to establish a mechanism under which consumers could borrow money, a proposal developed by Seidman in the 1970s (Seidman 1977, 123–28). A more attractive approach was to encourage individuals and families to save up funds to cover deductibles and cost sharing. This alternative would assure that consumers would be sensitive to the costs of medical care — they would make cost-benefit tradeoffs at the time they purchased care — while at the same time assuring that they would not be impoverished when high medical expenses were unexpectedly incurred.

As mentioned earlier, individual savings for health care costs had surfaced briefly as an idea for expanding access in the 1920s, only to be replaced by the idea of collective prepayment for health care through the Blue Cross plans. But in the 1970s the idea of individual savings reappeared. One of the earliest calls for HSAs, if not the earliest, was made in an article by Paul Worthington in *Inquiry* in 1978. Worthington had developed the concept together with Paul Hixson in 1974, when they worked together at the Bureau of Health Security in the Social Security Administration (which later became the Health Care Financing Administration and is now the Center for Medicare and Medicaid Services) (Bunce 2001). Worthington noted the by-now-familiar argument that the purchase of unnecessary services was encouraged by prepayment (which he distinguished from insurance, since it provided for the payment of services rather than the coverage of income losses) (Worthington 1978, 247–48). Worthington also argued that prepayment was perverse, because it used current income to cover what was in fact a capital expense, an investment in health capital (Worthington 1978, 249). It was more sensible, he argued, for such a capital expense to be covered by borrowing or from savings. He argued therefore for the creation of an account in which money would be invested to use against future medical expenses (Worthington 1978, 250–51). The holder of such an account would be cautious in purchasing medical services because he would be spending his own money, which could be withdrawn at death or upon termination of membership in the credit union in which the money was invested (Worthington 1978, 251–52). Worthington recognized that this solution might not work for the chronically ill poor, the handicapped, and the elderly, but considered it the most efficient solution on which to ground a system to pay for health care.

Other economists proposed HSAs at about the same time. In 1980 Edward Shapiro wrote an article proposing "individual health spending accounts," which would be funded by payroll taxes and administered by the federal government to cover individual health spending, with any balances left at death payable to the account holder's estate (Shapiro 1980). In the following year

Miron Sano published an article putting forth a proposal for mandated contributions to individual health accounts (with excess accumulations distributed to account holders once they had reached a high enough level), supplemented by a national health fund to cover those without accumulations or whose accumulations had been depleted (Stano 1981).

In the 1980s and 1990s the idea of MSAs took on added significance, as it first gained the sponsorship of policy advocacy organizations, then became a commercial reality, and finally was recognized by state and then federal legislation that offered tax subsidies for MSAs.

The Medical Savings Account Political Agenda

In the early 1980s Hixson interested John Goodman of the recently formed National Center for Policy Analysis in the idea of MSAs (Cohn 2005; Bunce 2001, 9). The NCPA, a free-market advocacy organization, had been founded in 1983 by Goodman with the encouragement of Anthony Fisher.[10] Fisher, a disciple of F. A. Hayek, had founded the Institute of Economic Affairs in London, which had significantly influenced Margaret Thatcher's economic policies in the UK, and was also instrumental in founding the Manhattan Institute and the Fraser Institute in Canada (Source Watch 2005). By the mid-1980s a number of free-market advocacy organizations were already actively promoting privatization and deregulation in the United States, and Goodman attempted to find a policy area that was not already well covered.[11] The area of health policy and the prescription of MSAs seemed ideal for the NCPA.

In 1984 John Goodman and Richard Rahm, then the chief economist for the U.S. Chamber of Commerce, put forth a proposal in the *Wall Street Journal* for privatizing Medicare through medical individual retirement accounts (Goodman and Rahm 1984). In 1990 the NCPA assembled about forty organizations, including the American Enterprise Institute, the AMA, the U.S. Chamber of Commerce, and the Hoover Institution, to develop a health policy agenda (National Center for Policy Analysis 1990). The resulting task force identified tax reform as the basis of health care reform, and proposed reforming the tax laws so that individually based health insurance, including medical savings vehicles, would enjoy tax benefits equal to those offered for group insurance. Specifically the task force proposed tax subsidies for Medisave accounts; individual MSAs; medical IRA accounts to encourage retirement MSAs that could subsidize and eventually replace Medicare; and no-frills catastrophic health insurance, free from state mandates, premium taxes, and risk pool assessments (Bowen 2005, 21). In 1992 Goodman joined with Robert Musgrave, a senior fellow at NCPA, to publicize the idea of MSAs further in their book *Patient Power*, republished in an abridged and popularized edition in 1994 by the Cato Institute as *Patient Power: The Free Enterprise Alternative to Clinton's Health Plan*. The abridged book was, according to Goodman, influential in building opposition to Clinton's health plan among Republican senators, and thus contributed to the demise of that proposal (Bowen 2005, 21). Goodman also published an article in *Health Affairs* in 1995 with Mark Pauly advocating MSAs (Pauly and Goodman 1995).

At the same time, MSAs began to become available as a commercial product. Dominion Resources, a Virginia utility company, offered its employees high-deductible policies coupled with contributions to a MSA as early as 1989 (Bunce 2001, 9). The MSA was launched as a commercial concept in earnest by Golden Rule Insurance Company. J. Patrick Rooney, the CEO of Golden Rule, had learned of MSAs from John Goodman in 1990, and became the nation's foremost policy entrepreneur promoting MSAs, as well as a board member of NCPA and a major donor to it (Dreyfuss and Stone 1996; Bowen 2005, 24). Golden Rule became a major promoter of high-deductible health plans (HDHPs) and MSAs, and began offering MSAs to its own employees in May 1993 (Bowen 2005, 24).

Rooney and Golden Rule also became major political players. According to one source, Rooney, his family, his companies, and their employees gave $3.6 million to political candidates, mostly Republican, including over $1 million during the 1993–94 campaign against Clinton's health plan (Scherer 2004). In addition, Rooney and his companies gave $2.2 million to Republican organizations (including $121,000 to assist the Bush recount campaign in Florida and $1.9 million to the Republican Leadership Coalition, which ran attack advertisements against Al Gore during the 2000 campaign) (Scherer 2004). Rooney also spent $2.2 million as a registered lobbyist. Rooney was in particular a generous supporter of Newt Gingrich and his GOPAC political action committee, and seems to have had significant influence on Gingrich's health policies (Dreyfuss and Stone 1996; Goodman and Musgrave 1994, xiii).

Rooney also established or recruited other lobbying groups to assist with MSA advocacy. In 1992 Golden Rule and thirteen other small to mid-level insurance companies, dissatisfied with the managed care emphasis of the Health Insurance Association of America, started the Council for Affordable Health Insurance (CAHI) to advocate for MSAs and state risk pools (Bowen 2005, 29).

The CAHI recruited Greg Scandlen, who has become a major advocate for MSAs, as its first director. Rooney continues to combine activism with HSA marketing, and has recently been marketing HSAs and HDHPs coupled with a membership in Freedom Works, a right-wing advocacy organization led by the former House Republican leader Richard Armey. Freedom Works has reportedly received over $600,000 and sixteen thousand members from the arrangement, even though some who bought the insurance were unaware they were signing up for the organization as well (Weisman 2006, A, 5).

The advocacy work of Rooney, Golden Rule, Goodman, the NCPA, and their allies soon began to bear fruit, first at the state level. Rooney worked with the American Legislative Exchange Council, a free-market advocacy organization of state legislators and businesses, to draft a model state MSA enabling act that was introduced in twenty-eight states and adopted in eight. Missouri in 1993 became the first state to enact legislation providing state income tax subsidies for employee MSAs (Bowen 2005, 32–33). Over the next five years, twenty-four more states adopted legislation permitting employers, and in some instances individuals, to make tax-subsidized contributions to MSAs (Bunce 2001, 10; Bowen 2005, 33–34). Three additional states adopted laws in the 1990s providing for Medicaid MSA demonstration projects (Bunce 2001, 10).

The first attempt to provide federal tax subsidies for MSAs was H.R. 5250, introduced in May, 1992 by Reps. Andy Jacobs (D-Ind.) and Bill Archer (R-Tex.) (Bunce 2001, 10). Nine MSA bills were introduced in the 102nd Congress and sixteen in the 103rd (Bunce 2001, 10). The Senate Labor and Human Resources Committee on 8 June 1994 became the first congressional committee to report out legislation supporting MSAs. MSAs proved intensely controversial, however, and were strongly opposed by many Democrats who thought they would undermine employment-related group insurance (Bunce 2001, 12). A compromise creating limited tax subsidies for MSAs was finally adopted into law as part of the Health Insurance Portability and Accountability Act (HIPAA) in 1996.[12]

HIPAA was an attempt to adopt into law the less controversial proposals that had been mooted in the discussion of Clinton's Health Security Act in 1993 and 1994. Though HIPAA has subsequently come to be identified with its health care data confidentiality and security provisions, at the time it was mainly recognized for its provisions dealing with access to insurance, including limitations on preexisting conditions clauses, guaranteed issue and renewal of health insurance for small groups, and limitations on discrimination based on health status in group health insurance. The MSA provisions proved among the most contentious addressed by the legislation, and Congress finally adopted a compromise.

HIPAA established a demonstration project allowing tax deductions for money contributed to and income earned on MSAs established by small employers and the self-employed where the MSA was coupled with HDHPs.[13] The demonstration project was limited to four years (to expire on 31 December 2000) and 750,000 participants. Though the expiration date of the project was extended several times, HIPAA MSAs never caught on, and only about forty to fifty thousand MSAs were established in any one year under the program (Bunce 2001, 13).

Though the results of the HIPAA demonstration project were disappointing, MSA advocates contended that the problem was not with the MSA concept but with the limits imposed by HIPAA. They repeatedly called for dropping those limits, and finally achieved success in 2003 through the Medicare Modernization Act (MMA). Most of the debate surrounding the MMA focused on its Medicare prescription drug benefit, but the MMA also rechristened MSAs as health savings accounts (HSAs), opening them to all those willing to purchase a HDHP, lowering the minimum deductible limits, and allowing tax subsidies for contributions up to the level of the minimum deductible or higher. Legislation adopted during the final hours of Republican control of Congress in 2006 further expanded tax breaks for HSAs. Attempts are also under way to use HSAs in Medicare and Medicaid.

As Congress was creating the HSA, the IRS created another health savings device, the health reimbursement account (HRA). In 2002 the IRS determined that existing legislation authorized the offer of tax subsidies for employer contributions to health savings vehicles fully funded by employers.[14] The HRA has proved attractive to employers because the accounts can be held as notional accounts and need not be fully funded, and because the funds in them also need not go with the employee if he or she leaves employment.

At the beginning of the twenty-first century, CDHC seems once again firmly established. Its supporters have moved beyond advocacy for MSAs and HSAs to examine other issues raised by CDHC. Regina Herzlinger, for example, who began writing about CDHC early in the 1990s, has focused much of her work on the supply side — in particular the question of how providers should be organized to optimize competition for consumers (Herzlinger 1991; Herzlinger 1994). Another major focus of the movement has been the provision of consumer information on the price and quality of health services necessary to run a consumer-driven health care system. This has in fact been a major contribution of the CDHC movement, and an area where important progress is possible (although the production and use of this information remain limited, as is discussed in the next two chapters).

The primary question that confronts us at this point is whether the political victories of the CDHC movement are good for consumers and good for the country. In the chapters that follow I will explore the theoretical, empirical, legal, and ethical issues raised by CDHC in an attempt to address this question.

CHAPTER 7

The Theoretical Foundations of Consumer-Driven Health Care

The Neoclassical Economic Belief System

As noted in chapter 2, the CDHC movement is founded upon a theory that purports to explain how health care systems operate and how health care consumers and providers behave. This theory is based on neoclassical microeconomics. To understand the CDHC movement, therefore, it is necessary to understand something about neoclassical economics, the assumptions on which it is based, and its role in contemporary America.

Neoclassical microeconomics plays three interconnected roles in the contemporary American academy, society, and polity. First, economics is a social science: it offers a positive (that is, descriptive) scientific theory that claims to both explain how people behave and allow prediction of how humans will behave under specified conditions. This theory permits the mathematical representation of human behavior, just as theoretical physics permits the mathematical representation of the behavior of physical phenomena (Mirowski 1989). It also permits the disciplined empirical study of human behavior. Health economists, for example, analyze patterns of consumer behavior when deductibles or co-payments are increased or decreased, calculating elasticities of demand for various products or services, and then projecting how consumers would respond if cost sharing were to be further increased (see chapter 8). Second, neoclassical microeconomics is also used to support a political and philosophical ideology, often referred to as libertarianism. Economics is used to promote, that is, a normative philosophical and political agenda. Finally, economics in a less formal sense presents a practical commonsense, or at least commonly held, understanding of how humans behave. In this incarnation it is often invoked by persons neither schooled in the science of economics nor committed to a libertarian ideology to argue for particular public policies that support private business and denigrate the role of government. CDHC advocates shift freely among these various categories of thought, often confusing political positions with scientific observations.[1]

Neoclassical economics originated in the last quarter of the nineteenth century (Dobb 1973, 166–210). It is founded on certain beliefs about human behavior. These assumptions are that individuals derive utility from products, services, and other conditions and outcomes; that an individual's preferences among these products and services reflect that individual's understanding of how best to maximize his or her own utility; that these preferences are innate and stable and the product of individual freedom of choice and thus inherently worthy of respect; that individuals maximize their utility by ordering their preferences and then proceeding to satisfy their ranked preferences within the limits of their available resources through expenditure of those resources; that individuals act rationally to satisfy their preferences in expending their resources; and that individual preferences can therefore most accurately be ascertained and measured by observing how individuals reveal their preferences in their expenditures (Rice 2002, 9–14). Sellers of goods and services, on the other hand, be they firms or individuals, are assumed to set prices for their products and services so as to maximize their profits in light of the cost of resources that they must use to produce these products and services (Rice 2002, 14–18).

By observing how individuals reveal their preferences through purchasing decisions, demand curves can be plotted that predict how much of any given product or service will be purchased at any given price. Similarly, supply curves can be plotted that predict how much of a particular product or service will be provided at any given price given the cost of the resources needed to produce the product or service. Assuming competitive markets, a market clearing price can normally be identified where the supply and demand curves cross, at which point the total utility of consumers is maximized and "rents," that is, extra-competitive profits, disappear (Rice 2002, 14–18, 70–74).

Neoclassical economics posits that revealed consumer preferences permit us to identify the optimal, or efficient, allocation of resources in society. "Welfare economics," that is, posits that we can identify the optimal allocation of resources to maximize utility in a society by summing the utility of all individuals in the society as identified through their revealed preferences (Dodd 1973, 213, 241–44). Welfare economics assumes that it is not possible to aggregate individual utility through any sum of cardinal measurements, because there is no standard of measurement that allows us to compare utility among different individuals (Rice 2002, 67). It posits, on the other hand, that we can observe ordinal or relative rankings of value, as revealed through the purchasing behavior of individual consumers, and thereby describe the allocation of resources that maximizes the welfare of each individual within society given the relative preferences of each member of society. We can then sum these rankings to describe the allocation of resources that maximizes the welfare of society as a whole. Any public policy must be judged solely by its effect on the total welfare of society, defined as the aggregated utility of individuals as judged by those individuals themselves and revealed in their purchasing decisions (Hurley 1998, 373–95, 375–76).

The goal of a society, according to welfare economics, is to achieve an efficient allocation of resources through trades so that all resources end up with the individuals or firms that value them most highly. The purest definition of allocative efficiency is Pareto optimality (named after Vilfredo Pareto), a condition that is achieved when no individual in society can be made better off without someone else being made worse off (Sen 1970, 21; Rice 2002, 21–23; Dobb 1973, 242–43). To achieve optimality, individuals must be allowed to exchange products and services that they value less highly to obtain those that they value more highly from other individuals who value more highly the goods and services that they receive in return. Although it is possible in theory to describe pure Pareto optimal situations, it is often not possible to achieve them in practice because opportunities for trading are constrained, and trades are not costless. Welfare economics, therefore, often settles for another form of efficiency, often called Kaldor-Hicks optimality, representing the allocation of resources that would result after the carrying out of all trades in which the gains of winners exceed the losses of losers if such trades were carried out (Sen 1970, 56; Rice 2002, 22). Kaldor-Hicks optimality is different from Pareto optimality in that winners need not compensate losers as long as the winnings of winners in aggregate exceed the losses of losers.

Neoclassical economists take a dim view of the ability of government to improve societal welfare. The dominant view of government held by CDHC advocates is the "public choice" model (Goodman and Musgrave 1992, 551–53; Farina and Rachlinski 2002). Public choice theory treats political institutions as markets in which "goods" such as legislation, regulations, and public benefits and subsidies are supplied and demanded according to the same economic principles that govern the supply and demand of other goods (Croley 1998). These regulatory goods are supplied by the state — which has a monopoly over supplying them — to interest groups who stand to gain from them (Croley 1998, 35).

The classic public choice story begins with the proposition that the primary goal of legislators is to retain their office, that to accomplish this goal they must raise campaign funds, and that to do this they must depend on interest groups (Stigler 1971, 11–13). In return for support from interest groups, legislators enact legislation that gives interest groups the opportunities to gain "rents" in the form of direct cash subsidies, control over market entry, price controls, and favorable contracts (Mitchell and Munger 1991, 520). In the modern administrative state, the power to dispense many of these rent-seeking opportunities is often not directly under the control of the legislature but rather delegated by legislatures to administrative agencies, whose behavior the interest groups also seek to influence (Posner 1969, 82–87). Neither legislators nor regulators promote the public interest as it is revealed through the preferences of consumers, but rather the welfare of narrower interest groups. Government therefore tends to impede the attainment of societal efficiency rather than to promote it.

The publications of neoclassical microeconomists are filled with mathematic formulas and appear very scientific.[2] Robert Evans, a Canadian health economist, however, notes that economists tend to view mathematics the way medieval scholars viewed Latin: as a language conferring special authority on statements written in it and allowing those who write in it "to get away with a good deal of nonsense by avoiding the vernacular" (Evans 1998, 492).[3] It is necessary in fact to look past the elegance and mystery of presentation to examine more closely the extent to which the assumptions and the conclusions of the discipline, which purport to explain human behavior, actually reflect the reality of human experience (Mirowski 1989).[4]

Imperfect Markets

As neoclassical economics has evolved, many complications and difficulties have been identified in the application of the theory. In many instances, economists have recognized these challenges and incorporated them into their models, though often at the cost of considerable added complexity and lost elegance (Becker 1976; Coase 1960; Demsetz 1972).[5] Other challenges are more fundamental, going to the basic assumptions about psychology, sociology, and philosophy on which the discipline is based. The responses of economists to these challenges differ — some humbly acknowledge the limits of their discipline, others react with a defensiveness and patronizing arrogance that suggests a basic insecurity in their models (Kuttner 1997, 41). In the main, however, the primary popular voices calling for CDHC base their public policy advocacy on simple economic models that do not acknowledge the complexity of the real world and the limitations of the neoclassical model. A review of the common criticisms of the neoclassical model can therefore contribute to an understanding of the limits of the policy prescriptions of CDHC. More complex and detailed elaborations of these criticisms are readily available for those who wish to pursue them further.[6]

Economics has long recognized the limitations imposed by its simplifying assumptions. One of these assumptions is that consumers have sufficient information to make choices that reflect their preferences. In fact, information is in many markets a scarce commodity (Stone 2002, 76–78). Sellers obviously have an incentive to produce information about the price and quality of their products and services, but this information, just as obviously, is intended to put their products or services in their best light and may not be accurate. There is little incentive in many markets for the production of independent, unbiased comparative information about price and quality. Such information is often a "public good": the consumption of information by one individual does not preclude others from using it, and indeed, there may be no way to exclude others from using the information.[7] It is often not possible to obtain adequate compensation for producing the information, and therefore information is often under-produced (Sage 1999, 1771–74; Pauly 1992, 46–48). Consumers must purchase many products on the basis of very incomplete information, and thus may find that the purchase does not increase their utility as much as they had hoped or expected. Finally, it is often in the interests of sellers to conceal information, such as information about future discounts, or to hide unfavorable purchase terms in fine print (Stone 2002, 77). CDHC is dependent on the assumption that health care consumers can become informed sufficiently to play a useful role in health care markets, and thus the problem of producing adequate useful information poses a challenge to it.

The costs attributable to obtaining information about products are an example of the larger category of transaction costs. Transaction costs often stand in the way of or increase the cost of achieving otherwise efficient trades (Coase 1960). Negotiating purchases often costs money, and the more complex negotiations can require costly legal services. Negotiations can also result in strategic behavior that stymies the conclusion of deals from which all the parties would have benefited, such as when bilateral monopolies are involved (Posner 2002, 60–61).

Another complication of simple economic models is the problem of externalities. Resource allocation decisions often result in external costs or benefits that have significant effects on total societal welfare but are not fully taken into account by the individuals or firms making production or consumption decisions (Stone 2002, 72; Rice 2002, 24–26). A firm producing a product may not take into account the external costs of air and water pollution caused by the production process and thus may produce more than is optimal. Products that confer a significant benefit on society may be consumed to a lesser degree than is optimal because consumption of the good may confer external benefits, and thus, even though the aggregate benefit of the product exceeds its cost, the actual benefit of the product to the purchaser may not exceed its cost to the purchaser. (Rice 2002, 37–43). CDHC, however, encourages consumers to consider only the costs and benefits that they incur as individuals, not the external costs or benefits that their decisions might entail to others or to society.

Finally, markets are often not perfectly competitive (Stone 2002, 71; Federal Trade Commission / Department of Justice 2004; Posner 2002, 273–86). The production costs of some products fall continuously as production scale increases (Rice 2002, 148–49). These products can therefore be produced least expensively by a single monopoly producer. It rarely makes sense, for example, to duplicate electric or water supply networks (though approaches have been found to make many utilities competitive without reproducing networks). More importantly, competitors often prefer not to compete but rather to achieve sufficient market power to earn "rents." Occasionally such market power can be achieved through predatory behavior, but more often it is achieved through manipulation of government authority (Federal Trade Commission / Department of Justice 2004, 5). Licensing, for example, permits the achievement of market power in some markets. Regardless of how market power is achieved, it limits the ability of markets to reach efficiency.

Information deficits, transaction costs, externalities, and anticompetitive behavior have long been recognized by economists as problems that necessitate elaborations on the simplest economic models, and have been accommodated by more complex models. Other challenges, however, are more fundamental.

Fundamental Defects in Neoclassical Economic Theory

The most basic assumptions of neoclassical economics are that the preferences of individuals are innate and immutable and that consumers can make rational choices that improve their own welfare. These claims have been subjected to several challenges.

First, it is far from clear that individual preferences are in reality innate and immutable — "the immaculate conception of the indifference curve" has been called into question (Boulding 1969, 2). At its most doctrinaire, neo-classical economics rejects the possibility that preferences may be created or manipulated through marketing, peer pressure, or propaganda, and thus may reflect the preferences of a government or of marketers rather than of individuals themselves. In the words of two prominent economists: "[T]astes neither change capriciously nor differ importantly between people. . . . [O]ne does not argue over tastes for the same reason that one does not argue over the Rocky Mountains — both are there, will be there next year, too, and are the same for all men" (Stigler and Becker 1977, 76).[8]

Yet there is overwhelming evidence that tastes are mutable and subject to manipulation (Rice 2002, 45–50), especially for consumer goods. Tens of billions of dollars are spent each year in the United States on marketing and are obviously not simply intended to help consumers satisfy their inherent tastes. Rather marketing is often aimed at creating or shaping consumer preferences, usually through the use of peer pressure or by suggesting that purchase of a particular product will enhance social status (Kuttner 1997, 15). Tastes themselves are usually shaped by habit or experience; indeed in some instances they are the product of an unwanted addiction (such as tastes for tobacco or narcotics) (Rice 2002, 48–49). Tastes are often also the product of misinformation, prejudice, or ignorance. Indeed one of the primary functions of education is to elevate our knowledge, judgment, and discernment, and thus to improve not only the information on the basis of which we make decisions, but also our tastes (Kuttner 1997, 42). Between 1965 and 1995 the proportion of Americans who smoked declined from 42.4 percent to 25 percent as television advertising for tobacco was banned (in 1971) and as the public became aware of the perils of smoking, largely through government education campaigns (Kuttner

1997, 43). The taste for tobacco (which surely is not innate in any genetic sense) has proved mutable, and the welfare of our society was improved because this taste was changed (Rice 1997, 418; Rice 2002, 62–63).

A second assumption of neoclassical economics is that consumer behavior is rational. The model of decision making assumed by neoclassical economists is a compensatory model in which all salient characteristics of all available products and services are taken into consideration, with each characteristic weighted for its relative importance, resulting in a decision to purchase the products and services that provide the greatest marginal utility per dollar spent (Korobkin 1999, 46–48). Behavioral psychology has called into question the extent to which this model of rationality accurately describes how consumers make decisions (Kuttner 1997, 44–48).

Most consumer products and services (and in particular health care products and services) face multiple competitors and possess multiple characteristics. Even if perfect information were available, it would not be possible for the human mind to absorb and process it all.[9] Individuals making decisions usually settle for decision making based on "bounded" rather than perfect rationality; decisions that "satisfice" rather than maximize welfare (Simon 1979, 502–3). Individuals select a very few salient characteristics, compare products or services based on what they can find out about those salient characteristics, and then decide (Korobkin 1999, 48–52; Schwartz 2004, 78). Alternatively, they assign "lexicographical" importance to one or a handful of characteristics, ignoring all other characteristics in the decision-making process. Often consumers avoid the difficult task of decision making altogether, basing their choices on loyalty to existing relationships (as with a particular neighborhood store or doctor), and making no effort to look elsewhere for a better price or higher quality (Stone 2002, 75–76). Adopting a satisficing strategy permits consumer decision making to achieve only a relative rather than an absolute maximization of consumer welfare.

Many consumer decisions — and again, particularly decisions in health care settings — are based on predictions made in situations involving considerable uncertainty. A consumer may need to decide which of several possible diagnoses of a mysterious medical condition is most likely to be accurate and which of several alternative drugs or therapies is most likely to be successful (and to what extent) in treating the condition. A great deal of research by behavioral psychologists into decision making under conditions of uncertainty has revealed that such decisions commonly rely on "heuristics" that cause "biases," which induce decision makers to assign too much weight to some risks, too little to others (Tversky and Kahneman 1982). The "availability" heuristic, for example, assigns undue influence to highly salient recent experiences (Tversky and Kahneman 1982, 11–14; Schwartz 2004, 56–61). Thus a patient may decide not to have a surgery performed at a particular hospital even though the hospital has had excellent outcomes for that type of surgery, because the patient's mother recently had a bad outcome at the particular hospital from a wholly unrelated type of surgery.

Decision makers who must make predictions in the face of uncertainty often rely on stereotypes or very limited personal experience, rather than on statistical data or fundamental statistical principles like regression to the mean or the unreliability of small samples (Tversky and Kahneman 1982, 9–11). In addition, the way risks are presented has a substantial effect on how risks are perceived (Slovic, Fischoff, and Lichtenstein 1982, 483).

Research into biases and heuristics has been very fruitful in recent years, expanding the number of recognized common heuristics and facilitating better understanding of human decision making under uncertainty (Gilovich, Griffin, and Kahneman eds. 2002). An underlying message of this body of research is that human decision making is often affective rather than rational.[10] Consumers making decisions in the face of uncertainty do not necessarily satisfy their own underlying preferences, and thus do not necessarily enhance their own utility.

Another branch of behavioral psychology — prospect theory — further challenges the assumption that we can maximize societal welfare by relying solely on the rationality of consumer decision making. Prospect theory reveals that decisions involving uncertainty and risk may come out differently depending on whether they involve a purchase or a sale, a risk of loss or a chance to gain. Experimental evidence indicates that individuals prefer a 10 percent chance of a $100 loss to a certain $10 loss, but they also prefer a certain $10 gain to a 10 percent chance at a $100 gain, even though mathematically (i.e. rationally) each gain or loss is precisely equivalent (Nyman 2003, 24; Kahneman and Tversky 1979). Individuals are also sensitive to endowment effects: consumers who would not spend $100 to purchase a bottle of wine are often not willing to sell the same bottle for $100 if they already own it (Schwartz 2004, 71–72).[11]

While behavioral psychology challenges the fundamental assumption of neoclassical economics (and of CDHC) that individual purchasing decisions (or a firm's production decisions) are rational, other evidence challenges more radically the assumption that consumer self-interest is the primary motivation of human behavior. Many factors other than individual material self-interest affect the welfare of individuals and societies. Family relationships, friendships, religious beliefs and worship, work, education, enjoyment of the natural and human environment, security and freedom from fear, respect for and from others—all of these contribute to human welfare and some may be more important than the accumulation of material goods (Sen 1987, 15; Sen 1982, 84–106; Rice 2002, 188–89). Much of human behavior is better explained in terms of community-building values such as cooperation, commitment, and loyalty than as reflecting individual selfishness (Schwartz 2004, 107; Stone 2002, 32–33).[12] Indeed one important goal of individuals and of society, distributional equity or justice, can be achieved only at the cost of material sacrifice on the part of individuals (Hurley 1998, 384–87). Finally, some preferences simply cannot be satisfied by markets. Polls show that many Americans want universal health insurance, but markets cannot provide it for us (Kuttner 1997, 42).

The multiple goals that individuals pursue are often in conflict (Aaron 1994, 15–16; Kuttner 1997, 46, 60–61). I may pay hundreds of dollars in the morning to enroll in a health club to lose weight, but that evening gorge myself on a chocolate sundae. Moreover the satisfaction of some desires — such as the desire to own, or to inflict pain on, another human being—is simply wrong. This is the teaching of millennia of theological and philosophical reflection. Indeed, theology and philosophy often counsel us to look beyond material desires. As Mark Sagoff (1986) notes, "Literary and empirical studies amply confirm what every mature adult discovers: happiness and well-being come from overcoming or outgrowing many of our desires more than from satisfying them" (304).

That the satisfaction of material desires cannot maximize the welfare of society is not only taught by religion and philosophy: it is also demonstrated by modern psychology and public opinion research. Reported levels of happiness or satisfaction vary from society to society and within the same societies from one moment to the next in ways that bear little relationship to material prosperity (Easterlin 1974; Frank 1985, 28–34). Once individuals or a society reach the point where basic needs are met, simply accumulating material things seems to do little to contribute additionally to individual or societal welfare.[13] And even insofar as individual satisfaction and happiness are correlated with material prosperity, they seem to be related more to relative prosperity within a society than to absolute prosperity (Frank 1985, 23–36). Satisfaction seems to be more closely related to having more stuff than your neighbors or fellow employees than to how much stuff you own in absolute terms (Schwartz 2004, 187–97).

Finally, defining the welfare of a society in terms of the satisfaction of its individual members is problematic because of the phenomena of adaptation. Those born into abject poverty or those with serious disabilities often adjust their expectations to their reality, still finding pleasure in life. That they can learn to live with their condition, however, should not necessarily limit the legitimacy of their claims to better treatment by society (Hurley 1998, 379; Sen 1987, 45–46). A just and good society may attempt to provide more even to those who do not demand more.

Economics of Health Care: Particular Limitations of the Model

These limitations in the neoclassical economist's view of the world have important ramifications for the CDHC debate. CDHC advocates claim that if we follow their prescription — in this case decreasing insurance coverage and increasing cost sharing — individuals will have greater freedom of choice, will be better enabled to direct their resources to maximize their utility, and thus ultimately the utility of all and the welfare of society will be increased. But if individual choices are not wholly rational and do not necessarily enhance individual welfare, and if societal welfare is not merely the sum of all individual purchasing decisions, then perhaps the structures and systems we establish for providing health care coverage should reflect other values, like maximizing health in some absolute sense or maximizing access to health care for all, or perhaps reducing disparity in access to health or health care.

As we narrow our focus from general limitations of the neoclassical economic model to more specific problems with applying the model to health care and to health insurance, we have even more reason for being skeptical of the prescriptions of economists. As noted at the outset, CDHC advocates identify one complicating factor in health care transactions: the problem of moral hazard caused by insurance, which is purchased excessively because of the incentives created by tax subsidies. While the presence of insurance means that consumers do not behave in health care markets as they do in markets for breakfast cereal, this distortion is readily understood by neoclassical economics. All we need do is eliminate tax subsidies for insurance and increase cost sharing, and health care markets will return to "normal." Other distortions found in health care markets, however, are not so easy to deal with.

First, information deficiencies are particularly prevalent in health care. As noted above, neoclassical economics assumes that consumers make purchasing decisions with information about both the price and quality of products and services. Individuals gain information about simple and frequently purchased products, such as groceries and household products, by evaluating their own experience with those products. Consumers rely on search strategies to purchase more expensive and less frequently purchased products such as automobiles, homes, and major appliances, relying on web-based rating services, consumer magazines, or even, for some large purchases, professional agents (Sloan and Hall 2002, 172–73; Korobkin 1999, 27–28). Although some health care consumers — in particular those with chronic diseases — have sufficiently frequent experiences with particular products or services to become quite knowledgeable, many encounters that consumers (including even consumers with chronic diseases) have with the health care system are unique. Health information web sites are common and proliferating, but health care remains very complicated; health care processes and outcomes are still difficult to evaluate, and search strategies still have limited value. In few (if any) places in the United States can one find meaningful, comprehensive, and objective risk-adjusted information comparing the treatment outcomes of individual doctors or dentists. Finally, many health care products and services are "credence" goods — even after having used them, the consumer cannot evaluate the experience. Perhaps the patient would have got well without the seemingly successful treatment or fared much worse without the seemingly unsuccessful treatment (Rice 2002, 88). The consumer can only believe that the treatment helped, and it is quite possible that the belief itself has an independent beneficial effect (Hall 2002, 478–82).

Not only is information on quality lacking in health care, but so is information about cost. Uwe Reinhardt describes the American health care system as resembling "a haberdashery in which shirts are stored in white boxes, each labeled 'shirt,' but without showing on the outside of the box any information on the shirt's size and material, let alone price. Several months after freely choosing one of these boxes, the customer is sent an incomprehensible bill, whose only understandable text is the red framed box containing the statement 'Pay this amount: $69.99' " (Reinhardt 2002, xii).

Doctors and hospitals are accustomed to billing on a fee-for-service basis, and the fee often cannot be determined until after the patient is seen. Hospitals bill for piecework and are reluctant to quote fees in advance (although they are paid by Medicare and by many insurers on a bundled per-case basis, and are thus capable of charging in this way). Price advertising is still professionally frowned upon in many health care markets, and some professional regulation of price advertising has stood up to antitrust scrutiny.[14] CDHC advocates consistently call for more information about quality and price, but it is still available only to a very limited extent, and implementing CDHC without it is a risky venture.

Even if consumers had better information on quality and price, it is still likely that health care purchasing decisions would differ from other routine consumer transactions. One reason for this is the problem posed by the time horizons of health care decisions. Behavioral research has shown that decisions resulting in immediate pleasure are more salient than those resulting in long-term benefits (Frederick, Loewenstein, and O'Donoghue 2004). Many health care decisions, particularly those involving preventive health care, yield little immediate utility but might prove very valuable in the long run.

Another problem is that many health care purchasing decisions are not made primarily by patients but rather by their professional advisors. Consumers usually decide whether to initiate contact with a physician, but once they do so, further decisions with respect to tests or specialist consultations to diagnose a condition, or the drugs, devices, or hospital admissions necessary to treat it, are usually made primarily by the physician. Indeed some of these decisions, such as the prescribing of a drug, may legally only be made by professionals. At the very least, physicians play a major role in shaping a patient's preferences, even when the patient ultimately decides on treatment alternatives (Stone 2002, 74; Schneider 1998, 58–59).

And yet physicians often face a potential conflict of interest when acting as agents in advising consumers. They are acting not only as the agents of their patients but as the sellers of services. If they are paid on a fee-for-service basis, they can often increase their own income if they can persuade their patients to consume more of their services. The issue of physician-induced demand is complicated and controversial, but a recent thorough review of the literature concludes, "[a]dding up the evidence, on obstetricians doing more C-sections, surgeons doing more bypass operations, physicians referring more frequently to their own labs, and other studies, makes a convincing case that doctors can influence quantity and sometimes do for their own purpose" (McGuire 2000, 517).

Medical treatment decisions are often also influenced by managed care organizations, which either themselves review treatment decisions through utilization review or shape physicians' treatment decisions through incentive structures (such as capitation arrangements) or network selection protocols. Like patients, managed care companies are influenced by the time frames of likely payoffs of their decisions. With enrollee turnover rates of 25 percent a year, they have little incentive to invest in preventive care that might not provide real payoffs for years, even decades (Sloan and Hall 2002, 179–80; Rice 2002, 62). Managed care companies do, however, offer a serious deterrent to physician-induced demand, and are in general in a better position than individual consumers to do so, from the perspective of both knowledge and bargaining power. Paradoxically, payment for professional services by individual patients from their own HSAs rather than by managed care companies could increase provider-driven moral hazard.

Consumers do, of course, play a role in medical decisions. They are supposed to give "informed consent" to medical procedures, and can refuse to fill a prescription offered by a doctor or demand an available generic substitute (in some states). But in the end, the role of consumers in medical decision making is often limited. Decisions regarding treatment are often made while the patient is suffering considerable fear and anxiety and is not fully able to rationally weigh alternatives (Hall 1997, 36–39). If the patient is unconscious, demented, or in traumatic shock, it is even more difficult to characterize the patient as a consumer (although someone in the patient's family may step in to fill this role). In any event, it is not clear that patients always want to choose; sometimes patients would prefer to have decisions made for them (Schwartz 2004, 29–33). Indeed, the professional-patient relationship is a fiduciary as well as a commercial relationship, and the ability of the consumer to trust the professional, even to make choices, is arguably vital to the healing nature of the relationship (Kuttner 1997, 149–50; Hall 2002; see also chapter 9).

Carl Schneider has concluded from his comprehensive review of empirical research and patients' narratives of their own experience that a significant number of patients would prefer not to have to make decisions about their own medical care (Schneider 1998, 35–46). Schneider identifies several reasons for this: patients may believe themselves less competent than medical professionals to make wise decisions, may be too debilitated to think clearly about their situation, or may "wish to cede decisional authority in order to be manipulated into courses of action they in some sense wish to pursue but find themselves resisting" (Schneider 1998, 48). He notes that medical information is complex, and that patients often fail to understand it. Moreover, "the patient's vision is often—usually?—clouded by the haze of fable, fantasy, and superstition we assimilate over a lifetime of inattentive reading, careless listening, forgotten science, and antique learning" (Schneider 1998, 60). Schneider further observes that really sick people not only have diminished capacity to make medical decisions but also often have more important issues to attend to with their limited energies (Schneider 1998, 63–64, 75–87). When patients do make medical decisions, Schneider has discovered, their decisions are often snap judgments, not decisions made according to the rational decision-maker model (Schneider 1998, 92–99). Schneider does not reject the model grounded in patient autonomy and informed consent, but he does recognize its considerable limitations and argues against forcing patients to make decisions when they would prefer that others make them. Schneider recognizes that patients face a range of different kinds of decisions, and that some patients are (or become) very competent to make some decisions. In the end, he advocates moving beyond a model of consumer choice to one focused on consumer welfare, recognizing that what most patients want above all is not the opportunity to be a consumer, but rather competence and kindness on the part of those who care for them (Schneider 1998, 206–27).

Finally, health care markets seem particularly sensitive to the presence of market power (Rice 2002, 143–46). Pharmaceutical and medical device companies are awarded monopolies over drugs and devices for a significant period through the patent laws. During this period they are freely permitted to earn monopoly rents. Because of this market power, and because of the very high fixed and very low marginal costs that attend the production of many pharmaceuticals, the production function for pharmaceuticals bears little resemblance to the traditional neoclassical supply curve (Evans 1998, 489–90). Market power is also present in other health care markets. In rural areas hospitals face little competition for services such as emergency care. In some urban areas a few hospital chains dominate the market. The market for health insurance is very highly concentrated in much of the United States (American Medical Association 2006). Finally, even though the market for physicians is much less concentrated, limitations on market entry imposed by licensure and professional constraints on advertising limit competition.

None of these problems are new to health care market advocates. They have been recognized at least since Arrow's seminal essay in 1963, and market advocates have been grappling with them at least since Mark Pauly's response to Arrow in 1968 (see chapter 6). Regarding the problem of information deficits in health care, for example, CDHC advocates argue that computers, car repairs, and investment instruments are also complicated, but that perfectly adequate markets function for them (Herzlinger ed. 2004, 14–17). Even if only a few consumers are able to master the difficulties of shopping for health care, advocates contend, providers will realize that they have to compete for these marginal consumers, and all consumers will benefit (Sloan and Feldman 1978, 57–131, 61). Even though physicians make many decisions as the agents for their patients, physicians are likely to get reputations for frugality or extravagance, and patients will go to more frugal physicians. If patients can be made more cost-conscious through cost sharing, both providers and independent information sources will find it in their interests to provide more and better information. Finally, and this is their most powerfully pressed argument, even if health care markets are problematic, there is no obvious second-best alternative to markets. In particular, government regulation only makes things worse.

These responses are not on the whole overwhelmingly persuasive. Health care is ultimately much more complicated than computers or car repairs. I have no idea how a computer works, but I have bought a number of computers, each time using a search strategy that narrows my focus to a handful of salient attributes and then simply compares prices. At times I have little idea what my mechanic is doing to my car (at other times I know exactly what he is doing and could do it myself if I had the time). I do know, however, that the mechanic will stay within the price range he quoted up front, and that this price makes sense in terms of the current value of the car. When I have a serious medical problem, on the other hand, I usually have no idea what needs to be done, and I certainly have no idea how much whatever needs to be done might cost. I depend upon my doctor to recommend the right specialists and to run the right tests and prescribe the right treatments, and am glad that I have insurance so that I do not have to decide case by case whether to have a CT scan or MRI, to take drug X or drug Y.

It is not at all clear that doctors who got reputations for being cheap will get an edge in the market if they do not also develop a reputation for quality. Indeed, consumers may well view a higher price as a marker of better quality. Doctors might compete for the marginal patient who is a particularly intelligent shopper, but it is not obvious that doctors have an incentive to share the price (or the attention) they give to that patient with other patients. Comparative price and quality information appears to be a public good, and it is not clear that private sources will produce enough, and sufficiently reliable, information. A great many initiatives are currently under way in both the private and public sectors to increase the availability of quality and price information in health care, but we still have far to go before health care markets are truly functional.

Enigmas Posed by Health Insurance

The economics of health insurance also presents complexities not fully examined by CDHC advocates. One of the mysteries that CDHC advocates do not fully explain is why health insurance is so attractive to consumers (and has long been: see chapter 5). In general, neoclassical economists celebrate consumer choice and argue for removing artificial impediments to realizing consumer choice. If a consumer wants to purchase something, and if the choice will not harm others, then nothing should stand in the consumer's way. But CDHC advocates do not trust consumer choice when it comes to the purchase of health insurance. As noted in chapter 3, to a remarkable degree CDHC advocates believe that consumers purchase too much health insurance, and should be discouraged from doing so through the provision of tax subsidies for high-deductible health plans.[15]

CDHC advocates argue that consumers insure because health insurance is offered to them by their employers at artificially low nominal prices that artificially inflate demand, and that the employers' provision of health insurance is in turn driven by inappropriate and ill-advised tax subsidies. If consumers had to purchase health insurance at full price, they posit, consumers would purchase much less health insurance.

This explanation finds only weak support in the history of health insurance in the United States, examined earlier. Americans purchased health insurance before employers contributed to its cost and before tax subsidies became a major factor.[16] Elderly Americans continue to purchase Medicare supplemental insurance policies without tax subsidies. Americans purchase health insurance in the nongroup market, often without tax subsidies, even though administrative costs are very high and the value of the policies is quite low. And citizens of all other developed countries have made certain that everyone (or virtually everyone) within their countries has access to health care, even though this results in substantial transfers of income from the wealthy to the less wealthy. Perhaps consumers really do want health insurance.

The recent work of the economist John Nyman goes far toward explaining why consumers purchase health insurance. Nyman presents several explanations of why health insurance is of value to consumers and why moral hazard as conventionally defined is less of a problem than CDHC advocates claim. Indeed, Nyman defines moral hazard as a positive as well as a negative feature of insurance: he recognizes that insurance can increase as well as decrease consumer welfare, and argues that "the efficient portion of this additional care . . . so dominates the welfare implications that overall, moral hazard increases welfare" (Nyman 2003, 2).

Nyman develops several complex arguments as to why insurance enhances consumer welfare. He begins by reexamining the nature of insurance. Traditionally, economics has understood insurance in terms of risk aversion: economists have posited that consumers prefer the certain loss of a fixed sum of money (paid as a premium) to assuming the risk of a much larger loss (Nyman 2003, 17). Consumers would rather, that is, pay a premium of $100 today than risk a 10 percent chance of losing $1,000 tomorrow. The problem with this understanding identified by Nyman is that according to prospect theory based on the research of behavioral psychologists (described above), people do not behave this way: most in fact prefer a risk of loss to a certain loss (Nyman 2003, 24, 54–55).[17] Nyman also notes that according to research by behavioral psychologists into the "framing" of decisions, people do not view insurance as a simple gamble. Subjects in an experiment were significantly more likely to spend $40 on "travel insurance" to guard against a 2 percent chance of losing $2,000 than they were to choose a certain loss of $40 over a 2 percent chance of losing $2,000 in a standard gamble (Nyman 2003, 56–58).[18]

Nyman claims that the prevalence of insurance is better explained by the declining marginal utility of money (Nyman 2003, 25–26). One of the basic premises of economics, understood at least since the work of Daniel Bernoulli in the eighteenth century, is that money, like everything else, declines in its contribution to utility as more of it is owned (Nyman 2003, 2). The receipt of an additional $1,000 means more to a person earning $10,000 a year than to a person earning $100,000 a year; Bill Gates's next million will enhance his welfare less than my next million will enhance mine.

One ramification of the declining marginal utility of money is that it makes sense to spend $100 today to assure the availability of the additional income necessary to cover a $10,000 medical procedure next week if it is required by the occurrence of injury or illness (Nyman 2003, 51–52). Although the premium cost imposes a current reduction of wealth, the amount of money needed to diagnose and treat an illness could be much greater, imposing a loss in the steeper area of the utility curve where money is more valuable (Nyman 2003, 52, 129–30). Insurance, that is, is simply an income transfer from those who remain healthy to those who are ill, but the value of the income to the ill exceeds the current cost of the premium to the healthy (Nyman 2003, 30; de Meza 1983). Indeed, insurance is so much more valuable than the cost of an actuarially fair premium that people are willing to spend an additional amount to cover the "load" of administrative costs and the risk premium that an insurer demands for a policy.[19]

The purchase of insurance is therefore not driven by risk adversity, though risk adversity may strengthen or weaken the desire for insurance (Nyman 2003, 128–36). I may be risk averse or I may be a risk preferrer, but I am still likely to purchase health insurance simply because of the declining marginal utility of money.

If the function of insurance is to protect against the diminution of individual wealth caused by the need for medical care, it would make most sense (as some CDHC advocates suggest) for health insurance to simply provide lump-sum transfers of income to those who need health care, allowing them to decide how to spend the money (Goodman, Musgrave, and Herrick 2004, 245; Herzlinger ed. 2004, 232–33). Nyman recognizes the cogency of this argument, but responds that such a system is impractical because of the risk of fraud and high transaction costs (resulting from the need to specify the schedule of payoffs for each disease and each possible level of severity, complications, and sequellae) (Nyman 2003, 31, 42). Though health insurance undoubtedly results in wasteful expenditures, including waste driven by provider-induced demand, the consumption of health care is inherently time-consuming, painful, and in most respects unpleasant, and most people are reluctant to make claims on their insurance policies through the purchase of health care unless they are actually ill (Nyman 2003, 170). Direct payments to health care providers also make it more likely that payments will be spent in meeting medical needs, and reduce the risk that some ill persons may spend insurance payments on something other than medical care and then become dependent on society to meet their medical needs (Nyman 2003, 43). (This is, incidentally, a real risk with HSAs, which can be spent on many products and services not covered by traditional health insurance.) Nyman asserts that the much greater prevalence in health insurance of "price-payoff" systems rather than lump-sum payments demonstrates that the administrative cost savings of price-payoff systems more than offset the increased cost caused by moral hazard (Nyman 2003, 42).

Characterizing health insurance correctly as cover for a potential loss of income caused by disease or injury also permits, Nyman argues, a more accurate consideration of the problem of moral hazard. Nyman acknowledges that insurance can result in excess expenditures for medical care (Nyman 2003, 2). But he argues that to correctly understand moral hazard, we should not focus on how much people spend on medical care when they are insured as compared to when they are not insured. Rather we need to consider how much people spend on medical care if insurance pays directly for that care as compared to how much they would spend if they simply received a lump-sum transfer equal to the cost of medical care once they became ill, and could then decide to spend it on medical care or on something else (Nyman 2003, 40–41).[20] Nyman acknowledges that some consumers would spend the lump-sum payment on things other than medical care, but he claims that many consumers, in particular those requiring otherwise unaffordable life-saving interventions, would clearly spend their money on medical care. They receive, therefore, substantial positive value from health insurance contracts (Nyman 2003, 41, 46).

Nyman also contends that estimates of moral hazard fail to take fully into account income elasticity of demand. This is a double-barreled argument. First, if insurance simply results in an income transfer in time of need (as Nyman posits), it necessarily results in an increase in income at that point, which tends to increase overall demand for consumption by the consumer, including the consumption of medical services. Thus increased spending on medical services is a necessary consequence of insurance, not an unavoidable inefficiency. Also, insureds necessarily pay premiums for health insurance at regular intervals (either directly or through their employer in the form of decreased wages). If consumers did not spend this money on premiums, their available income would increase and they would spend this money on other products and services, including health care, and again, the demand for health care would correspondingly increase (Nyman 2003, 82, 99). Moreover, health insurance does not cause a market-wide decrease in the price of medical care: it causes a decrease in price only for those who are ill (Nyman 2003, 82). For all of these reasons, it is inaccurate to estimate inefficient moral hazard, attributable to the price decrease in the cost of medical care caused by insurance, by simply comparing demand from the uninsured with demand from the insured (Nyman 2003, 116).[21] Rather one must compare the demand for health care by those who pay for insurance and consume health care received in kind when they are ill with the demand for health care that would exist in the absence of insurance if the income now spent on premiums were available (in part) for health care. More importantly, one must compare the level of demand that would result if insured persons received lump-sum payments when they were ill equivalent to the cost of medical care, dramatically increasing their income and thus their efficient demand for health care, with the level of demand that results from current insurance arrangements (Nyman 2003, 95–100). Nyman posits that price-reduction moral-hazard loss is still a factor, but much less of a factor than is claimed by CDHC advocates.[22]

Finally and most importantly, Nyman argues that the most significant contribution of health insurance, what he calls its "access value," has been largely ignored by prior analysis (Nyman 2003, 67). One of the basic problems that must be faced in organizing a health care system, as noted in the Preface of this book, is the remarkably skewed nature of health care costs. Each year a few people need very expensive medical care, care that would overwhelm the income and savings of most Americans and that can often not be covered through borrowing, because the medical condition makes the patient a poor lending risk (Nyman 2003, 23). The choice is not simply between purchasing this health care through insurance and purchasing it through other private funds, but rather between purchasing it through insurance and not purchasing it at all (Nyman 2003, 23). Yet this medical care has very high value. If it saves a life or adds productive years to a life, as it often does, the value of the health care can far exceed its cost.[23] This high-value health care is accessible with insurance; without insurance, loss of life or functioning would almost certainly often ensue.

Clinical evidence amply demonstrates that the uninsured forgo a great deal of medical care that is vitally important in reducing mortality and morbidity (Nyman 2003, 21–22). High-cost health care accounts for a large share of the health care purchased by health insurance, and the value of this health care greatly exceeds its cost (Nyman 2003, 70–78). Any consideration of the cost of health insurance, Nyman contends, must weigh in the balance the positive contribution of the "access value" of health insurance against the waste that insurance encourages through moral hazard. On balance, Nyman argues, the positive value of health insurance significantly outweighs its costs, which is why consumers persist in buying it. The waste caused by insurance-induced demand for designer sunglasses or full-body scans for healthy persons is greatly outweighed by the value of organ transplants, coronary artery bypass grafts, and treatments for severe traumatic injuries in children that insurance makes possible (Nyman 2003, 104–6). Indeed, Nyman notes that if cost sharing discourages welfare-increasing care as well as low-value care, increased cost sharing might well cause more harm than good (Nyman 2003, 146–51).[24] Nyman estimates that the welfare gains of insuring the uninsured would be greater than three times the welfare loss that results from moral hazard as conventionally understood (Nyman 2003, 114).

Nyman's argument about access value is related to a broader argument commonly made by health insurance advocates (and in particular by public health insurance advocates). One of the primary values of health insurance is the security that it gives to the healthy, including those who from year to year never file a claim (Marmor and Mashaw 2006, W-115–W-116).[25] Even if I persistently remain in robust good health and have no need to draw on my health insurance coverage, nevertheless I enjoy the present security of knowing that if I need it — if I have a major traffic accident on my way home from work tonight, for example — health care will be available. If I have adequate health insurance coverage, I can have confidence that I will be able to afford the health care I need and still make my house and car payments, still be able to take that summer vacation with the family that I have been planning, and still be able eventually to cover the children's college tuition.

Insurance serves two primary functions. First, it allows people to even out risk over a lifetime. Employment-related insurance in particular allows employees to continue to afford insurance, even as they age and perhaps contract chronic illnesses, as long as they remain employed. Second, it allows a pooling of risk among low-risk and high-risk insureds. The "evening-out" function can be fulfilled by CDHC, at least if an individual or family begins investing in an HSA when young. But CDHC does not really address the second, risk-pooling function, and indeed would seem to undermine it.

One of the reasons why insurance enjoys broad support is the widespread belief that a good society is one that takes care of those within it who suffer misfortune. Deborah Stone has argued that it is incorrect to understand insurance simply as forced savings. It should rather be seen as an institution for broadly sharing risk within society (Stone 1990; Stone 2002, 20, 102). The "risk-sharing" character of insurance is more important than its "evening-out" function. Mutual aid binds a community, and it is based on values of sharing and caring within relationships that vie with competition and the promotion of self-interest as motivators of individual and social action (Stone 2002, 20). It provides basic security to all within a society, regardless of their individual wealth. Actuarially based insurance — insurance that attempts to charge each individual based on his or her own risk—imposes tremendous administrative costs (it is not cheap to figure out each applicant's potential risk) and charges unaffordable premiums to those most in need of health care (Kuttner 1997, 146–49). In most societies, therefore, it merely supplements a basic public insurance system that covers all, regardless of health status or ability to pay.

In sum, the story that CDHC advocates tell about health insurance based on neoclassical welfare economics is too simple, and in many respects misleading. It is not entirely wrong—if tax subsidies for health insurance were abolished, some employers would drop insurance and many would provide less generous policies (Glied 2005, 39). In turn, many people currently insured would drop their health insurance or purchase policies with more cost sharing. With less insurance, consumers would purchase less health care. Some of this forgone health care would likely consist of services or products that contribute little to health, but much of it would be care that is in fact important. Those who lost health insurance altogether would in particular face the possibility of devastating threats to their health. It is wrong to assume that society would be better off under these circumstances.

Are Consumer-Driven Markets Our Only Choice?

Would consumers be better off with less health insurance and less health care? Nyman's argument suggests that consumers might well be worse off if they lost the access value of insurance. It also suggests that CDHC advocates underestimate the extent to which reductions in health insurance would reduce access to health care, and certainly that they overestimate the extent to which reduction would increase consumer utility. Consumers would continue to purchase insurance, even without tax subsidies, because the security that it brings is worth a great deal. They also might press for universal, publicly funded health insurance if the end of tax subsidies dramatically increased the number of uninsured. Consumers might also find that paying for their own health care did not really increase their utility—if they lacked the information necessary to make wise consumption decisions, or if they made irrational decisions because of heuristic biases.

Many economists respond to these challenges to the authority of their models by admitting that the models are not perfect, but insisting that they do a better job than any other models of explaining and predicting how humans behave. Further, they claim, markets do a better job of maximizing human welfare than any other institutions do. There is some truth in this. The general experience of humankind, as will be discussed further below, is that markets do a better job than governments of deciding how much steel should be produced or which styles of cars should be manufactured. But the case may not be as strong for allowing markets to govern access to health care. If maximizing health is our goal, perhaps we can better accomplish it by empowering health care professionals to make decisions as to how to allocate health resources than by asking uninformed lay consumers to make the decisions. Professional decisions could be informed by objective health services research. This is the approach taken by many other countries that establish public budgets for health care and then depend largely (but usually not entirely) on professionals to make resource micro-allocation decisions. Allocating resources on the basis of medical need might well result in a "better" allocation of resources than that achieved by simply attending to consumers' willingness to pay based on their ability to afford or their understanding of their needs (Reinhardt 2002, 21–23). If maximizing equity of access to health services is a societal goal, then government may well be more effective than markets in getting us what we want.

This brings us back to the role of government. As we have seen, neoclassical economists tend to be very skeptical of the possibility that government can make a useful contribution to an economy. In recent years their predominant approach to understanding government has been the public choice model discussed above. Although the public choice view of government is a useful tool for understanding some government behavior and resonates with the general suspicion that Americans have toward government, it is a view far from universally accepted (Rubin 2002; Kelman 1988; Kuttner 1997, 333–42). Legislators are not always rent seekers: they are often motivated by ideology and by the desire to serve their constituencies, and many represent "safe districts" and do not need to worry excessively about contributions from interest groups to finance reelection campaigns. Administrators also are often ideologically committed to the mission of their agency and to the public interest, either as they view it themselves in a Burkean sense or as they interpret it according to the desires of the average voter (Levine and Forrence 1990, 176–82). One can easily think of many public policy initiatives of the past half-century, including the rise of environmental regulation and the deregulation of a number of industries, that square very poorly with the public choice understanding of governmental behavior.

When one looks at the health care sector, it is clear that government has a constructive role to play, a fact that experts in health politics have long recognized (Marmor and Mashaw 2006). First, only government can redistribute income. Most economists agree that welfare economics does not require or justify any particular distribution of wealth, and most theories of justice call for redistribution of wealth under some circumstances (Elhauge 1994, 1473–93). Most health policy experts, including economists, recognize that some redistribution of wealth will be necessary if universal access to health care is to be achieved. If any approximation of evenly distributed health status is desired, even greater redistribution of wealth will be required, since the poor tend to be in worse health to begin with (Kuttner 1997, 153–54).

A government that chooses to permit access to health care for the poor can do so in several ways. First, it can simply transfer lump sums of money to the poor and allow them to decide whether to spend it on health care. This is the favored approach of many economists, because it would allow the poor themselves to use the money for the purpose that they value most (Rice 2002, 39; Gaynor and Vogt 1997, 482). But the poor face many immediate needs, some of which are likely to take precedence over health care in the short term, even though in the longer term health care might prove more important. Most countries provide health care, like education, in kind. This is because voters are more supportive of providing specific products or services to the poor through wealth redistribution programs than of simply providing cash (Rice 2002, 190–91; Reinhardt 1998, 38). Health care, like education, is also fundamental for assuring basic opportunity to participate in society and in the economy (Rice 2002, 195–96, 199; Stone 2005, 68) Further, direct provision of health care is not likely to create disincentives for productive work, as the provision of cash might (Elhauge 1994, 1486–92; Rice 2002, 192). Health care also provides positive externalities that benefit those who finance income transfers — it offers protection from contagious diseases to all, protects wealthier members of society from having to witness the visible suffering of their poorer neighbors, and helps to make workers more productive. And payments for health care also benefit health care providers, who provide a powerful and reliable lobby for health care funding.[26]

Alternatively, government could provide vouchers to the poor to purchase private health insurance. This would assure that the money was actually spent for health care (or for health insurance). It also would involve the private sector in administering the program, and could be structured so as to take advantage of market competition. Managed competition proposals often take this approach. Yet these proposals usually recognize that significant government regulation is necessary if health plans are to make subsidized insurance markets function properly (Enthoven 1980, 78–82, 114–72). Given the highly skewed nature of health care costs, the easiest way for insurers to compete is to pursue healthy applicants, and considerable regulation is necessary to make them focus instead on competing to manage costs (Enthoven 1980; Enthoven and Kronick 1989). Managed competition also imposes an extra layer of administrative costs — private administrative costs on top of public administrative costs — thus adding to the total cost of the program. Although the issue is disputed, there is considerable evidence that public health insurance programs operate with much lower administrative costs than private insurance plans (Woolhandler, Campbell, and Himmelstein 2003). The Medicare Advantage program (and its previous incarnations) costs much more than the Medicare fee-for-service program (Biles, Nicholas, Cooper, Adrion, and Guterman 2006; Berenson 2006).

Many countries have found that the most effective way to provide access to health care for all is through direct government financing of health care (White 1995; Jost 2003). Direct government payment for health care allows much greater control over costs than private sector funding does. Government financing of health care has advantages and disadvantages, discussed fully in chapter 10, but in real life (rather than within the confines of the economist's blackboard — or Power Point slides) government financing of health care has not proved inferior to private sector financing.

Government can make other contributions as well. It can produce public goods that are under-produced in the private sector because of the difficulty of restricting the benefits of the product or service to those who will pay for it. Most of the dramatic gains in longevity over the past two centuries have been due to better public health, sanitation, nutrition, and living conditions, and many of these improvements have been due to government activity (Kuttner 1997, 111; Easterlin 2004). The provision of some forms of information, such as reliable comparative information on quality, also partake of a public good nature, as noted above. Regina Herzlinger, otherwise a strong advocate of markets, argues for the creation of a government agency to provide this form of information (Herzlinger ed. 2004, 797–810). Government protects us from harm, not only by offering police protection from violent crime but also by protecting us from invasions of the privacy of our health care information and assuring the solvency of insurance companies. Government can also in some instances protect us from making foolish or dangerous decisions, or protect us from fraud and deception. Under some circumstances, that is, government "paternalism" may be appropriate (Rice 2002, 80–81). The Food and Drug Administration, for example, exists to provide assurances that drugs and devices marketed in the United States are "safe and effective" consumer options, and although it has come in for criticism recently because of issues of regulatory capture, it still enjoys wide support for its mission. Finally, the role of government in funding and facilitating research in health care has been absolutely central. One of the most significant strengths of the American health care system is its creativity and innovativeness, much of which is attributable to public research funding (Kuttner 1997, 217–18). Government funds have also paid for the training of research scientists, who have made the American health care system the most innovative in the world.

It is important, moreover, to remember that not all decisions in health care are made by individual consumers or government bureaucrats. Most health care decisions, as noted above, are made by professionals, primarily physicians. This is often wholly appropriate. While experts are subject to many of the same biases as lay people, they are not necessarily subject to biases to the same degree, and often are better able to correct biased thinking (Schneider 1998, 103–4). Experts are experts precisely because they have experience — tacit knowledge allowing them to intuitively recognize patterns and prototypes that lay people do not see (Schneider 1998, 57, 104–5). Experts are also trained to make immediate, intuitive judgments that are much more likely to be accurate than those of lay people (Gladwell 2005, 107). They are able to understand and explain their judgments much more accurately than untrained consumers can (Gladwell 2005, 176–86). Medical professionals are less emotionally involved in medical conditions than their patients are, and thus less subject to the distortions in judgment that emotions can bring (Schneider 1998, 103). Finally, medical professionals operate under the constraint of professional and societal norms that constrain them from taking advantage of their patients even when economic incentives might tempt them to do so (Arrow 1968).

Experts also have access to a knowledge base not shared by the lay patient, "a large and sophisticated literature which subjects standard medical reasoning to statistical and logical scrutiny" (Schneider 1998, 105). Most serious medical problems are now subjected to the scrutiny of several professionals, who bring to bear multiple perspectives and discuss and analyze problems collectively (Schneider 1998, 105). Professional guidelines based on research into actual outcomes may permit experts to make even more reliable and accurate decisions in the face of uncertainty (Dawes, Faust, and Meehl 2002). If "rational choice" in health care is our goal, therefore, trusting lay consumers may be less likely to get us there than turning to professional experts or to health services research. Correspondingly, cost-control strategies aimed at changing the incentives and thus refocusing the decision-making skills of providers of health care services, such as capitation payments for physicians, might be more effective than those aimed at controlling consumer demand (Rice 2002, 110).

Obviously, consumers have their own expertise complementing that of professionals — for one thing, they have a better understanding of their own needs and limitations. But in the end, unless we are to lapse into complete nihilism, we must acknowledge that modern medicine does offer some useful knowledge of the human body and its malfunctions; that pharmaceuticals, surgeries, and other medical treatments can make a real contribution toward improving the condition of human bodies that are not functioning properly; and that health care professionals, who have the benefit of up to a decade of higher education and often years of practice, do know more about the human body and its malfunctions than lay consumers do, even consumers who have spent hours visiting health care web sites. Most doctors also know more about medicine than most economists do.

Economics as Ideology

CDHC advocates are not convinced. They remain very skeptical about the role of government in health care systems and about trusting experts (other than themselves, of course) to make decisions for consumers (see chapter 3). Their skepticism illuminates an important truth about economics. Although the practitioners of neoclassical economics understand it to be a science, in reality, at least as generally practiced in the United States, it is based on a particular philosophical ideology that drives the assumptions on which its models are based, and its conclusions are often used to support a particular political agenda. Economics, that is, often plays a normative as well as a positive role (Evans 1998, 467–75). Economists tend to get confused, believing that their normative beliefs are scientific conclusions (Culyer and Evans 1996).

This is not to say that all practitioners of economics have the same politics. The political alignments of American academics who write about health economics, as revealed through their policy assumptions and prescriptions, span the ideological and political spectrum, from Vicente Navarro to Uwe Reinhardt and Thomas Rice, to Joseph Newhouse and Henry Aaron, to Mark Pauly and Patricia Danzon, to Stuart Butler and John Goodman. Health economists from other countries, such as Canada, the United Kingdom, and the Netherlands, also tend to reach health policy conclusions very different from those of mainstream American health economists. Nevertheless, the writings of neoclassical economists, and in particular those who advocate CDHC, tend toward a particular ideological position: a libertarian one that places a high value on individual freedom of choice and envisions a very limited role for the state (Hayek 1960; Nozick 1974, 160–64).

Neoclassical economics meshes neatly with a libertarian ideology for a number of reasons. To begin, neoclassical economics privileges individual over collective preferences. Indeed, it conceptualizes the welfare of a society as merely the sum of the preferences of its individual constituents as revealed by their spending, thus depriving collective preference of any meaning other than as the aggregate of individual preferences. Neoclassical economics also views individual preferences as inherent and as accurate indicators of individual welfare, and thus places a very high value on the freedom of individuals to satisfy their preferences. Finally, neoclassical economics views individual preferences as most clearly and properly reflected in purchasing decisions, as opposed to voting behavior or opinion polls, for example. Nonmarket decision-making processes, such as the legislative and regulatory processes, are viewed as suspect; indeed they are viewed as inefficient and thus inferior approaches to promoting the public welfare.

One ramification of viewing social welfare as the sum of revealed individual preferences is that it privileges the wealthy over the poor. If preferences are revealed through purchases, only the preferences of those who have money to make purchases count (Dobb 1973, 34–35). The welfare of the rich, that is to say, takes precedence over the welfare of the poor, because the rich have more purchasing power. Uwe Reinhardt illustrates this point with the example of two families, one a wealthy family with a healthy baby, the other a poor family whose baby has numerous health problems (Reinhardt 2002, xiv–xv). If social welfare is defined as an aggregation of individual preferences as revealed through willingness to pay, more pediatric visits will in all likelihood go to the wealthy, healthy baby than to the poor, sickly baby. An "inefficient" allocation of health care that gave more health care to the sick baby, one could argue, might make more sense, and be more just. But economics would view a distribution which gives more resources to the wealthy, healthy baby as more efficient.

Neoclassical economists admit that economics as a science cannot tell us how wealth should be distributed in society.[27] They recognize that allocative efficiency does not address the question of the original distribution of wealth in society. There are an infinite number of Pareto-optimal possibilities corresponding to the infinite number of possible original distributions of resources within societies (Arrow 1963, 943; Kuttner 1997, 27–28). As Amatya Sen has observed, "An economy can be [Pareto] optimal . . . even when some people are rolling in luxury and others are near starvation as long as the starvers cannot be made better off without cutting into the pleasure of the rich. . . . In short, a society or an economy can be Pareto-optimal and still be perfectly disgusting" (Sen 1970, 22).

Kaldor-Hicks optimality is even more problematic. A trade that ends up making a poor person worse off while improving the lot of a rich person is "efficient" under this definition if the rich person could compensate the poor person for the poor person's loss and still come out ahead, regardless of whether he or she in fact does so. Uwe Reinhardt refers to this as the "punch-in-the-nose criterion," because it would allow one person to punch another in the nose without compensation if the utility to the puncher would exceed the disutility to the punched (Reinhardt 1998, 31).

Almost by definition, a discussion of social justice requires a judgment of the distribution of wealth in society as reflected by markets, not simply an acceptance of the individual interests revealed in market transactions (Rice 2002, 175–76). A society in which a few people control almost all the wealth and live in great luxury while others are starving is not one that commends itself to most people. Indeed there is considerable, though controversial, evidence that less equal societies are less healthy and have less happy populations (Rice 2002, 50–55; Kawachi 2005, 29–33).

Yet in general economists are wary of wealth redistribution (Reinhardt 1998, 36), for several reasons. One is a concern that the recipients of redistribution would have less incentive to be productive. Economic productivity is driven in the neoclassical model by the desire for wealth, and if people are given resources without producing anything, they have little incentive to be productive (Stone 2002, 80; Rhoads 1985, 88–89). Second, economists are concerned about the impact of redistribution on the productivity of those from whom resources are taken. There is always a trade-off between earning money and enjoying leisure, and economists believe that when income is taxed, productive activities become less attractive and leisure more attractive (Rhoads 1985, 91–97; Rice 2002, 39). Further, in the view of many economists taxes encourage wasteful and unproductive tax-avoiding activities that do nothing to increase social welfare. Indeed, government redistribution almost inevitably involves government interference with individual choices over the use of resources, which in turn interferes with the achievement of efficiency (Stone 2002, 80). And redistribution necessarily requires a government bureaucracy —taxation agencies, welfare departments, administrative appeal agencies, and courts for sorting out conflicts over taxes and payments. This bureaucracy is a deadweight loss: it uses resources that could otherwise be used for productive purposes (Stone 2002, 82).

Redistribution is inevitably difficult politically, as it requires the transfer of resources from the wealthy to those with less wealth. In a polity in which the wealthy are more likely to vote and are certainly more capable of making campaign contributions and of lobbying legislators, redistribution is an uphill battle (Kuttner 1997, 28). As Robert Kuttner observes, "The more powerfully entrenched the market model becomes, the less appetite have its custodians for redistributing its prizes" (Kuttner 1997, 35). Most economists, it would seem, acknowledge the need for redistribution in theory but do not see themselves as responsible for taking on the battle to bring it about. Their job, they believe, is to provide advice as to how to achieve allocative efficiency given a particular wealth distribution. Advocating the redistribution of wealth to achieve equity is someone else's job, perhaps that of philosophers, theologians, or political scientists.

The ideological nature of health economics comes into clearer focus when observed through the lens of health policy contributions by scholars in other disciplines. Political scientists have long observed that health care markets are not independent and self-sustaining but rather are political creations, dependent upon political institutions for their implementation and regulation (see Morone 1993; Brown 1993; Marmor and Boyum 1993). Markets are also ideological in nature, and favor some political values over others. Health politics scholars have offered persuasive arguments for alternative approaches to financing health care based on public insurance (Marmor and Mashaw 2006; Stone 1993). They have also illuminated the "faddishness" of health policy movements like CDHC (Marmor 2007). Finally, the writings of health politics scholars are useful in exposing the ideology and the limitations of CDHC in particular (Oberlander 2006; Hacker 2006, 149–53). Much of what is said in this book builds on the challenges that political scientists have posed to the politics of markets in health care.

Economics as Common Sense

Even though the foundations and conclusions of neoclassical economics as a science are questionable and the ideological inclinations of the discipline render its normative prescriptions suspect, economics retains great influence on policy making in the United States, more so than any of the other social sciences. The political success that CDHC advocates have enjoyed in recent years illustrates this influence. The power of economics is no doubt in large part due to the tendency of its descriptions of human behavior to accord with common sense, or at least with American common sense.

It is our common experience, and probably the common experience of most of humankind, that people do respond to financial incentives, that people are most productive and creative when the fruits of their labor are likely to be enjoyed by them and their families, that people do spend their resources on things that they value, and that governments seldom increase the efficiency of markets and are often unproductive, if not corrupt. The example of the Soviet bloc socialist states in the 1980s is a powerful example (though the counter-example of the experience of Russia with market capitalism in the 1990s tends to be ignored). We do understand "that love is scarce, and that consequently we had better try to get along without it, organizing our affairs to take advantage of the abundant selfishness instead" (McCloskey 1990, 142–43).[28] People may derive satisfaction from nonmaterial things, and their behavior is not wholly explained by response to material rewards, but material rewards are important.

Americans also seem to have a particularly strong belief that creative and hardworking people are likely to become wealthy, that pleasure and satisfaction can be obtained from material things, that private business tends to be productive and creative, that government bureaucrats tend to be bumbling incompetents, and that taxation is evil. We have a common vocabulary of stories, metaphors, and symbols — about welfare queens and slippery slopes and $630 toilet seats — all of which reinforce support for markets and challenge the positive contribution of government (Stone 2002, 82–84). Americans therefore find the message of neoclassical economists particularly sympathetic. Economic individualism is strong in the United States, while the sense of social solidarity that animates social welfare systems in most European and some Asian nations is largely lacking. The large role that money plays in political campaigns and in efforts to lobby legislatures and regulatory bodies, the weakness of the left and of workers' unions, and the lack of a tradition of a strong and independent civil service render the American political system particularly liable to control by the wealthy and by business interests (Jost 2004, 437–39). All of this makes Americans particularly susceptible to the message of libertarian economists.

While we are susceptible, we should also be skeptical. As noted above, economics is based on certain assumptions and beliefs that are open to question — or at least qualification — and that are amenable to being used to promote a particular political agenda.[29] The objective and scientific language of economics can be used to mask policies that are clearly aimed at achieving particular agendas that would probably not be politically acceptable if stated more baldly. If "consumer-driven health care" were advertised as a proposal to shift the weight of health care spending from healthy Americans to the shoulders of the chronically ill it would probably not sell (Reinhardt 1998, 15).

Moreover, although the socialist economies of the Soviet empire provide ample evidence of the problems that can result when governments run economies and entrepreneurs are discouraged, the growth in productivity of western European economies through most of the second half of the twentieth century, a growth that roughly paralleled our own, demonstrates that higher taxes, greater involvement of the government in the economy, and more generous social welfare benefits (including universal public health insurance) are not inconsistent with economic growth (Lindert 2004). Indeed, from the 1940s through the early 1970s the United States enjoyed unprecedented economic growth and prosperity, even though we had more government involvement in the economy and much higher and more progressive taxes then we have today (when taxes are low and free enterprise is largely untrammeled, but nonetheless economic growth is sluggish by historical standards) (Kuttner 1997, 209–18). Finally, with respect to health care at least, ordinary Americans are not wholly sold on the virtue of markets. Opinion surveys demonstrate that political élites are more convinced of the value of individual responsibility for health care and less concerned about equal access than the general public is outside the Beltway (Schlesinger 2005, 110–12).

Although Americans are predisposed to listen to economists, Americans are also pragmatic, and are unlikely to support ideologically based policies that do not really work. The primary question therefore is whether CDHC will, and does, work in practice. To this question we turn next.

CHAPTER 8

But Does It Work? The Evidence for and against Consumer-Driven Health Care

The Empirical Question

While the arguments for CDHC are ultimately based on economic theory, CDHC proponents also point to an impressive body of empirical evidence to support their position that consumers use less health care and get more value from the health care they purchase when confronted with greater cost-sharing obligations. There is considerable evidence that demand for health care is elastic: if the price of health care as experienced by the consumer goes up, demand for health care will go down. On the basis of this evidence, CDHC advocates argue that if more of the costs of health care can be shifted to the consumer through higher deductibles or other forms of cost sharing, consumers will moderate increases in the cost of health care.

The empirical arguments for (and against) CDHC are based on research conducted over the past three decades in a number of countries. Most of these studies have either used econometric models to analyze survey or administrative data or have analyzed what happened to demand when particular insurance programs added or removed cost-sharing obligations. The most important and ambitious study of the effects of cost sharing on consumer demand was undoubtedly the Rand Health Insurance Experiment (HIE) of the late 1970s and early 1980s, a large experiment that randomly assigned participants to a variety of plans with different levels of cost sharing, and then followed not only their expenditures but also their health decisions and their health status over an extended period. The HIE definitively established that consumer demand for health care is elastic (Newhouse and Insurance Experiment Group 1993, 40–43, 56, 68–71, 82–83). But the HIE also found that when faced with higher cost sharing, consumers are unable to distinguish between more essential and less essential health care services and are equally likely to forgo highly effective and less effective services. It also discovered that some consumers, particularly poorer consumers, have worse health outcomes when they face higher cost sharing. Subsequent studies have confirmed the major findings of the HIE.

The HIE and similar studies looked only at the effects of high cost sharing. Contemporary consumer-driven products couple HDHPs with health savings accounts (HSAs), which wholly or partially cover the consumer's cost-sharing obligations. Consumers with HSAs can be expected to behave somewhat differently from consumers who must cover cost-sharing obligations out of pocket. CDHC products also often attempt to provide decision support to their enrollees to improve the quality of their health care decisions. CDHC plans, therefore, might have results different from those of the cost-sharing plans used in the HIE. A growing body of studies looks at how HSAs, health reimbursement accounts (HRAs), and medical savings accounts (MSAs) are performing, who is adopting them, how they are being used, how consumers experience them, and how they are affecting health care expenditures. Moreover, several countries, notably Singapore, China, and South Africa, have extensive and growing experience with MSAs, which has to some extent been studied.

This chapter first reviews empirical research examining consumer response to cost sharing, focusing particularly on the HIE and examining the costs as well as the benefits of cost sharing. It then considers available evidence on the effects of HSAs, looking at foreign as well as domestic experience.

The Rand Health Insurance Experiment

As described in chapter 7, the economic understanding of moral hazard on which the current CDHC movement is based emerged in the late 1960s and early 1970s. This theory posited that demand for health care services was elastic—as the price of health care services increased, consumer demand for those services would decrease.

A number of studies at that time confirmed this assumption. These were primarily studies based on natural experiments (Ginsburg and Mannheim 1973). One study examined changes in service consumption when Stanford University's prepaid health plan changed from free care to 25 percent coinsurance in 1967 (Scitovsky and Snyder 1972). Another study looked at changes in use when the United Mine Workers (UMW) health plan instituted cost sharing in West Virginia in 1977 (Sheffler 1984).

These studies found significant elasticity of demand for services. But as was true with other early studies, it was unclear to what extent their findings could be projected to determine the effects of cost sharing generally. The UMW study, for example, covered a short period during which it was rumored that the cost-sharing arrangement was only temporary. Consumption of services, therefore, may have simply been delayed rather than forgone (Rice and Morrison 1994, 249). Some of the studies also involved situations where insureds who preferred to avoid cost-sharing obligations could shift to other health plans, thus confounding the effects of moral hazard and adverse selection (Rubin and Mendelson 1995, 2–88). Finally and most importantly, the studies tended to look only at how cost sharing affected the consumption of services, not at how it affected the health or welfare of those required to pay deductibles or coinsurance.

The Rand Health Insurance Experiment (HIE) was designed to determine comprehensively the health policy ramifications of increased cost sharing. It attempted to accomplish this through a controlled experiment, well designed to avoid the problems that had limited the validity of the results of earlier studies. Though the HIE has been widely cited by advocates of a market-driven health care system, the experiment itself was in fact funded by the federal government to determine what role, if any, cost sharing should play in the newly created Medicaid program and in future public health insurance programs (Newhouse and Insurance Experiment Group 1993, 3–4).

The HIE ultimately involved about two thousand families and about seventeen thousand person-years of experience (Newhouse and Insurance Experiment Group 1993, 8, 140). Six experiment sites were chosen to assure diversity by region and by size of urban area, as well as variation in the availability of medical resources (Newhouse and Insurance Experiment Group 1993, 15–17). The experiment lasted for periods of three to five years for each family, spanning from 1974 to 1982 (Newhouse and Insurance Experiment Group 1993, 15). The HIE excluded people over sixty-five and those who earned more than $25,000 a year in 1978 dollars ($80,312 in 2006 dollars), but otherwise randomly selected people who were representative of the general population in terms of their economic and health status. Participants were assigned randomly to several cost-sharing plans, including one that provided free care and others with coinsurance obligations of 25 percent, 50 percent, and 95 percent.[1] The 95 percent plan was essentially a high-deductible plan, as the participants bore virtually all the costs of services until they met an expenditure cap. This cap was generally $1,000 for a family (roughly $4,384 in 2006 dollars when the experiment began in 1974 and $2,139 in 2006 dollars when it ended in 1982), but for poorer families it was limited to 5 percent, 10 percent, or 15 percent of family income (Newhouse and Insurance Experiment Group 1993, 8–9). Finally, the HIE assigned one group in Seattle to membership in an HMO, the Group Health Cooperative of Puget Sound, to examine the comparative ability of HMOs to reduce health care costs.

All participants in the experiment were compensated for their participation, so that none were made worse off than they would have been had they maintained their existing insurance arrangements (Newhouse and Insurance Experiment Group 1993, 12, 408). The HIE also assured that participants would not be penalized by waiting periods or preexisting condition requirements when they returned to their prior insurance at the end of the experiment.

The most important contribution of the HIE was that it examined not just how elastic the demand for health services was but also which services were reduced by cost sharing — that is, whether the reduction was primarily in less or more effective services, and whether the reduction in consumption of services had an effect on the health of consumers. CDHC advocates, of course, posit that consumers are able to identify and to reduce their consumption of ineffective services if they have incentives to do so, and that reduction of these services will not harm (and perhaps will improve) their health. The HIE set out to determine whether this was true.

The HIE determined conclusively that elasticity of demand for health care services exists. Participants assigned to the free care program consumed many more services than those assigned to the 25 percent coinsurance plan, and in general those assigned to the 25 percent coinsurance plan used more services than those assigned to the 50 percent or 95 percent plan. Price elasticity of demand is expressed as a number representing the percentage of reduction in services that will result from a 10 percent increase in price. Thus an elasticity of -.2 means that for every 10 percent increase in price, use is reduced 2 percent. The HIE determined that on average the elasticity of demand for health services moving from free care to the 25 percent coinsurance level was -.17 (Newhouse and Insurance Experiment Group 1993, 121). Per capita expenses on the free plan were 45 percent higher than those on the plan with 95 percent coinsurance (Newhouse and Insurance Experiment Group 1993, 40). Elasticity varied little from service to service, though it was greater for mental health services (Newhouse and Insurance Experiment Group 1993, 93, 338–39). The HIE found no price response for the use of inpatient medical care for children (Newhouse and Insurance Experiment Group 1993, 47). The study found income elasticity of demand as well: poorer participants were more likely to reduce use of most health care services than wealthier participants in the face of higher cost sharing.[2]

Most of the reduction in use of services resulted from a reduction in the number of initial contacts with the health care system, not in the number of services used after the patient saw a doctor. Once patients saw a doctor or entered a hospital, their course of treatment and subsequent expenses were quite similar to those of patients receiving free care (Newhouse and Insurance Experiment Group 1993, 42, 45, 82, 98–99). Variations in drug expenditures among the plans, for example, were based on the rate of visits to health care professionals, not on the expenditures on drugs per visit (Newhouse and Insurance Experiment Group 1993, 168).

The HIE also examined whether the services forgone in the face of cost sharing were more or less essential. Expert physicians categorized services covered by the plan into those that are generally regarded as highly effective (treatment of pneumonia, trauma fractures, or diabetes), quite effective (hemorrhoids, hay fever), less effective (varicose veins of lower extremities), or rarely effective (headaches, constipation) (Newhouse and Insurance Experiment Group 1993, 161–64). The HIE found that in general, consumers were not able to discriminate between more and less essential services, but simply reduced use of all services across the board (Newhouse and Insurance Experiment Group 1993, 162). The proportion of appropriate and inappropriate hospital admissions also did not differ by level of cost sharing (Newhouse and Insurance Experiment Group 1993, 162–165, 173). Poor children, however, were much more likely than nonpoor children to undergo a reduction in effective care (Newhouse and Insurance Experiment Group 1993, 164–65). Only with respect to the use of emergency departments and antibiotics was there evidence that participants reduced inappropriate use more than appropriate use (Newhouse and Insurance Experiment Group 1993, 156–57, 170). The HIE established, therefore, that cost sharing is a very blunt tool for eliminating the greatest inefficiency in health care: the overuse of ineffective health care services and the underuse of effective services (Rice 1992).

Because the HIE found that participants reduced essential as well as non-essential services, one could assume that participants in the cost-sharing arms of the study would suffer ill health effects compared to those who received free care. This was only partially true. The HIE found that lower-income persons with free care had better controlled blood pressure and better corrected vision than those on the cost-sharing plans (Newhouse and Insurance Experiment Group 1993, 201, 204). Higher cost sharing increased the risk of mortality for poor persons with elevated blood pressure (Newhouse and Insurance Experiment Group 1993, 339). Participants with free care also reported less pain for certain conditions, and poor persons with free care reported fewer serious symptoms at the conclusion of the study (Newhouse and Insurance Experiment Group 1993, 208, 219). Dental cavities were more likely to be filled on the free plan (Newhouse and Insurance Experiment Group 1993, 243). Poor children on the free plan were less likely to have anemia at the conclusion of the experiment and more likely to have received effective dental care (Newhouse and Insurance Experiment Group 1993, 251, 259). But most participants, including higher-income participants in general, suffered no ill-health effects from reducing their use of health care services.

Why did participants in high cost-sharing plans not suffer greater ill-health effects from their reduced use of "essential" services? A number of explanations have been offered for this finding. Some explanations question the HIE's effectiveness categorizations. One possibility is that the HIE categorizations were either faulty or so vague as to be of limited use in categorizing services. The HIE, for example, listed treatment of strep throat as highly effective and of throat pain as ineffective (Feldman and Dowd 1991, 193–200). A second possibility is that persons with truly serious medical problems were in fact able to get all the care they needed for free once they exceeded the maximum expenditure level (which was lower for poor families) (Feldman and Dowd 1991, 257). A third is that within each category of service there is a range of effectiveness, and the study categorization captured only the average for each category. Participants chose services based on marginal rather than average utility of services, and thus those who chose not to use "essential services" were in fact forgoing services that in their particular situation were marginally of little value. Conversely, those who used "less effective" services were perhaps using those services in situations where they were in fact of great value (Peele

1993, 205–8). Free care may also have led to a harmful overuse of some services, causing iatrogenic injury in the free care group (Peele 1993, 170).

Other explanations focus on the HIE's health outcomes findings. The HIE examined only a very limited range of possible health outcomes, and might have missed serious problems (Donaldson and Gerard 1989, 241–42). It is also quite possible that the study's time frame of three to five years failed to capture the long-term effects of forgone health care: 70 percent of the participants were part of the experiment for only three years (Newhouse and Insurance Experiment Group 1993, 15; Donaldson and Gerard 1989, 242). Finally, the study took place thirty years ago, and health care was much less effective in the 1970s than it is today (Cutler 2004). Treatment of congestive heart failure and of mental illness, for example, has made dramatic strides over the past quarter-century. Elimination of effective care today might have a much larger impact on health outcomes than it did in the 1970s.

The HIE remains the gold standard among studies of the elasticity of demand for health care services. Market advocates welcomed it as definitive proof of the high level of welfare loss caused by excess health insurance, which was estimated to be as high as $109.3 billion in 1984 dollars ($212 billion in 2006 dollars) by economists who extrapolated from the RAND findings (Feldman and Dowd 1991). Virtually every book or article advocating CDHC still mentions the HIE.

From the outset questions were raised about the validity of the study's findings, and over time these questions have persisted. One source of concern is that the rates of refusal to participate in the study and attrition rates (the rates at which participants left the study before its end) were much higher for participants in the high-cost-sharing plans than in the free plan (Newhouse and Insurance Experiment Group 1993, 18, 19–26). Although the investigators recognized this problem and claimed that those who refused to participate or who ceased participating were sufficiently like those who participated as not to threaten the validity of the results, doubts linger. If a significant number of those who left the high cost-sharing arm of the study were subsequently hospitalized, for example, the study might have seriously understated the total costs of those participants and thus overestimated the reduction in costs brought about by high cost sharing (Nyman 2003, 94). Another potentially significant problem is that although providers billing for free care had to submit claims to get paid, there was little incentive for providers serving participants in the 95 percent cost sharing plan to submit claims. Though the investigators concluded that under-submission of claims for the high-cost-sharing group was not a problem, it could have easily distorted the conclusions of the study if it did occur.

More significant questions have been raised as to the external validity of the study—the extent to which its results can be generalized to the health care system more broadly. For one thing, the study did not include participants over the age of sixty-five or receiving Social Security disability. Mortality rates are much higher among the elderly than among the study population, and health care expenditures are heavily concentrated in the last few months of life (Evans and Barer 1995, 377). The elderly and disabled are also generally in worse health and more subject to chronic diseases, and in many cases have limited mental capacity. The HIE tells us little about how the elderly might respond to cost sharing. The HIE also did not look at the differential access of ethnic minorities, an issue that has emerged as vital in more recent health services research.

Other challenges can be raised to the predictive value of the HIE for determining the effects of high cost sharing on the entire health care system. HIE participants represented a small portion of the caseload of the health care professionals and institutions in each study site location. If high cost sharing became general, on the other hand, providers might well adjust their practices to protect their incomes (Chalkey and Robinson 1997, 25; Stoddart, Barer, and Evans 1993, 26; Rice and Morrison 1994, 247–51). They might, for example, order more follow-up tests or services, or charge higher prices to their more fully insured patients. There is some limited evidence from other studies that providers do this. One study of the mineworkers' experience, for example, found that multi-specialty group medical practices in Pennsylvania dependent on mineworker patients experienced increased use by their other patients when their miner patients cut back on use in response to cost sharing. Similarly, a Canadian study found that increased cost sharing province-wide resulted in less use of services by lower-income groups but increased use by higher-income groups, suggesting a supply response by physicians (Stoddard, Barer, and Evans 1993, 20, 27).

Another important limitation of the HIE is that it tells us little about the financial impact of cost sharing on low-income families, an issue that it did not address. It is likely that low-income families participating in the HIE experienced much milder effects than do low-income families subject to high cost-sharing under contemporary HDHPs. Recall that although the maximum out-of-pocket ceiling for the HIE was set at $1,000, lower ceilings based on percentage of family income were imposed on low-income participants. Over 40 percent of poor families on the 95 percent coinsurance plan exceeded these lower limits, compared to only 27 percent of wealthier families who exceeded the absolute $1,000 expenditure limit (Newhouse and Insurance Experiment Group 1993, 255). Low-income families were also protected by the payments they received for participating in the project (Newhouse and Insurance Experiment Group 1993, 407–8). Finally, health care costs were much lower in comparison to family income in the late 1970s than they are now, and thus were less likely to have had as devastating an effect on low-income households as they do today.

Indeed, in the quarter-century since the HIE much has changed in our health care system and economy (Rubin and Mendelson 1995, 2-100–2-103). The clear message of the HIE was that cost sharing decreases medical expenditures, and one of the immediate effects of the study was that many employers and insurers raised cost sharing in the 1980s (Newhouse 2004, 109–10). Paradoxically, these increases in cost sharing were accompanied by some of the greatest increases in health care expenditures in the history of the country. Between 1985 and 1990 health care expenditures increased from 10.1 percent to 12 percent of the GDP (National Center for Health Statistics 2005, 30). In response, the United States moved very rapidly in the late 1980s and early 1990s to managed care (see chapter 5). The HMO arm of the HIE study had demonstrated that a traditional HMO could reduce health care costs to the same extent as high cost sharing. This cost-saving potential of HMOs was also demonstrated by independent contemporaneous research (Luft 1978), and managed care was embraced in the late 1980s as the best solution to growing health care costs.

During the mid-1990s, as managed care was replacing traditional health insurance, health care cost increases declined sharply, as did the utilization of health care services, particularly of inpatient hospital services, the most expensive form of health care. Moderation in health care cost increases was also encouraged by the shift of first Medicare and then other payers from cost- and charge-based payment for hospitals to diagnosis-related, group-prospective payments (a change that Medicare made in 1983), which dramatically decreased the length of stay in hospitals and promoted the transition from inpatient to outpatient treatment. Hospital admissions for the elderly dropped 23 percent between 1980 and 1986 (Newhouse and Insurance Experiment Group 1993, 344). The past quarter-century has brought further developments in the progress of medicine. In particular pharmaceutical innovation has reduced the need for hospitalization, particularly for the mentally ill (Cutler 2004, 32–46). Pharmacy use has gone up as hospital use has gone down.

It is quite possible, therefore, that if the HIE were conducted today, it would discover less significant decreases in the consumption of services. It is also likely that decreases in consumption of the magnitude found a quarter-century ago would have a greater impact on health outcomes if they occurred today. In sum, it makes no sense to just take the elasticity of demand figures that emerge from the HIE and use them in mathematical formulas to predict the effects of cost sharing today.

Before leaving the HIE, two further observations are in order. First, the absolute and income-related caps that the HIE imposed on health care expenditures assured that catastrophic events suffered by the participants were fully covered by insurance. Indeed, most patients needing inpatient care (and in particular those with 95 percent cost sharing obligations) quickly exceeded the cap and from then on were fully covered. A patient facing high health care expenses also usually had the option of leaving the study and returning to prior health insurance coverage. The HIE investigators were very clear that their findings of lack of serious health status effects from cost sharing did not mean that insurance was unimportant. One of their conclusions was that "the largest gains in welfare will probably result not from adding to initial cost sharing, but from extending insurance coverage to those who currently have none" (Newhouse and Insurance Experiment Group 1993, 141). Subsequent research has consistently demonstrated that the uninsured suffer much worse outcomes than the insured across a wide range of medical conditions, and ultimately suffer much higher rates of mortality (Institute of Medicine 2002a; Institute of Medicine 2002b). The investigators who led the HIE argued for national health insurance with cost sharing, not for the elimination or substantial curtailment of health insurance coverage.

Second, the HIE found absolutely no evidence of ex ante moral hazard — that people engaged in more risky behaviors because they faced lower cost sharing. The HIE monitored health behaviors and found no evidence that free care resulted in more smoking, more alcohol consumption, less beneficial physical activity, or diminished use of seat belts (Newhouse and Insurance Experiment Group 1993, 200–201, 208). Indeed it found that participants facing higher cost sharing were less likely to make use of preventive care. The argument of CDHC advocates that increased cost sharing will encourage better health behaviors, therefore, finds no support in the HIE.

The Ongoing Debate

The RAND HIE has not subsequently been duplicated, and it is unlikely that any-one will ever conduct such an ambitious experiment again. Research has continued, however, involving various attempts to address moral hazard (Farnsworth 2006, 257–67). Debate continues regarding what the findings of these studies mean, as well as what the HIE means.

International observers tend to be quite skeptical about the value of cost sharing, which they usually call "user charges." In a series of articles and reports, Robert Evans, Morris Barer, Greg Stoddart, and other Canadian economists have denounced user charges as a mechanism for shifting resources from poor and unhealthy people to wealthier people (who benefit from tax cuts when the expenses of public systems are cut) and to providers, who gain extra income from user charges (Evans, Barer, Stoddart, and Bhatia 1993; Stoddart, Barer, and Evans 1993; Evans and Barer 1995). There is a long history of opposition to user charges in the UK, where they have been characterized as "a tax on illness" (Eversley and Webster 1997). International observers also view cost sharing as less effective than provider incentives in controlling health care costs (Creese 1997; Birch 2004).

In fact, different countries impose different levels of cost sharing for different health care services; some countries impose quite high levels of cost sharing, others little cost sharing (Chalkey and Robinson 1997, 18–22). There does not seem to be any obvious correlation between cost sharing and national health expenditures (Chalkey and Robinson 1997, 19). Japan, for example, has long imposed cost sharing at fairly high levels for primary care, but has had the highest level of annual doctor visits in the OECD (Chalkey and Robinson 1997, 15, 19; Campbell and Ikegami 1998, 93–94). Japan raised co-payments for insured employees from 10 percent to 20 percent in 1997 and from 20 percent to 30 percent in 2003, yet claims data analysis found no effect on total expenditures.[3] Germany in 2004 imposed a co-payment of 10 Euros on the first doctor visit in each quarter, but the charge had no significant effect on the probability of visiting a doctor (Augurzky, Bauer, and Schaffner 2006). The United Kingdom provides most services free at point of service (although it imposes some cost sharing for pharmaceuticals and dental care), but spends less than half as much per person as the United States does (Chalkey and Robinson 1997, 22).

Studies in the United States, on the other hand, continue to demonstrate that demand for health care services is reduced when cost sharing is imposed (Rubin and Mendelson 1995, 2-83–2-95, 2-110–2-116; Ringel, Hosek, Vollaard, and Mahnovski 2002). A literature review published recently by Michael Morrisey for the National Federation of Independent Business (NFIB) Research Foundation affirmed the HIE conclusion that demand for health services is moderately elastic, although it found greater variation in elasticity of demand for services than the HIE did (Morissey 2005). Unlike the HIE, however, the NFIB's summary pays little attention to the adverse health impacts of higher cost sharing. It also fails to consider the financial effects of health care cost sharing on the poor.

A significant body of literature does exist examining the health and economic impacts of cost sharing. First, a number of studies have confirmed the HIE finding that cost sharing is as likely to depress appropriate care as it is to depress inappropriate care (Rubin and Mendelson 1995, 2-113–2-114). Studies have also confirmed the HIE conclusion that increased cost sharing can have adverse health effects. Most of these studies have examined pharmaceutical usage, for which cost sharing is very common. One study found that members of the Medicare + Choice plan whose benefits were capped had 31 percent lower pharmacy costs, but also had more emergency department visits, non-elective hospitalizations, and deaths; that they were less likely to comply with drug treatment regimens; and that they had total medical costs essentially equal to those of beneficiaries whose benefits were not capped (Hsu, Price, Huang, Brand, Fung, Hui, et al. 2006). A Canadian study found that pharmaceutical cost sharing resulted in increased use of physician services and more hospital admissions per month (Anis, Guh, Lacaille, Marra, Rashidi, Li, et al. 2005). Another found that the introduction of pharmaceutical cost sharing was accompanied by higher use of emergency departments and more serious adverse events among the elderly and welfare recipients (Tamblyn, Laprise, Hanley, Abrahamowicz, Scott, Mayo, et al. 2001). A study of the effects of drug co-payments in Italy found an immediate reduction in the use of essential drugs, and thus, potentially, an increase in hospitalization and mortality rates (Atella, Peracchi, Depalo, and Rossetti 2005). That study was of particular interest because it involved drugs for treating hypertension, since long-term compliance is essential but noncompliance may not result in immediately palpable symptoms. A recent survey of twenty-five pharmaceutical cost-sharing studies concluded that cost sharing indeed reduces drug expenditures, but that "in most studies reviewed, cost sharing leads to patients foregoing essential medications and increases in use of emergency services, nursing home admissions, and serious adverse events" (Lexchin and Grootendorst 2004, 118).[4] Finally, a study of increases in cost sharing in the Oregon Medicaid program in 2003 found that the increases led to a steep decline in enrollment, which in turn led to decreased access to health care and increased financial distress for former enrollees (Wright, Carlson, Edlund, DeVoe, Gallia, and Smith 2005). One-third of adults subject to co-payments reported unmet medical needs because of cost, as did one-quarter because they did not have the co-payment, and one-sixth because they owed their physicians money (Artiga and O'Malley 2005, 17).

The adverse financial effects of high cost-sharing obligations have also come into much sharper focus in recent years. Whereas the HIE capped cost-sharing obligations as a percentage of family income for poor families, contemporary high-deductible policies do not. For many Americans, out-of-pocket health care costs amount to an unsustainably high proportion of family income. This often has devastating consequences in terms of access to health care and family finances.

Over one in seven American families spent 10 percent or more of their income (5 percent or more if low income) on out-of-pocket medical costs in 2001–2 (Merlis, Gould, and Mahato 2006, 3). These families are more than twice as likely not to obtain needed medical care and half again as likely to delay or have difficulty finding needed care than insured Americans generally (Merlis, Gould, and Mahato 2006, 10). Another study found that adults with health problems with deductibles above $500 (and particularly those with incomes below $35,000 a year) are much more likely than those with lower deductibles not to fill a prescription, not to get needed specialist care, to skip a recommended test or follow-up visit, or to have a medical problem for which they have not sought medical care (Davis, Doty, and Ho 2005, 10). Patients with high deductibles are also much more likely to have problems with medical bills or medical debt (Davis, Doty, and Ho 2005, 11). Nearly half of "underinsured" adults were contacted by a collection agency about medical bills in the year before a recent survey, while more than one-third said that they had to change their lives significantly to pay for medical bills.[5] (Schoen, Doty, Collins, and Holmgren 2005, W5–295). Medical debt is one of the most important contributors to bankruptcies in the United States (Himmelstein, Warren, Thorne, and Woolhandler 2005). Bankruptcy of health care consumers is of course also bound to affect providers, who will often be creditors in bankruptcy proceedings.

Cost sharing causes particular problems for Medicaid recipients. One study found that Utah's imposition of Medicaid co-payments of $2 to $3 per service or prescription caused "serious" financial hardship for four out of ten affected recipients (Ku and Wachino 2005, 7). Another study found that Medicaid recipients already spend a higher proportion of their income on medical costs than do insured adults with incomes more than twice the poverty level (Ku and Broaddus 2005, 2).

Indeed, Sherry Glied has demonstrated that high-deductible policies have very little value for low-income uninsured people, because the bankruptcy laws and the uncompensated-care policies of hospitals already provide considerable protection for high-cost events (Glied 2002). The uninsured would find much more valuable a zero-deductible policy with low out-of-pocket maximums, which would provide them access to primary care and pharmaceuticals that are not otherwise readily available.

This does not mean, of course, that all cost sharing is likely to have adverse health or unacceptable financial effects. Wealthier Americans are quite capable of bearing cost sharing at the levels found in many HDHPs, and indeed many might find these policies attractive because of the tax benefits that they offer when coupled with HSAs, or because they offer less financial exposure over all than do low-deductible, high-coinsurance policies with high out-of-pocket limits. But the disadvantages as well as the advantages of cost sharing must be taken into account, something overlooked by many CDHC advocates. The reduction in expenditures that is caused by high cost-sharing obligations may result in lower expenditures on health care over all, at least if providers are not able to shift utilization elsewhere or raise prices. But if high cost sharing also leads to worse health care outcomes or to financial catastrophe for many Americans, we have not made an advance in health policy.

Do Account-Based Plans Solve the Problem of High Cost Sharing?

If the effects of health care plans with high cost sharing are reasonably well understood, the effects of HSAs are less so. Supporters of CDHC argue that account-based health plans solve the financial and health access risks that attend high cost sharing, while preserving the efficiency-enhancing effect of cost sharing.

In the United States we have had experience with three forms of tax-subsidized, consumer-driven, account-based health plans: medical savings accounts (MSAs), which were created by the Health Insurance Portability and Accountability Act and lasted until 2004; health reimbursement arrangements

(HRAS), recognized by a Revenue Ruling in 2002; and health savings accounts (HSAS), established by the Medicare Modernization Act of 2003 (Government Accountability Office 2006, 7–10).[6] MSAS, HRAS, and HSAS and the legislation and regulations that established them have already been described in chapter 2.

MSAS were available on only a limited basis and never really became popular (Minicozzi 2006, 259). HRAS and HSAS, on the other hand, have spread rapidly and may soon have a noticeable effect on our health care system. What we know about them will be discussed below, but it can be summarized by saying that for the moment, our experience is too recent to allow definitive conclusions as to their effects. As noted earlier, Singapore, South Africa, China, and several other countries have had longer experience with account-based health plans. We will examine their experience more closely at the end of this chapter.

For many account holders, particularly before an account balance can be built up, there will be a gap between the amount held in the account and the health plan deductible. The account holder must cover this gap out of pocket, as well as any further cost-sharing obligations (coinsurance or co-payments) imposed beyond the deductible. Finally, CDHC accounts are coupled in theory, and often in reality, with health care decision-making tools, including information on cost and sometimes quality, to permit account holders to make better-informed health care purchasing decisions. These tools remain quite primitive — providing information on the average prices charged by providers, for example, rather than specific prices for specific services — though considerable effort is going into improving their sophistication and usefulness.

Issues Raised by Consumer-Driven Health Plans

Consumer-driven health plans (CDHPS) — plans that combine HDHPs with MSAS, HRAS, or HSAS — present several research questions. First, who will choose them? CDHPs are now available as an option in almost all states in the individual market. An ever-increasing number of employers, small and large, offer them as an option as well. Advocates argue that they will be attractive to virtually all potential purchasers. Low-income individuals and families, including many of the uninsured, will find them attractive because of their low premiums. Persons with chronic illness will find them attractive because they offer choice of treatment and provider. Higher-income persons will sign up because HSAS offer tax advantages.

CDHC skeptics believe that CDHPs will attract primarily the wealthy and healthy and thus will fail to make health care available to those who need it most. As discussed in chapter 2, the tax advantages of HSAs to individuals in high tax brackets are considerable. Skeptics also believe that the healthy (including younger persons) will choose CDHPs, because the healthy face little risk of out-of-pocket costs. According to some scenarios, as the young, healthy, and wealthy move to consumer-driven plans, the cost of CDHPs will go down while the cost of traditional plans, chosen by poorer, older, and unhealthier people, will correspondingly go up. As premiums go up for traditional plans, these plans will see further desertions by those in marginally better health. Ultimately, traditional plans will enter the "insurance death spiral," becoming unaffordable to anyone (Zabinski, Selden, Moeller, and Banthin 1997, 207).

A second policy question is whether CDHPs will actually save money, and whether they can do so without adversely affecting the health or welfare of their enrollees. The HIE as well as subsequent research has demonstrated that high cost-sharing obligations reduce expenditures, but can also lead to adverse health consequences for low-income families. More recent research, discussed above, has also shown that high cost sharing can have serious financial consequences for low-income individuals and families. CDHC advocates claim that health accounts coupled with high-deductible plans preserve the advantages of high cost sharing while mitigating its adverse consequences.

CDHC advocates believe that account holders will treat HSAs as their own personal funds rather than as "free" insurance money, and therefore will not purchase health care products or services unless they value those products or services as much as they value alternatives that they could purchase with the same amount of money. HSA owners will spend their funds carefully, both to avoid having to spend their post-tax dollars in the "donut hole" if they exhaust their HSA before reaching their deductible, and because of the lure of accumulating a tax-subsidized nest egg that can be withdrawn at the age of sixty-five. Nevertheless the availability of health care accounts will, in this view, assure that account holders have sufficient funds to purchase needed care. Account holders with chronic diseases will be able to afford necessary care using their HSAs. Lower-income account holders will be less likely to face financial hardship because of high out-of-pocket spending than they would if they simply had an HDHP without an HSA. No one will need to scrimp on preventive care, for which HDHPs can give first-dollar coverage under the MMA. CDHC advocates also believe that consumers (empowered with the decision-making tools that the health plan makes available) will shop carefully for products and services that have low cost and high quality, thus further improving the efficiency of the health care system. Finally, advocates contend that the use of health care accounts will eliminate the administrative costs of processing health care bills, further reducing health care spending.

Critics of CDHC, on the other hand, claim that CDHPs will have little effect on health care spending growth, but will expose the poor and those with chronic diseases to dangerously high health care expenditures and greater economic insecurity. To begin with, CDHC skeptics claim that the concentration of health care expenditures described in the Preface will undermine the effectiveness of CDHC (Halvorson 2004). Remember, 10 percent of the population is responsible for 70 percent of health care expenditures, half the population for only 3 percent. This concentration of expenditures has three primary ramifications for consumer-driven health care.

First and most importantly, it means that many health care expenditures are not affected by the incentives that are created by HSAS or HRAS. Once an HDHP enrollee hits the deductible, incentives for controlling expenditures are considerably reduced, and once the out-of-pocket maximum is reached (which will happen after a few of days of hospitalization for most), all further health care is free (Parente, Feldman, and Christianson 2004b, 1192–93). Indeed, high-cost enrollees face reduced incentives to spend their HSA carefully as soon as they realize that they will soon hit the deductible, and thus even within the deductible range health care services may be treated as essentially free.

Second, the concentration of expenditures means that CDHC products will prove particularly onerous to people with chronic health care problems who will year after year exhaust their HSAS and HRAS and then have to spend large sums of money out of their own pockets before reaching the deductible. This is particularly a problem for the poor with chronic illnesses.

Third, the concentration of health care expenses suggests that much of the money contributed by employers to HSAS is likely to go, at least in the first instance, to employees who would not otherwise incur health care expenses (Trude and Conwell 2004). Employers will continue to cover much of the cost of premiums for HDHPs, and thus the expenses of high-cost employees, but will now additionally be contributing to HSAS for employees who previously incurred virtually no health care costs at all. Regardless of whether these employees spend the money on health care products or services not covered by insurance or simply save the funds, employers will be spending money that they were not spending on traditional insurance.[7] The risk is still greater if enrollees in HSAs coupled with HDHPs have an annual opportunity to switch to low-deductible plans. Employees may choose low-deductible plans in years when they expect high costs (for example, when they plan to have a child), and high-deductible plans in years when they expect few expenses.

CDHC supporters respond by claiming that even though most health care costs are attributable to a very few people, a high proportion of health care costs — including some of the costs of high-cost individuals and virtually all the costs of low-cost individuals — still fall within the deductible range of higher-deductible HDHPs and are thus influenced by cost-sharing incentives. An even higher proportion of costs fall under the HDHP out-of-pocket maximum range and can be controlled to some extent through cost sharing. A plan, for example, with a deductible of $1,050 and 20 percent coinsurance up to an out-of-pocket maximum of $5,100 would continue to affect consumer behavior until the costs incurred reached $21,300, influencing more than 60 percent of the medical expenditures of fully-insured, non-elderly individuals (Cannon and Tanner 2005, 20). Further, many people who end up incurring large expenditures for health care may not anticipate these expenditures, and thus may spend HSA funds carefully until the deductible is met.[8] It is also possible that HSA owners will develop good purchasing habits such as searching for low-cost providers or services, forgoing unnecessary outpatient visits, or switching to generic drugs, and will continue these good habits once they hit the deductible, again reducing above-deductible expenses.

While this may happen, one finding of the HIE was that once participants reached the deductible (which was also the out-of-pocket maximum) they spent even more money on health care than did those who received free care from the first (Newhouse and Insurance Experiment Group 1993, 117). The extent to which CDHC will influence high-expense cases remains, therefore, to be established.

Another question raised by CDHC skeptics is how account holders will in fact view their accounts — as tax-subsidized funds to purchase health care or rather as savings to be accumulated for later use. Behavioral economics, discussed in chapter 7, teaches us that people generally have a hard time forgoing present consumption in favor of future consumption, and Americans in particular have a dismal record of saving for the future (Hibbard 2003, 9). That funds in accounts can be used to purchase items and services not covered by traditional insurance presents the possibility that account holders will increase their expenditures for health care over those of the traditionally insured.

Even more problematic is that HSAs operate largely on the honor system. Expenditures of flexible spending accounts and HRAs are closely monitored by employers and account managers to assure that funds are spent only for qualified health care services. By contrast, HSA account managers have no obligation to monitor HSA expenditures (Lyke 2006, CRS-10). Rather, HSA owners are responsible for keeping records, risking a minuscule chance of being audited by the IRS.[9] HSA fraud is not only possible, but likely.

Another concern raised by CDHC skeptics is whether CDHC will really result in better, or even less expensive, health care decisions. Research on consumer decision making discussed in chapter 7 raises real questions as to whether consumers are capable of making accurate health care purchasing decisions. So little information is currently available, even with respect to comparative health care prices (let alone health care quality) that it might be difficult for health care consumers to make good comparative shopping decisions even if they were psychologically equipped to do so. Skeptics also believe it unlikely that CDHPs will result in either negotiations for lower prices or reduced claims processing costs. If consumers do not learn the price of a service until after the service has been rendered, or if providers simply bill the insurer for the product and service and the insurer subsequently deducts the money from the consumer's HSA or HRA, the consumer will have no opportunity to bargain for (or even shop around for) a lower price, and there will be few, if any, administrative cost savings.

Yet another question is how consumers will contend with the potential confusion and the risks attendant to CDHC. A survey by the Kaiser Family Foundation after the State of the Union Address in 2006 found that only 29 percent of Americans polled knew what an HSA was (Kaiser Family Foundation 2006a). Research has also shown that consumers have a difficult time understanding how CDHPs operate (Hibbard 2003, 4). Almost 70 percent of Californians who earn less than $35,000 a year are not confident that they understand what a deductible is, and over 75 percent are not sure that they understand what coinsurance is (California Healthcare Foundation 2003, 3).

Consumers may not understand that not all medical expenses will count against the deductible. As the Treasury Department has interpreted the HSA law, insurers can, if they choose, refuse to count against the deductible part of payments to out-of-network providers or payments for services provided without pre-authorization (U.S. Department of the Treasury 2004, 11). Payment for non-covered products or services will certainly not count against the deductible, even though they are qualified health expenses that can be paid for out of an HSA or HRA. Enrollees will be responsible for proving that they have met the deductible before their insurance will cover further expenses, and in cases where providers do not bill insurers directly, this might involve keeping track of a lot of receipts.

Consumers are likely to be surprised if they exhaust their HSA on expenses that do not count against the deductible and find themselves still facing a high deductible. On the other hand, if providers bill the insurer directly, and the insurer then withdraws funds from the HSA or HRA, enrollees may have a hard time keeping track of their account balance, and may be surprised when it is exhausted.

Understanding how to use CDHPs and the information they provide is likely to be a particular problem for people with limited literacy, numeracy, or comprehension. Approximately 21 percent of American adults are functionally illiterate, and another 27 percent have marginal literacy skills (Hibbard 2003, 10). As many as 57 percent of Medicare beneficiaries have difficulty interpreting simple data displays (Hibbard 2003, 10). It is hard to believe, therefore, that many consumers will take charge of the health care system in the ways that CDHC advocates predict.

Early Evidence

Time will tell whether CDHC lives up to its promises or is fatally flawed. CDHPs are still relatively uncommon. Yet we do have some empirical evidence on the performance of CDHC.

To begin, there is some evidence of favorable selection to consumer-driven plans, but the evidence is far from conclusive (Buntin, Damberg, Haviland, Kapur, Lurie, McDevitt, and Marquis 2006, w519). Several studies have shown that persons with higher incomes and higher occupational status tend to choose CDHPs (Parente, Feldman, and Christianson 2004a; Parente, Feldman, and Christianson 2004b, 1198; Christianson, Parente, and Feldman 2004; Tollen, Ross, and Poor 2004, 1178; Minicozzi 2006, 263–264). For example, 20 percent of enrollees in HSA-qualified plans sold by a large online insurance broker had incomes of $100,000 or more (Ehealthinsurance 2006). Indeed, some people use HSAs solely as tax-subsidized retirement savings vehicles, paying for health care costs out-of-pocket (Government Accountability Office 2006, 5, 17). Surveys have also shown that CDHPs are more likely to be chosen by better-educated people (Government Accountability Office 2005,

13). Enrollees are also more likely to be white, and less likely to be African American or Hispanic, than conventional insurance enrollees (Kaiser Family Foundation 2006).

On the other hand, CDHPs are often chosen by purchasers over forty, who might be attracted by their low premiums or by their retirement investment feature (Sullivan 2005; America's Health Insurance Plans 2006, 4). CDHPs are also chosen by many low-income purchasers, probably because of their low premium costs (Cannon 2006, 16). A significant proportion of enrollees in CDHPs are also persons who were formerly uninsured. America's Health Insurance Plans (AHIP), the health insurance trade organization, reported that 31 percent of new enrollees in the nongroup market as of January 2006 were previously uninsured, while 33 percent of enrollment in combined HSA-HDHP plans was in small companies that had not previously offered coverage (America's Health Insurance Plans 2006, 1). Blue Cross also reported in 2005 that a higher proportion of its CDHP enrollees were formerly uninsured than enrollees in conventional plans (Sullivan 2005). But the uninsured are a primary market for nongroup policies, which make up the insurance market of last resort, and one would expect that any new enrollees in the nongroup market would be disproportionately uninsured. There is also a constant stream of small businesses starting up, and the AHIP data do not reveal to what extent the small businesses offering HSA-HDHPs that it identifies as "not previously offering coverage" in fact did not even previously exist (Park and Greenstein 2006, 11). In addition, many small employers are making HDHPs available to their employees as the only benefit plan option and not offering a contribution to an HSA, in effect just offering a catastrophic plan (Regopolous, Christianson, Claxton, and Trude 2006, 770). One recent survey found that 42 percent of CDHP enrollees and 54 percent of high-deductible plan enrollees did not have a choice of health plan (Fronstin and Collins 2006, 14). Another found that when employees do have a choice, they overwhelmingly do not choose a CDHP (Gabel, Pickreign, and Whitmore 2006, 2).

It is not clear that CDHPs are disproportionately chosen by healthier persons, as many predicted. Several studies have found that employees choosing a CDHP are those who had much lower prior-year health services usage or claims, while other studies show that employees choosing a CDHP are less likely to be mentally ill, to have chronic health problems, to have recently seen a physician, or to be nonwhite (Tollen, Ross, and Poor 2004, 1179; Lo Sasso, Rice, Gabel, and Whitmore 2004, 1082; Fowles, Kind, Braun, and Bertko 2004, 1146).

Several studies have found that persons reporting "excellent" or "very good" health disproportionately chose a CDHP product (Government Accountability Office 2005, 13; Fronstin and Collins 2005, 6).

Other studies using different measures have not found favorable selection (Parente, Feldman, and Christianson 2004a). A Blue Cross report on its HSA and HRA enrollees found their self-reported health status to be similar to that of enrollees in its traditional plans.[10] In fact, the attractiveness of a health plan to persons with high health care expenses is determined by several factors in addition to the size of the deductible. The most important of these might be the size of the out-of-pocket limit. Choice of provider, the richness of the benefit package, and the size and applicability of co-payments and coinsurance are also important. An HDHP that offers free choice of provider, a generous benefit package, and a low out-of-pocket limit might be much more attractive to a person with chronically high health care costs than a low-deductible, high-coinsurance, high-out-of-pocket-limit, tightly controlled PPO plan.

Cost-sharing obligations have been steadily on the increase in recent years in traditional PPO, conventional, and even HMO health plans, and thus the choice is rarely between HSA-HDHPs and insurance that provides free access to services (Remler and Glied 2006). Further, there are relatively few people who face high health care expenses year after year and thus would never benefit from the investment feature of a CDHP. Although health care expenses are highly concentrated in any one year, they are much less concentrated over time (Monheit 2003). A significant proportion of those facing the highest cost in any one year die during that year or the year following, and thereafter cost very little. Others at the high end of the cost distribution are experiencing one-time high-cost events, such as a traumatic injury or a complicated delivery of a child. Even for people who have chronic conditions, expenses tend to regress toward the mean over time. Some individuals do experience high health care costs for years and then die expensive deaths, while others remain healthy all their lives and quietly and inexpensively slip away (Roos, Shapiro, and Tate 1989). But the vast majority of us, even those who have serious conditions such as cancer or heart disease, end up somewhere in the middle over time. One study projects that over a lifetime 80 percent of employees who contribute $2,000 annually for an HSA coupled with an HDHP that has a deductible of $4,000 and an out-of-pocket maximum of $4,000 will end up with at least 50 percent of their total contributions, although 5 percent will end up with less than 20 percent (Eichner, McClellan, and Wise 1996, 23–24).

This presumes, however, that persons invest in HSAs year after year so that they can build up balances to take them through bad years. Experience with HIPAA MSAs demonstrated that many people held accounts for only short periods and exhausted their accounts for current expenditures, although over time a growing number did build up their account balances (Minicozzi 2006, 261).[11] The current HSA is structured quite differently and experience with it may differ accordingly, but there is anecdotal evidence of low contribution rates to HSAs, and it is still too early to tell how consistently account holders will contribute (Government Accountability Office 2006, 17–18). One study found that almost half of account holders spent their entire account during the study year, with expenses surging in November and December (Lo Sasso, Rice, Gabel, and Whitmore 2004, 1076). A report by the Government Accountability Office (GAO) found that 36 percent of single coverage enrollees and 58 percent of family coverage enrollees spent all their HRA funds in 2004 (Government Accountability Office 2006, 16). It is likely that a considerable number of HSA holders will never in fact accumulate substantial savings in their HSA.

It is also not clear yet to what extent HSAs will save money. Some surveys have shown that CDHPs are very successful in holding down health care costs (United Health Group 2006). They report, for example, that premiums for consumer-directed products are going up much more slowly than premiums for traditional insurance products, and that companies offering CDHPs are saving a great deal of money (Deloitte Center for Health Solutions 2006). The Kaiser Family Foundation / Health Research and Educational Trust *Survey of Employer Health Benefits* (2006) found that premiums and employer contributions for HSAs coupled with HDHPs were lower than those for other plans, although not significantly lower when employer contributions to the HSA were added on (Kaiser Family Foundation / Health Research and Educational Trust 2006, 5).[12] It also found that employee contributions for HSA-qualified family HDHPs were significantly lower than employee premiums for health plans overall (although they were not lower for individual HDHPs) (Kaiser Family Foundation / Health Research and Educational Trust 2006, 5).

It is hard to know what these data mean. Lower premiums for CDHPs usually reflect thinner benefits in addition to higher cost sharing. Only about one in twenty MSA-HSA nongroup policies, for example, covers a normal delivery, compared to virtually all nongroup HMO and POS plans (America's Health Insurance Plans 2005b, 26, 27). CDHP data, moreover, often report only premium costs, not total costs including those borne by enrollees, and thus the data are not really comparable to the costs of lower-deductible plans, which shift fewer costs to enrollees.

Also, early adopters are by definition outliers, and we need to know much more about the employee populations of companies that have changed in whole or part to CDHPs, about individuals who sign up for CDHPs in the nongroup market, and about the persistence of favorable experience to understand to what extent reported experiences are generalizable. Reports of the success of CDHC plans in holding down premiums compared to premiums for conventional plans, for example, could be attributable to several factors, some of which are problematic. One obvious factor is favorable selection, which seems quite clearly to have played an important role in some instances (Lo Sasso, Rice, Gabel, and Whitmore 2004, 1079, 1082). It is easy to keep premium costs low with healthy subscribers. Another factor may simply be that costs are normally low in the first year or two of a new insurance plan. This is particularly true if the plan is underwritten based on the health of applicants or if there is any element of favorable selection by applicants. Over time, as initially healthy members of the new plan experience higher health care costs, premiums will rise (Brink, Modaff, and Sherman 1993). The low costs experienced by new plans almost inevitably regress to the mean. This is the basis of the well-known phenomenon of durational rating: the practice of charging low rates for new plans or enrollees and then sharply raising rates over time (Hall 2001).

Therefore, just because an employer experiences significantly lower premiums in the year or two following a change by some of its employees to a CDHP tells us little about the comparative advantages of that plan for the long term. Indeed, one independent study that found dramatically lower costs in the first year after a consumer-driven plan was introduced also found that costs crept up in the second and third years, and by the third year hospitalization rates were higher among the HDHP members than among those who stayed with traditional plans (Parente, Feldman, and Christianson 2004b, 1201).

Yet another factor in slowed premium growth may be that premium costs for CDHPs were set too high initially by insurers unfamiliar with the potential costs of these plans, and thus have not had to rise as much as other plans (Government Accountability Office 2006, 27). There has been surprisingly little initial difference in premiums, often only 15–20 percent, between high-deductible plans and traditional plans, suggesting that CDHPs might have set their premiums too high initially and are now simply becoming more realistic

(Maxwell, Temin, Zaman, and Petigara 2005, W5-237). A lower premium may also reflect the purchase of a less valuable insurance policy rather than a declining price. A report from eHealthInsurance in late 2005 on experience with high-deductible plans noted that premiums had decreased since 2004 (17 percent for individuals and 6 percent for families), but also that consumers were moving dramatically to higher-deductible plans, which should cost less (eHealthInsurance 2006). Finally, premium savings may represent a one-time gain and not a mitigation of upward trends over the long term (Buntin 2005, 8). And the gain will be much smaller for HDHPs coupled with HSAs than the gain would be from a move to HDHPs alone (Buntin, Damberg, Haviland, Kapur, Lurie, McDevitt, and Marquis 2006).

We also do not know yet to what extent CDHP holders are successfully shopping for lower cost or better quality of care. According to one survey conducted in 2005 of health insurers that offered CDHPs, only 56 percent published comparative cost data, only 28 percent published information on both physicians and hospitals, and only 17 percent published information for specific services with specific hospitals or physicians. Few adjust cost data for severity of illness (Reden and Anders Ltd. 2005, 27). A more serious barrier to shopping for services based on price is that enrollees typically do not know what a provider has charged for services until their insurer has processed the provider claim and made a withdrawal from the HSA or HRA (Government Accountability Office 2006, 24). There are also frequent press reports of misunderstandings and excessive billings to persons with CDHPs (Dorschner 2006).

Further, information about costs is not very helpful without information about quality. In a recent survey of Americans, 90 percent of respondents stated that they would give more weight to quality than cost in choosing a provider for open heart surgery or cancer, and over 70 percent claimed that they would consider quality over cost for immunizations or a physical. (Helman, Mathew Greenwald & Associates, and Fronstin 2006, 2). Indeed consumers report being reluctant to choose lowest-cost providers for fear that lower cost is associated with lower quality (Business Week Online 2002). According to one study of CDHPs, only 44 percent of the plans published information on quality, and even fewer — 18 percent — published information on physicians (Reden and Anders Ltd. 2005, 26, 27). Indeed, one survey found that members of comprehensive plans were significantly more likely than members of HDHPs or CDHPs to report that they received information on quality from their plans (Fronstin and Collins 2006, 29). As noted above, most of the tools made available by health plans to compare prices are still quite crude, and information on quality is even less sophisticated. It also seems that few members of CDHPs are using the internet to compare prices (Kaiser Family Foundation 2006c). As of yet, there is little evidence of competition among providers to bring down prices outside areas of traditional price competition, such as vision care and cosmetic surgery.

There is also evidence that information put out by CDHPs has little effect on purchasing. Reports indicate that persons enrolled in CDHPs do tend to seek information before purchasing health care and to consider costs in making health care decisions (Fronstin and Collins 2005, 20; Kaiser Family Foundation 2006c, 3; Buntin, Damberg, Kapur, Lurie, McDevitt, and Marquis 2006, w525). They are more likely to ask their doctors to prescribe generics or lower-cost drugs (Fronstin and Collins 2006, 33). But cost-conscious behavior is not remarkably different for CDHP members than for members of comprehensive plans (Fronstin and Collins 2006, 33). And although consumers are interested in comparative quality information, few are using it to make purchasing decisions (Hibbard 2003, 8). Consumers still make health care purchasing decisions subjectively and with little consideration for available information about quality (VHA Inc. 2003, 18–20). In particular, consumers do not seem to be using information provided by health plans (Agrawal, Ehrbeck, Packard, and Mango 2005, 11; Christianson, Parente, and Feldman 2004, 1133; Buntin 2005, 22). Finally, there are of course questions as to the capacity of really sick people to make reasonable consumer decisions (Cassell, Leon, and Kaufman 2001).

To date managed care organizations have had a greater effect than competition among providers for consumers' business in holding down the costs of health care to CDHP participants. According to one survey, 95 percent of managed care organizations with HDHPs have made their network provider discounts available to their HDHP members, giving HSA holders the bargaining clout of big purchasers in spending their HSA funds (Reden and Anders Ltd. 2005, 17; Cannon 2006, 18). The disadvantage of their doing so is that claims continue to be processed through the insurer, diminishing cost transparency and the possibility of savings in processing costs (Government Accountability Office 2006, 11). HSA administrators also usually charge their account holders initial setup and ongoing management fees — administrative costs that are not charged for processing insurance claims.

There are of course positive reports on the effects of CDHC. Enrollees in

CDHPs report that they are using doctors and emergency rooms less often, are switching to generic drugs, are searching for information on providers, are carefully following treatment regimens for chronic conditions, are taking necessary medications, and are not forgoing preventive care (United Health Group 2006; Agrawal, Ehrbeck, Packard, and Mango 2005, 6–9; Buntin 2005, 25: Cigna Health Care 2006). Consumers even report a willingness to travel further to save money on health care (Agrawal, Ehrbeck, Packard, and Mango 2005, 7). All this is good news for CDHC advocates and supports an argument that cost savings will be achieved in the long term.

We must not just look at the positive effects of CDHC, however, but also at its potential problems. The HIE tells us that attempts at stinting on health care costs can have adverse effects on some populations. One study found that people with CDHPs "were significantly more likely to report that they had avoided, skipped, or delayed health care because of costs than were those with more comprehensive insurance, with problems particularly pronounced among those with health problems or incomes under $50,000" (Fronstin and Collins 2005, 1, 15). Other studies have also shown that consumers in HDHPs forgo necessary care (Lee and Zapert 2005, 1202–3), or preventive care such as colon cancer screens or Pap tests (Fronstin and Collins 2006, 26). Still other reports raise concern about the financial effects of CDHPs on low-income families, including patterns of delaying or avoiding needed care and not filling prescriptions or skipping doses (Fronstin and Collins 2006, 29). On the whole, evidence about the effect of CDHC on quality is mixed (Buntin, Damberg, Kapur, Lurie, McDevitt, and Marquis 2006, w523–w525).

Quality of CDHPs themselves is also an issue that must be considered. There is some evidence of dissatisfaction on the part of members of CDHPs as compared to enrollees in other plans, some of which seems to be due to frustration with a lack of support for consumer decision making (Agrawal, Ehrbeck, Packard, and Mango 2005, 10–11; Fronstin and Collins 2005, 9; Fronstin and Collins 2006, 11). Members of CDHPs are also more likely to feel vulnerable to high costs and less likely to feel "well protected" by their plan (Kaiser Family Foundation 2006c, 5). Other surveys have found reasonably high levels of satisfaction, and reenrollment in consumer-driven plans seems to be high (Christianson, Parente, and Feldman 2005; Lo Sasso, Rice, Gabel, and Whitmore 2004, 1079; Government Accountability Office 2005, 14).

Finally, a particularly troubling concern is that CDHPs may be sold in two discrete markets, that CDHC may look very different to the wealthy from how it looks to the poor. Purchasing an HDHP does not mean that one has an HSA to cover the deductible. According to some estimates only half of HSA-eligible HDHP enrollees actually open an HSA (Government Accountability Office 2006, 5). The EBRI / Commonwealth Fund survey in 2006 found that 32 percent of employees with a CDHP received no employer contribution toward their accounts, while another 22 percent received employer contributions under $500 (Fronstin 2006, 18). It also found that one in five CDHP members contributed nothing to their account (with individuals having a household income of under $50,000 contributing nothing at twice the rate of those with higher incomes); 23 percent had rolled over nothing in their accounts at the end of the previous year; and 30 percent had less than $200 in their account at the time of the survey (with 14 percent not knowing how much they had in their account) (Fronstin and Collins 2006, 18).

Another survey found that employer contributions toward employee HSAs averaged only 28 percent of the average HSA-HDHP deductible for family coverage and 34 percent for single coverage, and that 37 percent of employers contributed nothing at all to their employees' HSAs (Kaiser Family Foundation / Health Research and Educational Trust 2006, 5).[13]

It appears that higher-income persons, one CDHP market segment, are accumulating tax-sheltered funds in their HSAs, supported by employer contributions, and in some instances are not even using their HSA funds to pay for health care. At the same time, in another market segment, lower-income persons have HDHPs either through their employment or purchased in the nongroup market, but without employer contributions and without personal accumulations in the HSAs. They simply have catastrophic insurance.

Members of the wealthier group will make, or try to make, sound health care decisions to protect their HSA balances and will have enough money to cover health care expenses up to their deductible. Poorer participants will forgo important health care and encounter financial troubles when they fall ill. If this occurs, CDHC will simply be one more device to further divide an already badly divided American health care system — to further erode solidarity. We need to know more before CDHC can be endorsed as a solution for the problems that ail the American health care system.

Lessons from International Experience with Consumer-Driven Health Care

That then leaves a final question: What can we learn from the experience of others? All three nations that have had extensive experience with medical savings accounts — Singapore, South Africa, and China — have health systems, cultures, and economies radically different from those of the United States. While it may be possible to implement policy innovations developed in one system in a very similar system, it is dangerous to conclude that policies with a successful record in one health care system can be implemented in a radically different system, at least unless a pattern has emerged from a significant number of systems (Marmor 2001). Even if the experience of other countries strongly supported CDHC, therefore, the question would still remain whether we could learn from that experience. In fact, however, it is far from clear that the experience of these nations supports the claims of the CDHC movement.

Singapore has had the longest experience with CDHC. Since 1984 all Singaporeans have had to pay 6 percent to 8.5 percent of their income into a "Medisave" account that in some respects resembles an MSA (Hanvoravong-chai 2002, 12). Money is accumulated in these accounts to be used to pay for inpatient care and expensive outpatient care (Hanvoravongchai 2002, 11–12). "Medisave" accounts are supplemented by "Medishield" insurance, a voluntary catastrophic insurance fund, and "Medifund," a government fund that provides a safety net for the poor (Hanvoravongchai 2002, 12–13). Singaporeans also pay out of pocket for health care at levels that are very high compared to those in other countries (Lim 2004, 86). Singapore is a developed country that provides modern medicine at costs that are very low by international standards and thus, not surprisingly, has been held up as a model of what can be achieved through the use of CDHC (Lim 2004; Schreyögg 2004, 693–95).

On closer inspection, however, the Singapore picture blurs. In fact Medisave payments account for only about 8 percent of health care payments in Singapore. Employer benefits and private insurance cover 30 percent of health care costs, and public payments and subsidies cover 25 percent (Lim 2004, 86). In Singapore the main choice that consumers face seems to be with respect to hospital accommodations, the lowest-cost of which are six-bed wards that have no air conditioning and open wards that have more than six beds, conditions hardly typical of the choices for which American consumers are beating down the door (Lim 2004, 87).

Though health care costs as a proportion of GDP in Singapore are growing slowly, this is largely because GDP has grown very rapidly in Singapore in recent years (Hanvoravongchai 2002, 21–26). There is also a real debate as to how much cost control in Singapore is attributable to CDHC and how much to supply-driven strategies that Singapore has concurrently pursued, such as controls on the introduction of technology, price caps on services in government hospitals, restrictions on the number of government hospital beds, and restrictions on the number of doctors (Barr 2001, 716–19). Commentators have also raised the concern that the Singapore health care system offers little help to the poor and to those with chronic diseases (Barr 2001, 722–23).

China's public health insurance system largely collapsed in the 1980s, and since then China's health care system has been characterized by rapid growth in costs and radical inequities. In late 1998 China announced the implementation in urban areas of a system combining MSAS (to which 3.8 percent of employees' wages are contributed) and a social insurance fund (to which 4.2 percent of wages are contributed) that takes over once a deductible equal to 10 percent of a worker's annual wage is met (Liu 2002, 139–40). Social insurance coverage is capped at four times the annual wage. MSAS have been accompanied by regulatory controls, including a restrictive drug formulary and a prospective payment system, so it is unclear to what extent cost controls are due to the MSA program rather than to regulation (Yip and Hsiao 1997, 244–51). The new system, moreover, is replacing one in which most health care expenses were out of pocket rather than insured, so whatever success China has had in controlling costs cannot be attributed to increased cost sharing.[14]

In South Africa, the success of MSAS in the private sector in holding down costs has been widely proclaimed by CDHC advocacy groups. The situation in South Africa is complex, and I have explored it in depth elsewhere (Jost 2005). South Africa's radical inequities are mirrored in its health care system, with the vast majority of the medical resources concentrated in a private sector serving the small segment of the population that controls most of South Africa's wealth. Within the small privately insured population, MSAS are widely available. Depending on how one interprets the evidence, they have either successfully controlled some forms of medical expenditures or allowed private insurers to skim the insured population to attract the best risks and thus keep expenditures low for those groups. The data are consistent with both hypotheses. CDHC advocates within the United States favor the former version; insurance regulators in South Africa seem to put more stock in the latter.

In conclusion, although international experience can be seen as supporting the claims of CDHC advocates, further analysis of the experience weakens that support. In addition, the countries in which CDHC has been used are so different from the United States that it is not clear whether we can learn anything from their experience. International evidence therefore adds little to the preliminary and contradictory evidence that is available domestically. We clearly need to know much more before we turn to CDHC as a solution to the pressing problems of our health care system, and we should attend to the danger signals we see as well as the positive evidence. We also need to ponder the effects of CDHC on the relationship between professional and patient, the subject of the next chapter.

CHAPTER 9

Legal, Ethical, and Regulatory Issues
Presented by Consumer-Driven Health Care

From Professional and Patient to Merchant and Consumer

The CDHC revolution will undoubtedly bring about significant changes in the relationship between patients and health care professionals and providers. These changes raise important legal and ethical issues—issues that are only beginning to be identified and may not be resolved for some time. These issues are largely ignored by CDHC advocates, but they make the CDHC enterprise risky for both providers and patients and must be considered in a thorough evaluation of the advantages and disadvantages of CDHC. CDHC also raises important regulatory questions that are being addressed by the federal government and will ultimately need to be addressed by the state governments, which have traditionally been responsible for regulating health insurance. In the end CDHC might not result in the unregulated markets that CDHC advocates long for. Any consideration of CDHC is incomplete without a discussion of these issues and potential problems, which this chapter examines.[1]

Holly Smith has become increasingly worried about what appears to be a serious internal infection. She has family coverage through an HDHP that she purchased in the nongroup market, which has a deductible of $5,000 and imposes 20 percent coinsurance until an out-of-pocket maximum of $10,000 is reached. She has an HSA, to which she has been able to contribute only $200 so far this year. Ms. Smith is examined by her internist, Dr. Miller. She tells him right up front about her insurance arrangements.

Having examined Ms. Smith, Dr. Miller suspects that she does have an infection, but one that he believes is minor and easily treated. But there is a slight chance that she has a much more serious condition that presents with similar symptoms. This possibility can be definitively ruled out if Ms. Smith is tested using a newly available blood test. Dr. Miller does not know how much the test costs but suspects that it will be in the range of $500. Alternatively, the more serious condition can be largely, though less definitively, ruled out by an older blood test, which probably costs about $50. The standard of care adhered to by most doctors would be to order at least the cheaper test, but although no data are available, it is possible that most doctors would currently order the more expensive test for a person presenting with Ms. Smith's symptoms. Dr. Miller, an internist, could also refer Ms. Smith to a specialist, who could more definitively diagnose her condition. Dr. Miller has no idea how much a specialist would charge, especially if the specialist decided to run additional tests.

Assuming that Ms. Smith has the less serious condition, it can be treated most effectively by a relatively new brand-name drug, still under patent and therefore without an exact generic equivalent. Although Dr. Miller does not know exactly how much it costs, he believes that a thirty-day supply probably costs about $300. The infection can also be treated by a generic drug that is much less expensive but also less effective for some patients, and that has unpleasant side effects for a significant minority of patients. Dr. Miller believes that whatever course of action he pursues, he should see Ms. Smith again in two weeks to see how her treatment is going.

Dr. Miller does not know exactly what his fee is for an examination. He just checks a code on a billing form, which initiates a bill sent out by his billing service. The charge depends on the extent of the examination, plus whatever additional specific services (such as an injection or minor surgery) are rendered and whatever tests are run at the time of the service.

Dr. Miller is also worried about a second patient, James Johnson, who has been in the hospital for two days for a lung infection. Dr. Miller would like to keep him in the hospital another day, but Mr. Johnson, who has a policy similar to Ms. Smith's, has exhausted the $2,000 balance of his HSA, has run up an additional personal obligation for $3,000, and is now accruing a bill in excess of $500 a day for coinsurance charges for the hospitalization.

If Ms. Smith and Mr. Johnson had traditional Blue Cross–Blue Shield or commercial indemnity policies of the sort that was the norm in the late 1970s and early 1980s–the glory days of fee-for-service medicine–Dr. Miller might well have ordered the expensive test, prescribed the expensive drug, and told Ms. Smith to come back in two weeks. He would also have kept Mr. Johnson in the hospital for another day, or two, or three.[2] If Ms. Smith or Mr. Johnson belonged to a restrictive HMO in the mid-1990s, Dr. Miller might have hesitated before ordering the more expensive test or drug, or the additional day of hospitalization—he might not even have mentioned the more expensive alternative (Krause 1999, 281–305).

If Ms. Smith or Mr. Johnson belonged to a modern managed care plan, however, Dr Miller's practice might well have been much the same as it would have been under fee-for-service medicine (J. C. Robinson 2002). Ms. Smith would probably have had to pay a bit more for the more expensive drug in a two- or three-tier pharmacy benefits plan, and might have been liable for a $50 co-payment for the more expensive test, but these added costs would probably not have been enough to steer her toward the cheaper option, and Dr. Miller would have been unlikely to understand the cost-sharing structure of Ms. Smith's managed care plan in any event, because it would probably have been only one of many that he had contracts with. Indeed, Ms. Smith might very well have had only a vague notion of how the cost-sharing structure of her plan worked, and would just have paid the bills when they arrived (California Health Care Foundation 2003, 3). Dr. Miller might have had to fax a form to a toll-free number to justify to a concurrent review program Mr. Johnson's additional day of hospitalization, but coverage would in all likelihood been been approved.

The Traditional Model

There was of course a time—as recently as the first half of the twentieth century (discussed in chapter 4), before health insurance became common—when patients and doctors faced situations similar to those that Ms. Smith, Mr. Johnson, and Dr. Miller now face under CDHC. But tests and treatments were simpler and options more limited, drugs were relatively inexpensive (and ineffective), treatment generally involved urgently necessary acute care rather than long-term chronic care, and physicians, on the whole, saw their duty as doing what they thought best for their patients (Alexander, Hall, and Lantos

2006). The primary cost that most patients faced was the doctor's bill, but doctors were expected to charge less or to provide services for free to impecunious patients, and it was up to the doctor to decide how much to charge.

Under traditional "aspirational" medical ethics, Dr. Miller has an obligation to do whatever best meets the medical needs of his patients (Alexander, Hall, and Lantos 2006). "It should not be the physician's responsibility to eliminate [diagnostic tests] on cost grounds if the physician believes on balance that the procedure is even infinitesimally beneficial to patients" (Veatch 1981, 285). This principle may have been plausible in the time of fee-for-service medicine and first-dollar insurance coverage, when the interests of the patient in the most effective treatment and the financial interest of the physician were largely aligned. It fit less comfortably with the more rigorous forms of managed care, particularly under capitation or other physician-incentive systems, which confronted physicians with incentives to practice conservatively and to limit the amount of care provided to their patients. The conflicts of interest presented by managed care loosed a torrent of legal and ethical scholarship, and provoked legislation, regulations, and at least one Supreme Court decision (Sage 1999; Jacobson 2002; Pegram v. Herdrich).[3] Although there have been a number of egregious anecdotes about managed care companies that denied care to patients, however, there is little evidence that the quality of care over all has been worse under managed care, or even that patients' trust in their doctors has been significantly diminished because of managed care (Hall, Dugan, Zheng, and Mishra 2001, 624–26; Hall 2002, 505–7). The most common form of physician payment throughout the managed care era remained discounted fee-for-service, which left the interests of physicians and patients largely aligned. Physicians often ended up serving as advocates for their patients against managed care companies to secure coverage, sometimes even misrepresenting their patients' conditions to obtain coverage (Wynia, Cummins, VanGeest, and Wilson 2000).

Under CDHC the incentives change once again. The patient is the consumer, the doctor or health care institution a merchant. Yet the relationship is not simply one of buyer and seller, governed by the law of caveat emptor. A physician does not become a used car dealer with a white coat (Mariner 2004, 494–95). The physician remains a professional; the health care institution is in many cases a "charity" (or at least presents itself as one to the Internal Revenue Service). The relationship between professional and patient remains a relationship of trust (Mehlman 1990; Schuck 1994, 921).

The Fiduciary Relationship

There are several reasons why the physician-patient relationship has been understood to be a relationship of trust (Hall, Dugan, Zheng, and Mishra 2001; Mechanic 1998). First, the physician is often an agent for the patient. A doctor decides (in consultation with her patients) which tests to order, which drugs to prescribe, which specialists to consult, even which services she herself should provide. In doing so she has power and authority over her patients, which she must exercise, putting her patients' interest first and foremost. Second, the patient encounters the physician in a condition of particular vulnerability. The patient is often weakened by disease or injury, anxious, and unsettled. The patient is dependent upon the physician for information, both to understand the medical condition and to know how to respond to it. The patient must trust the physician or provider not to take advantage of this vulnerability. Trust is also necessary if the patient is to disclose confidential information to the physician and to cooperate with the treatment plan proposed by the physician (Morreim 2001, 66; Hall, Dugan, Zheng, and Mishra 2001, 629). Finally, trust may be essential to healing itself — healing may be to a greater or lesser degree dependent on the ability of the patient to entrust himself to the care of a healer (Hall 2002, 478–82).

The law has long recognized this trust relationship by regarding physicians as fiduciaries with respect to their patients (Mehlman 1990). As fiduciaries, physicians (and other health care professionals) are supposed to hold information gained from their patients in confidence and to refrain from taking advantage of their patients for their own financial gain.[4] Physicians must also disclose conflicts of interests to their patients under some circumstances. In Moore v. Regents of the University of California,[5] the court recognized an obligation on the part of a physician involved in clinical research to disclose to a patient "personal interests unrelated to the patient's health, whether research or economic, that may affect his medical judgment" (793 P.2d at 485). Providers are limited in their ability to require their patients to waive claims or remedies for liability for substandard care.[6] Physicians also have a general obligation to treat their patients fairly (Mehlman 1990, 393–401). Punitive damages can be imposed on physicians who breach their fiduciary obligations to their patients.[7]

The physician's fiduciary obligations are limited. The law recognizes that in many instances the physician will have conflicting obligations, and therefore does not demand an absolute allegiance to the patient (Rodwin 1995; Bloche 1999). The obligation to keep confidences is subject to many limitations, because of a recognition that disclosure of information may be necessary to protect the public's health, to protect the public safety or fisc, or even to assure that the physician gets paid.[8] Statutes and rules prohibiting financial conflicts of interest and self-referrals on the part of physicians and providers are subject to a host of exceptions (Furrow, Greaney, Johnson, Jost, and Schwartz 2000, 637–55). Finally, although courts recognize that physicians have a fiduciary obligation, they prefer to look to tort rather than fiduciary law when remedying situations in which physicians have injured their patients, thus seeking guidance under the "standard of care" observed by physicians generally rather than imposing an absolute obligation of faithfulness to the patient's interests.[9]

What obligations does the fiduciary relationship impose on Dr. Miller with respect to Ms. Smith or Mr. Johnson? Must he still do everything possible to protect and restore their health, or can he just do what they are willing to pay for? How much information must he give them about financial costs in addition to the information he must give them about health risks and benefits? If his patients cannot afford the treatment he thinks most appropriate for them, what should he do?

In considering these questions, we should remember that other professional relationships are also relationships of trust, although they too are usually structured as buyer-seller relationships without the intervention of third-party payment. Attorneys, accountants, and counselors are often paid for in cash on a fee-for-service basis, yet their relationship to the client is viewed as fiduciary, not governed strictly by the law of caveat emptor. A lawyer, for example, can withdraw from representing a client who does not pay the lawyer's fees, but must first give reasonable warning and take necessary steps to protect the client's interests.[10]

But what, in particular, are the implications of a doctor's fiduciary relationship with his consumer-patients? Moreover, what obligations does a doctor have to consumer-patients under tort law — what is the "standard of care" in a consumer-driven relationship? In particular, how does the obligation to obtain "informed consent" change in CDHC? And what are the responsibilities of Ms. Smith and Mr. Johnson, as empowered consumers, and how do their responsibilities relate to those of Dr. Miller? What, moreover, are the contractual obligations that govern the provider-patient relationship under CDHC?

Legal Ramifications

To begin, Dr. Miller arguably has an obligation in the era of CDHC to take into account the financial situation of Ms. Smith and Mr. Johnson. First, as their agent in deciding which tests, drugs, and procedures they should purchase, he may be responsible for taking into account not only their physical needs but also the financial burden that recommended treatment will impose upon them (Alexander, Hall, and Lantos 2006).[11] As chapter 8 made clear, the financial effects of medical treatments in a consumer-driven environment can be devastating. Ignoring the financial situation of the patient might very well affect compliance with treatment, and thus affect the patient's health directly. If Dr. Miller prescribes the more expensive drug, but Ms. Smith fails to fill the prescription once she determines that she cannot afford it, she may be much worse off than she would have been had Dr. Miller prescribed the less expensive drug. Moreover, financial disaster can itself be indirectly harmful to the patient's health if it affects the patient's nutrition or housing, for example.

For nearly half a century the law has recognized the doctor's obligation to inform the patient of the risks and benefits of a proposed test or treatment, and the alternatives to it, and then to secure the patient's consent before proceeding.[12] This obligation is imposed under the law of negligence, but the standard of care in many jurisdictions is measured by the reasonable patient's "need to know" rather than by the professional standard of care that normally governs medical negligence (Furrow, Greaney, Johnson, Jost, and Schwartz 2000, 313–15). In a CDHC environment, one of the things that a patient "needs to know" is the cost of a treatment or the relative cost of possible alternative treatments (Morreim 2006, 1214–16, 1218–21). The obligation to inform has always extended to information on risks, and out-of-pocket costs would seem to be a risk under CDHC. Even those jurisdictions that measure a professional's duty to disclose by the standard of care observed by other professionals rather than by the patient's need to know may come to recognize a duty to provide information as to cost once CDHC becomes widespread.

The obligation is far from clear, however. In Arato v. Avedon the court stated that a "physician is not the patient's financial advisor."[13] In that case the question was whether the doctor had an obligation to disclose to the patient information known to the doctor that might have assisted the patient in making other financial arrangements. The patient's estate claimed that the doctor's failure to disclose the patient's statistical risk of death from cancer kept the patient from getting his estate in order. When financial information directly affects the patient's choice of treatment, on the other hand, the doctor's obligations may well be higher.

This is also true because the patient has, at least in some jurisdictions, a right to "informed refusal." Even if Dr. Miller believes that Ms. Smith will not be able to afford the more expensive test or drug, he may have an obligation to tell her that it is an option.[14] The doctor will in all likelihood rarely be able to tell the patient exactly how much a procedure costs, but in most instances the doctor will have, or should have, some notion as to relative cost among alternative procedures, and probably some information as to the magnitude of the difference in cost (Morreim 2006, 1219–20).[15] Dr. Miller should tell Ms. Smith what he understands to be the relative costs of the various treatment options.

If the treatment that the patient needs is clear, on the other hand, but the patient cannot afford it, the health care provider must consider carefully how to proceed. Under some circumstances a health care institution may have an obligation to treat regardless of ability to pay. The Emergency Medical Treatment and Active Labor Act requires hospitals that have emergency departments and that participate in Medicare to screen patients who present in an emergency and to stabilize their condition before discharge or transfer.[16] Institutions may have additional obligations under the Hill-Burton program or under the law of tax-exempt organizations to offer free or reduced-cost services to those who cannot afford care (Furrow, Greaney, Johnson, Jost, and Schwartz 2000, 509–35).[17] Health care providers are prohibited in most instances from refusing services to Medicaid recipients who cannot afford to cover the co-payments authorized under the federal Medicaid statute.[18] Finally, there is limited judicial authority for an obligation on the part of health care providers to assist patients in identifying funding sources for needed treatment.[19]

A physician has no general obligation to take on a particular patient, and can refuse to treat those who cannot afford his or her services. But once a physician begins treatment, the physician cannot precipitously abandon a patient. In the leading case of Ricks v. Budge,[20] a malpractice claim was upheld against a physician who refused treatment to a patient in an urgent medical situation because of an unpaid past bill. The court held that the physician must give a patient notice of termination and a reasonable opportunity to seek care elsewhere before terminating care (Hall 1993, 650–52). In the interim, the physician must provide treatment that meets the professional standard of care.

The standard of care has always had a fair amount of wiggle room in it, because doctors often disagree on how to best treat various conditions.[21] In particular, there is authority for concluding that if the physician is otherwise skillful in treating the patient, the determination of the standard of care may take into account the resources available for the treatment (Hall 2006). Dr. Miller will probably be protected in recommending the less expensive test and the generic drug if Ms. Smith follows his recommendations and suffers injury.

What if Dr. Miller recommends the more expensive treatment or drug, however, and Ms. Smith refuses or fails to carry through with the recommendation for financial reasons, or Dr. Miller recommends that Mr. Johnson spend another day in the hospital and Mr. Johnson decides to go home because of cost? Dr. Miller has several defenses to a claim of liability if injury ensues. The "assumption of risk" doctrine, for example, holds that a plaintiff cannot hold another liable for the eventuation of obvious risks that the plaintiff took on voluntarily.[22] Assumption of risk has been accepted as a defense in several cases involving patients who sought out unconventional treatments for cancer and refused conventional lifesaving treatments.[23] Courts have also applied the doctrines of contributory negligence and comparative negligence to absolve doctors from liability for injuries that ensued when patients refused to follow medical advice,[24] for example when a patient failed to comply with a doctor's orders for follow-up visits or continued monitoring, or failed to comply with post-treatment instructions.[25] A physician can expect a patient to follow medical advice, and has no obligation to force the patient to comply.[26] Even when a patient's failure to comply with proper instructions does not altogether preclude damages flowing from the negligence of a provider or professional, the damages may be reduced to the extent that the consequences of the professional's negligence could have been avoided if the patient had complied with the instructions (Murphy 1991, 162–64). Finally, a patient in a malpractice case must show that a doctor's negligence proximately caused an injury, a showing that will be difficult if the patient's failure to follow through on prescribed treatment was the real cause of an injury (Murphy 1991, 166–70).[27] But defenses such as assumption of risk and comparative negligence will only be available to a physician who fully informs the patient of the reasons for a recommended treatment and the risks of rejecting it.

Finally, CDHC brings to the forefront the question of what a patient owes for health care products and services. For the past two decades, under managed care, this has seldom been an issue. Providers have negotiated prices or payment schemes with managed care organizations, which have in turn specified how much was owed by the patient. Under CDHC, however, the obligation to pay arises directly within the patient-provider relationship.

Providers and patients rarely negotiate ahead of time a contract under which the patient agrees to pay a particular price for a particular service. More often, the patient undertakes a vague obligation to pay a provider's "charges" or does not take on an explicit obligation at all. The courts will normally hold that patients are bound by any agreement to pay that they sign with a health care provider, regardless of the circumstances under which the obligation was assumed.[28] If there is no express contract, courts will still hold patients responsible to pay under a quasi-contract or unjust enrichment theory for the value of services they have received from health care providers.[29] Some courts limit the obligation of patients who have not agreed to pay a specific sum to the "reasonable value" of services provided, which seems to be measured by the going cost of services in the community.[30] Alternatively, patients have been held liable under the principle of an "account stated" if they were billed by a provider and did not protest the amount of the charge within a reasonable time, or the principle of "voluntary payment" if they paid a bill without protesting the amount.[31]

Attempts by patients to challenge high hospital charges in recent federal litigation under a host of theories, usually centered on the obligations of hospitals as charitable organizations under federal tax law, have largely failed (Cohen 2006). State class actions, on the other hand, under state consumer fraud or fair trade practices laws have survived early motions to dismiss (Cohen 2006, 135–37).[32] Yet as a practical matter, claims by health care providers rarely result in appellate litigation. They are commonly resolved through collection agencies or end up in small claims courts. Alternatively, they end up in bankruptcy courts, where the amount of the claim is presumed valid and the debtor has little incentive to argue with any creditor over the amount of the debt.

In sum, CDHC is likely to complicate relationships between professionals and patients in ways that are difficult to foresee. Health care providers and professionals are likely to have new responsibilities to their patients, and will need to consider their financial as well as their medical condition. In some circumstances providers may have an obligation to provide care that patients cannot afford, while in other circumstances patients may have to forgo care that they cannot afford, at their own peril. Courts will have to confront the question of whether a doctor can provide "second-best" treatments when the resources to provide the very best are lacking. Disputes about what is owed for health care are likely to become more common and contentious. But how exactly things will work out is far from certain — note the number of times that the word "probably" has been used in this discussion. All that can be said for certain is that the relationship between patients and providers will change in ways that are not now fully predictable and that professionals and patients may not like.

State Regulation of Consumer-Driven Health Care

Throughout the last half-century, both the federal and state governments have played a major role in regulating health insurance in the United States. Their respective jurisdictions have evolved over time, and a variety of approaches to sharing and allocating authority have emerged (Krause 2003). A dominant theme — arguably the dominant theme — has been federal deference to state regulation. Since adopting the McCarran-Ferguson Act in 1945,[33] Congress has recognized that insurance regulation is principally the domain of the states. Although Congress in the Employee Retirement Income Security Act of 1974 (ERISA) preempted state laws affecting employee benefit plans, it left in place state regulation of insured health benefit plans.

With the CDHC provisions of the Medicare Modernization Act (MMA), Congress has taken a quite different approach. The remarkable aspect of the MMA's provisions regulating HSA-HDHPs is the indirectness of its regulatory strategy. The MMA does not require insurers to offer HDHPs. It does not require states to require insurers to offer HDHPs. It does not even require the states to allow conforming HDHPs. It simply makes it clear that tax subsidies are only available for HSAs coupled with an HDHP, and that states that prohibit HDHPs will deprive their residents of access to a generous federal tax subsidy. Although HSAs are one of the major federal health policy initiatives of our time, states may completely block or fail to implement them if they desire, by not permitting HDHPs.

Health insurance is one of the most heavily regulated industries in the United States. A new form of insurance is therefore bound to raise a host of regulatory issues. In order to understand these issues, Professor Mark Hall and I conducted a series of interviews over a three-month period in the spring of 2005 with state regulators, representatives of the insurance industry, and specialists in consumer-driven health care. All told we spoke with thirty-three people, who included representatives of nineteen regulators and regulated entities, as well as individual experts. The remainder of this chapter is based on those interviews.[34]

Most public discussion of state regulatory issues affecting HSAs and HDHPs to date has centered on three issues, and all three came up frequently in our interviews. The first of these is the one issue specifically addressed by the federal government: the problem of state mandates that bar high deductibles for particular services. HSAs only qualify for tax subsidies under the MMA if they are coupled with HDHPs that have minimum deductibles of at least $1,000 for individuals and $2,000 for families, adjusted each year for inflation.[35] At the time the MMA was adopted, a number of states mandated coverage of specific health services (as defined by federal law), either without a deductible or with a low deductible. Examples included a Florida law that prohibited insurers from charging insurance deductibles or co-payments to victims of violent crime and laws in Maryland and Pennsylvania that prohibited applying a deductible to certain home health visits for recently delivered mothers and newborns. The IRS gave the states until the end of 2005 to revoke or amend their conflicting requirements so as to allow their residents to take advantage of the HSA tax subsidies.[36] Most states quickly followed suit. According to a survey conducted by America's Health Insurance Plans (AHIP), by May of 2005 the legislatures of all but four states with impediments had passed laws removing them (America's Health Insurance Plans 2005a).

A second widely recognized issue is whether HMOs can offer an HDHP. Most insurers structure HDHPs as PPOs (Jost and Hall 2005, 405). But some insurers also want to make HDHPs available through HMOs, although the traditional understanding of an HMO is that it offers comprehensive health care in exchange for a fixed premium. An HMO with a deductible of $1,000, or, to stretch things further, $5,000 or $10,000, seems therefore to raise definitional problems. Many states have resolved the inconsistency either by explicitly allowing HMOs to have deductibles or by stretching their state law definitions of HMOs to allow HDHPs. In a few states, however, state law prohibits or limits HMO deductibles. In a number of other states, moreover, regulators expressed to us some concern about how high HMO deductibles can go. In sum, most states are trying to permit HMOs to offer HDHPs that comply with the MMA, but there may be limits to how far they are willing to go.

The third major issue is state tax subsidies for HSAs. Twenty-seven of the states (and the District of Columbia) simply use the federal definition of taxable income and therefore automatically recognize all deductions and exclusions available under federal law for state income tax filers, including HSA-related deductions. Another eight states do not have a state income tax, and thus are not in a position to offer income tax incentives. But the fifteen remaining states needed a specific law if they wanted to single out HSAs for favorable treatment. In the wake of the MMA, many states have amended their state tax laws to conform to the new federal provisions. But as of 2006 six states apparently had not done so, and therefore currently provide no state tax subsidies for HSAs (National Conference of State Legislatures 2004–6).

These three issues have been the primary ones raised by insurers and regulators, but they do not exhaust the range of those that may arise. First, administration of HSAs may raise several questions of state regulation. One of the essential functions of insurance regulation is to assure that insurers have sufficient capital and reserves to meet their obligations as those obligations become due. Because funds in HSAs can be carried over from year to year, insurers that administer HSAs could potentially accumulate large sums of money for which they are responsible. Most insurers, however, have little experience functioning as banks.

Under the MMA, an HSA may be administered by a bank, an insurance company, or "another person who demonstrates to the satisfaction of the Secretary [of the Treasury] that the manner in which such person will administer the trust will be consistent with the requirements of this section."[37] Banks are regulated by the Federal Deposit Insurance Corporation (FDIC), the comptroller of the currency, and state banking regulators. Administrators other than banks and insurers are regulated by the federal government in the same way that 401(k) administrators are, and as such are subject to a reasonably thorough regulatory process. But most states do not appear to have a regulatory mechanism that oversees insurers offering financial services. If HSA funds are kept separate from the insurer's other funds, they are not regulated. The first time HSA holders (or providers who expect to be paid by HSAs) encounter major problems in getting an insurance administrator to honor checks or debit card transactions, questions will undoubtedly surface about state regulatory oversight. Why did insurance regulators allow the problem to arise? Will state insurance guaranty funds cover the obligations of insolvent insurers under their HSAs, or only under their HDHPs? Do unfair claims practice laws cover HSA claims? We found little evidence in our interviews that insurers or insurance regulators are considering these issues.[38]

A second issue that HSAs raise is how state statutes and regulations regulating managed care will apply to HSA transactions. Managed care uses a number of tools to control health care utilization and prices, including provider networks, utilization review, and provider payment incentives. Perceived excesses in the application of these tools have resulted in extensive state regulation of managed care. Although state laws clearly apply to the portion of services that the HDHPs insure, it is unclear whether they apply to covered services below the deductible or to other services paid from HSAs but not covered by the HDHP.

All the HDHP insurers with whom we spoke make their negotiated network discounts available to HSA holders. Insurers also use their standard claims processing systems, including utilization review, to determine when the policy deductible (and ultimately the out-of-pocket maximum) has been met for any subscriber. In general only insured expenses can be counted against a deductible. If a subscriber with a $3,000 deductible receives an outpatient surgery costing $2,500, insurers are unlikely to credit the cost of the surgery fully against the deductible without determining whether the surgery was a covered expense, whether $2,500 was a reasonable charge, and whether the subscriber received pre-approval for the surgery if required under the policy. In short, even while spending their own money from HSAs, subscribers will be subject to managed care controls to the extent that they later attempt to claim expenses against their insurance deductibles.

This raises a host of questions. If an insurer refuses to credit the cost of the surgery fully against the deductible because it was not medically necessary, can the HSA holder appeal the decision under the state's claims review laws?[39] If a network provider is treating an HSA holder and that provider's contract with the HDHP is terminated, must the provider continue to offer the HSA owner the HDHP-negotiated discount for the period of time that a state's continuity-of-care statute requires the HDHP to cover services from the provider? Do state any-willing-provider statutes apply to HDHP networks for HSA-covered services as well as for HDHP-funded services? In sum, does the whole panoply of managed care regulatory statutes also apply to HSA expenditures, at least insofar as they are applied against HDHP deductibles?

The answer to these questions in general seems to be yes. Virtually all regulators and insurers we talked to assumed this to be the case, but this assumption has not yet been challenged or tested, as it might be if, for instance, a particular provider insisted that it was not bound by the restraints in its managed care contract for services paid directly by patients through their HSAs (Cross 2004). Even if the current understanding holds, it means that HDHPs will face a regulatory environment no less restrictive than that of conventional managed care plans. Because many people believe that regulation mortally wounded managed care, this realization might cause states to consider whether some aspects of existing regulation will deter appropriate development or operation of HSAs and HDHPs (Hall 2005, 427).

Another traditional focus of state insurance regulation has been improving access to health insurance for the uninsured by controlling insurers' underwriting and rating practices, primarily in the small group market but in some states also in the individual market. The goal of these laws is to open the insurance market to higher-risk insurance applicants and small groups that might otherwise be excluded. This goal is manifest in laws that require forms of community rating and the offer of standardized policies, and that establish high-risk pools.

A number of commentators have expressed a concern that HDHPs might further fragment insurers' risk pools by attracting mainly low-risk subscribers, leaving high-risk subscribers in separate risk pools with ever-increasing premiums for conventional insurance (Shearer 2004, 1164–65; Mariner 2004, 511; Fuchs and James 2005, 24–28). If HDHPs end up attracting only low risks, then the goals of rating reforms will be eroded even if insurers charge each person an actuarially fair rate for the type of policy that he or she purchases. Accordingly, states concerned about access to coverage by sicker people might choose to regulate HDHP premiums to assure that lower prices for these policies reflect only their leaner benefits and not the better inherent health of the people who choose to purchase these policies.

Most of the regulators whom we interviewed felt that risk segmentation was not a pressing problem. Those who had actuarial expertise said, however, that so far their rating rules had not required insurers to spread risk between HDHPs and more conventional health plans. Most felt that it was appropriate, and actuarially fair, to instead base the premiums for each policy type on the health care costs and utilization generated by each policy's benefit structure and risk pool. One reason why regulators may have refrained from scrutinizing rating practices for HDHPs is the growing disillusionment with traditional approaches to expanding access to coverage, which we detected in several quarters. Regulators seemed very sensitized to the "zero-sum" logic that for every high-risk subscriber whose rates are lowered by regulation, several lower-risk subscribers must pay higher rates, which at the margin may deter some of them from purchasing any insurance.

Over all, the states' initial response to the MMA has been quite remarkable. Most states have responded affirmatively to the latest federal legislation, despite its lack of explicit compulsion, by removing any regulatory barriers to qualified HDHPs. Some states have gone further, adopting or modifying state income tax laws to supplement the federal incentives with state incentives for the purchase of HSAs and HDHPs.

Perhaps the experience with managed care regulation has caused most states to lose their taste for insurance regulation; or perhaps the receptive regulatory response is attributable to the newness of the HSA-HDHP product and thus a lack of experience with the problems it might cause. Whatever the explanation, the new approach to federalism in insurance regulation evidenced by the MMA appears to have accomplished its goals. At least for the moment, the lure of tax incentives has been sufficient to launch HSA-HDHPs successfully in most states without the need for either direct preemption of state law or direct federal regulation of insurance, thus avoiding all the friction and controversies that have accompanied these strategies under ERISA. Yet it is too early to know for sure what the full regulatory impact of HSAs and HDHPs will be. We may be at much the same place we were in the late 1980s with respect to managed care, when we were still quite innocent of the problems it posed. A few years later, the managed care backlash hit and state legislatures responded with a host of new regulatory statutes. A decade from now, if HSAs and HDHPs take off with the speed and force that their advocates predict, we may see a very different regulatory environment, one that bears little resemblance to the free and unregulated market promised by consumer-driven health care.

It may be possible, moreover, that even if insurers that offer HSA-compliant HDHPs largely escape state regulation, they may not totally escape legal troubles. A prominent hope of the CDHC movement is that insurers will be one of the primary sources that consumers can turn to for information about health care providers. Insurers that offer CDHC products are in fact offering information on providers' prices and quality (see chapter 8). Presumably, consumers will rely on this information. But what will happen when a patient is injured negligently by a physician, and it becomes clear that information provided by the insurer about the competence of that physician was incorrect, indeed was negligently provided? Could the insurer be liable for the damage suffered by the consumer? Other providers of information — accountants or lawyers for example — have been held liable to persons who have been injured by reliance on information provided by those professionals (Dobbs 2000, 1351).[40] The consumer revolution depends on information — on reliable information. Who will be responsible when consumers rely on insurer-provided information that is faulty remains to be established.

Are Consumers Our Only Hope? How Other Countries Organize Their Health Care Systems

A World of Alternatives

One of the primary claims of the CDHC advocates is that their model for financing health care is superior not only to the current health care financing arrangements in the United States but also to those of every other country in the world, at least every country that has not adopted a consumer-driven model (Adam Smith Institute 2002). John Goodman, one of the leading advocates of HSAs, has published two books criticizing in some detail the health care systems of other countries, while market-oriented advocacy groups such as the National Center for Policy Analysis (NCPA), the Heritage Foundation, and the Galen Institute regularly issue "policy briefs" criticizing the health care systems of other countries (Goodman, Musgrave, and Herrick 2004; Goodman 1980a). They are joined in this criticism by pro-market advocacy groups in other countries such as the Fraser Institute in Canada.

CDHC skeptics, on the other hand, proclaim that other countries offer universal access to health care at lower cost than the United States, which would be wise to move toward the models used by those countries (White 1995). It is therefore necessary to ask how other countries organize their health care systems, and how successful they have been at addressing issues of access, quality, and cost. This chapter describes how the health care systems of other countries function, analyzes the performance of those countries, and finally considers what we can learn from their experience.

There are 192 countries in the world, more or less, and each of these countries has a health care system. But the vast majority of these countries are so different from the United States, either in the size of their population or in their level of economic development, that there is little we can learn from their experiences. It is highly unlikely that a new model for the American health care system will emerge from a study of health care financing in Monaco or Burkina Faso (although advocates of CDHC claim that we should model our system after that of Singapore) (Marmor 2001). We are most likely to learn from the experiences of a handful of developed countries—approximately twenty—with mature health care systems. Most of these countries are European, though they also include Japan, Australia, New Zealand, and Canada.

Most comparative health policy analysis found in the American media or directed at general audiences focuses on the experience of the United Kingdom and Canada, both English-speaking countries closely associated historically with the United States and very familiar to Americans. This is particularly true of CDHC advocates. Typically, Robert Moffit states: "Ultimately, members of Congress have two choices: They can adopt a government-run health care system along the lines of the British, Canadian, or Clinton-style model or they can eliminate the distortions in the U.S. health insurance market and recreate a sound market in the financing and delivery of health care. There is no third way" (Moffit 1999, 46). Less sophisticated American commentators used to lump together the health care financing systems of all other countries under the rubric "socialized medicine," but now are more likely to use the phrase "single-payer," by which they mean the same thing. In fact, however, the world's health care systems are remarkably varied. Each country's system is the unique product of the history, culture, and politics of that country (Oliver, Mossialos, and Wilsford eds. 2005) Each system is also, like our own, continually changing.[1]

Most attempts to categorize the world's various systems begin with a division between social insurance and national health service models (Saltman and Dubois 2004, 22–26; Chinitz, Wismar, and LePen 2004, 158). The former systems are usually referred to as "Bismarck model" systems after Otto von Bismarck, who is largely credited with creating the German social health insurance system in the 1880s. The latter systems are often referred to as "Beveridge model" systems, after Lord Beveridge, the author of the Beveridge Report

(1942), which called for creation of a national health care system in Britain at the end of the Second World War. The most distinctive characteristic of national health services on the Beveridge model is that they have centralized funding from general revenues, such as general income or consumption taxes. Social health insurance programs, on the other hand, were historically employment-based and funded by employer and employee contributions, essentially payroll taxes (Mossialos and Dixon 2002; Normand and Busse 2002).

Other features also characterize these alternative models. The government tends to play a much more prominent role in managing national health services, and although general practitioners are usually independent contractors, hospitals and other health care institutions tend to be government-owned.[2] Social insurance programs were historically managed by quasi-public social insurance funds which operated within general "framework laws" set down by the government (Chinitz, Wismar, and LePen 2004, 155–69). Institutional providers are more likely to be nonprofit or religious entities (or even for-profit entities) in social insurance countries. National health service systems are found in the United Kingdom, Canada, Australia, Scandinavia, Iberia, and southern Europe. Germany, France, Austria, Belgium, the Netherlands, Switzerland, and Japan, as well as a number of eastern European and Latin American countries, are identified as social insurance countries.

This traditional approach to classification is problematic. First, there are many countries that do not fit perfectly within either model—the UK, the archetypical Beveridge-model country, pays for about 10 percent of its health care system through national insurance contributions, while Switzerland and Belgium, archetypical Bismarck-model countries, pay for a significant share of their health care systems from general revenue funds (Mossialos and Dixon 2002, 11; Busse, Saltman, and Dubois 2004, 33–47, 50). More importantly, there is tremendous variation among countries not captured by either model.

It is therefore more useful to classify countries along a more complex grid, recognizing a number of variables. One of these is certainly the distinction illuminated by the Bismarck and Beveridge classification: What is the primary source of funding of the system? Most mature health care systems are funded in large part through general revenues, earmarked social insurance contributions, or some combination of both. In all systems, however, health care services are also funded in part by private health insurance. Private health insurance plays a different role in each country (Mossialos and Thompson 2004; Maynard ed. 2005; Jost 2001). In Canada it funds services not covered by the national health program such as nonsurgical dental care and optical care. In France it covers cost-sharing obligations that would otherwise be borne by the patient. In Germany private insurance covers persons who because of their wealth or occupation are not obligated to participate in the social insurance plans. In the UK and Sweden persons with private health insurance can jump to the head of queues in which they would otherwise have to wait for publicly funded services. In a few countries, such as the Netherlands and Switzerland, residents are required to purchase heavily regulated quasi-private insurance, which effectively operates the public system. Finally, in each country health care services are funded to a greater or lesser extent through out-of-pocket payments, which cover deductibles, co-payments, and coinsurance obligations; services not covered by the public system (such as over-the-counter drugs); and payments made to providers (often under the table) in excess of those payments made by the public system (J. C. Robinson 2002).

Allocation among these sources of income varies considerably, and sometimes surprisingly, among the reference countries. Most Beveridge countries do not have social insurance funding, but many Bismarck countries rely in part on general revenue funds, at least to pay for coverage for the poor. France has in recent years changed the funding of its social insurance system from a payroll tax to a general income tax, and has also extended universal coverage to all lawful residents, regardless of employment status or insurance contributions (Bellanger and Mossé 2005, S122–S123). Although we often describe Canada as a single-payer system, 30 percent of Canadian health expenditures are private, including 12.3 percent covered by private insurance (Marchildon 2005, 72–85). Cost-sharing obligations are quite high in the Scandinavian countries, even though those countries are often thought of as having the most socialized health care systems (R. Robinson 2002, 165–70).

A second important way in which countries vary is with respect to the role of government in operating the health care system. As noted above, in Beveridge countries the government tends to play a central role in managing the health system. This is clearly seen in England, which despite a quarter-century of rhetoric about markets and decentralization continues to operate one of the most centralized health care systems in Europe (Giaimo 2002). Government tends to play a lesser role in Bismarck countries, although the long-term trend has been toward greater government involvement. The German government, for example, has exerted tighter control over the health care system in recent years, although the social health insurance funds and the corporatist providers' institutions are still independent and still collectively exercise considerable power over the system (Giaimo 2002, 131–47).

A third key variable with respect to governance is federalism. In many Beveridge systems, such as those of Canada and Sweden and to a lesser extent Australia, regional governments (provincial, state, and county) play a key role in operating a health care system supported by federal funding and subject to broad federal guidelines. In some social insurance systems as well, including the Swiss and the German, regional governments also play a role, at least with respect to some forms of care. In Germany the states (Länder) are responsible for providing capital funding for hospitals and operate many of the hospitals. The corporate provider and social insurer organizations are organized at the state level (Busse and Riesberg 2004, 33–36, 72–73, 104–5).

A fourth variable, already mentioned, is how health care delivery is organized. Most countries have some mix of public and private provision — general practitioners are usually independent contractors (who may be organized in union-like corporatist organizations), while hospitals are usually government-owned or nonprofit organizations that employ the professionals who practice within them. Public hospitals are more likely to be owned by local or regional governments (or to be independent public entities) than to be owned by national governments. In some countries religious hospitals are common, and in others so are, increasingly, for-profit hospitals. In Germany, 53 percent of acute-care beds are in public, 39 percent in nonprofit, and 8 percent in private hospitals; in France 65 percent are in government, 15 percent in nonprofit, and 20 percent in private, for-profit hospitals; and in the United Kingdom 95 percent of beds are in public hospitals and 5 percent in private hospitals (though some public beds are available to private patients) (Grosse-Tebbe and Figueras 2004, 61). Pharmaceutical companies, pharmacies, and dental practices are usually private entities. Long-term care facilities are also mostly private in many countries.

Yet another organizational variable is how the utilization of health care is controlled. In a number of systems, such as the British, a patient must first be seen by a primary-care professional (general practitioner) before he or she may gain access to a hospital or specialist, except in emergencies. Other countries, including Germany, generally permit patients to self-refer directly to specialists. A number of countries are also beginning to use disease management programs to bring down the high costs of chronic disease (Busse 2004, 56–57). Finally, some countries monitor the utilization of services, often in the aggregate (statistically) rather than individually, to tackle the problem of provider-induced demand.

The approach that different countries take to paying for the services of professionals and providers is another important variable. In most countries professionals in the ambulatory sector are simply reimbursed for their services on some basis, usually fee-for-service. This is generally true, for example, of physicians in Canada (Marchildon 2005, 53). In some countries, such as Japan, the government regulates professional fees (Campbell and Ikegami 1998, 145–65). In other countries, such as Germany, professionals are corporately organized and contracts exist between the government or corporate organizations of health insurance funds on the one hand and corporate provider organizations on the other (Busse and Riesberg 2004, 177–82). In a few countries, such as Finland, professionals are largely integrated into public clinics and are paid a salary (Häkkinen 2005, S102). In most countries hospitals and other health care institutions are paid on a negotiated budget or prospective payment system.

A final, closely related variable is the role of markets within the system. Countries in which private insurance or cost sharing plays a large role obviously rely to some extent on market forces. A number of countries have attempted to integrate market elements within their public insurance systems as well. Germans are largely free to choose among social insurance funds, which to some extent compete for their business (although reallocation of costs through a risk-sharing pool limits the disparity in insurance fund premiums) (Wörz and Busse 2005, S137–S138). Competition among insurers is emphasized even more strongly in the Netherlands and Switzerland, whose systems are structured so as to encourage competition. In Sweden and the United Kingdom there is some competition among providers for patients, though it is not clear that this competition has led to an improvement in quality (Fotaki and Boyd 2005). Finally, under recent decisions of the European Court of Justice, patients in each European country are free to seek services in other countries, subject to certain evolving limitations (Hervey and McHale 2004, 124–38). Thus all European countries compete with each other for selling their services to patients within the European Union.

Commonality among Diversity

Despite the remarkable diversity among the world's health care systems, most are similar in two respects. First, the health care systems of virtually all developed nations are based on an underlying commitment to solidarity. Solidarity is not a fuzzy notion about the common good, but means that a health care system is organized and managed on the basis of universal access, without risk selection, and financed through a system based primarily on income-related premiums or taxes, with no significant differences in the benefit package based on income. There is no relationship in a solidarity-based system between the premium paid and access to the insurance entitlement (Stone 1993). Solidarity is fundamentally a rejection of markets as the best means to distributing health care goods and services, although solidarity-based systems often incorporate internal market mechanisms and leave room for substantial private markets for health care.

True solidarity is solidarity with the stranger. Unlike the ancient and Christian concept of *caritas*, solidarity among strangers is not voluntary but rather institutionalized by means of law. This concept of compulsory solidarity reflects a political choice based on social justice to redistribute resources in order to guarantee equal access to health care. The level of redistribution of resources varies considerably among health care systems, as indeed does the extent of equity of access to health care services (or to health). Not every country covers all possible medical services, and some do not cover the entire population, leaving wealthier citizens to purchase private insurance. But solidarity is the fundamental principle in the design of the health care systems of all other mature health care systems.

Second, in all other mature health care systems the public insurance program exercises control over the cost of the health care system. No equivalent program for health care cost control exists in the United States, although Medicare, Medicaid, and private insurance programs attempt to control their own costs through prospective and negotiated payment systems and managed care. In Beveridge countries like the UK, costs are generally controlled through a health care budget. The government decides how much it intends to spend on health care and then attempts to control the cost of goods and services purchased from the health care budget through administered payment systems or by imposing budgets on, or negotiating budgets with, providers. This is often a multilevel process, with central governments (or, in federal systems, state or provincial governments) allocating funds to regional or local health authorities (primary care trusts in England, county governments in Sweden), which in turn pay providers. Bismarck-model countries like Germany are more likely to set or cap health insurance premiums, and then leave to the social insurers the job of determining the amounts paid to providers of goods and services, again usually through administered pricing systems or negotiated budgets. In many systems pharmaceutical prices are set through price or profit controls, and in some systems, such as that of Japan, price controls are also imposed on the cost of services (Mossialos and Mrazek 2002, 154–58; Campbell and Ikegami 1998, 16–18).

In most countries costs are also addressed through a system that screens new technologies to decide which will be covered by public health insurance (Jost ed. 2005). In many systems market or pseudo-market controls are also used to control cost increases, including reference price systems for drugs and competition among social insurance funds. In some systems, as is described below, cost controls are tight enough to result in visible rationing. In other systems, rationing is not a major issue. In every system, however, governments intervene to control costs. Indeed government attempts to control costs follow inevitably from government guarantees of access to health care — no nation on earth is wealthy enough to guarantee health care access to all without regard to cost.

How Does the United States Measure Up?

Descriptions of solidarity-based health care systems in CDHC literature caricature them as bureaucratic, insensitive, technologically backward systems that deliver inferior care. Overwhelmingly, this literature highlights waiting lists for services as the inevitable result and defining feature of government financing of health care. More sophisticated analyses point to genuine problems in equity of access, technological innovation, and ready availability of care in solidarity-based systems. No health care system is perfect, and solidarity-based systems certainly have their problems, although the nature and severity of these problems varies considerably from system to system. Many fail to provide care as rapid, technically sophisticated, and luxurious as is available to wealthy, fully insured Americans. Also, in no other system are professionals and providers as consistently well compensated as they are in the United States.

But on the whole, solidarity-based systems provide care of reasonably high quality and technical sophistication, reasonably quickly, to all who need it. In none of these systems is any significant number of poor people uninsured. In none do poor persons encounter the barriers to care that they face in the United States (though in none are the poor likely to be as healthy as the affluent). But in none is health care perfect.

The material that follows compares the performance of the American health care system with those of other developed countries that have sophisticated health care systems with regard to several key health policy variables. These include cost, access to care, equity of care provision, availability of new technologies, delays in accessing services (waiting lists), and quality of care. As to each of these features, the story that emerges is quite different from that found in the CDHC advocacy literature.

Other Countries Spend Less on Health Care

The most striking characteristic of the American health care system is its cost. By any measure, the United States has the most expensive health care system in the world. In 2003, when the United States spent 15 percent of its GDP on health care, the United Kingdom spent 7.7 percent, Germany 11.1 percent, and Canada 9.9 percent (Anderson, Frogner, John, and Reinhardt 2006, 819–31). If cost is measured by health expenditures per capita, expressed in "purchase parity–adjusted dollars," the United States fares just as poorly. This approach looks at how much money is spent per person on health care, adjusting expenditures not simply for exchange rates but also for the actual purchasing power of local currencies, recognizing that most goods and services usually cost less in less wealthy countries. In 2003 the United States spent $5,635 purchase parity–adjusted dollars per capita, compared to $3,003 for Canada, $2,996 for Germany, and $2,231 for the UK (Anderson, Frogner, John, and Reinhardt 2006, 820).

If one looks not at the absolute level of health care costs but rather at the rate at which they are growing, the United States also stands out, though not so remarkably. From 1993 to 2003 the proportion of the GDP devoted to health care in the United States grew at an annual rate of 3.4 percent (Anderson, Frogner, John, and Reinhardt 2006, 820). This rate is equal to the average of countries belonging to the Organization for Economic Cooperation and Development (OECD). But if one compares expenditure growth in the United States only with growth in OECD countries that have mature health care systems (that is, if one removes from the mix countries like Korea and Poland that saw very high growth in health care spending during this period as their economies modernized), growth in the United States, at 3.4 percent, was well above the 3.1 percent rate of growth of the other countries. Expenditure growth in the United States would surely have been greater were it not for the fact that the mid-1990s saw some of the slowest growth rates in American health care costs in recent history, as managed care achieved its maximum cost-control effectiveness, while other developed countries such as the United Kingdom and Canada were consciously trying to increase inadequate expenditures on health care. Indeed, if one looks at expenditure growth over the longer term, the exceptional nature of the United States comes into sharper focus. Between 1970 and 2003 health expenditures grew from 7 percent to 9.9 percent of GDP in Canada, from 4.5 percent to 7.7 percent in the UK, but from 6.9 percent to 15 percent in the United States (Organization for Economic Cooperation and Development 2005, 150).

Why does health care cost so much more in the United States than elsewhere? One factor accounts for much of the difference: the greater wealth of the United States. The relationship between health expenditures per capita and GDP per capita among developed nations is nearly linear — wealthier nations simply spend more on health care (Goodman, Musgrave, and Herrick 2004, 77). The United States is one of the wealthiest nations on earth, and thus, not surprisingly, spends more than anyone else on health care.[3] But while almost all the other developed nations cluster very tightly along a line when health expenditures and GDP per capita are graphed against each other, the United States is far above that line, spending $1,962 more on health care per person than would be predicted if we simply followed the pattern seen in other developed nations (Anderson, Frogner, Johns, and Reinhardt 2006, 821). In other words, this relationship explains much of the difference, but far from all of it.

What then explains the "surplus" costs in the United States? Although population aging is often suggested (and often rejected) as a cause of health expenditure growth worldwide, it cannot explain higher costs in the United States, which has one of the youngest populations of any OECD country (a characteristic that makes the higher costs stand out even more). The difference also cannot be explained by pointing to higher resource use in the United States: we use no more physicians, hospitals, or drugs per person per year than other countries. In fact Americans spend fewer days in the hospital annually than do the residents of virtually any other developed country (Anderson, Reinhardt, Hussey, and Petrosyan 2003, 89–105). Many commentators believe that medical malpractice litigation is more of a problem in the United States and explains some of our excess costs. But malpractice claims account for a very small part of our total health care expenditures, less than half of one percent (Anderson, Hussey, Frogner, and Waters 2005, 903–26). Medical negligence litigation is also not uncommon in other countries, and evidence for defensive medicine as a major cost factor is weak.[4]

Rather, higher American costs seem to be attributable primarily to three causes. First, we spend far more on the administration of our health care system than other countries do (Woolhandler, Campbell, and Himmelstein 2003). Our highly fragmented health insurance system requires health care institutions and professionals to hire numerous personnel for billing and claims processing who are unnecessary in unitary systems. Our private insurance premiums must also cover advertising, sales commissions, underwriting, lobbying, and profit, expenses that do not exist in public systems. Even in the United States, the administrative costs of the Medicare program are a fraction of those of private insurance.

Second, new medical technologies are generally adopted earlier and diffused much faster in the United States than in other countries (Technological Change in Health Care Research Network 2001, 25–42). For example, in 2002 the United States maintained 8.6 magnetic resonance imaging (MRI) units per million inhabitants, compared to 6.6 in Belgium and 6 in Germany. In 2003 we had 13.1 computed tomography (CT) scanners per million compared to 10.3 per million in Canada (Anderson, Frogner, Johns, and Reinhardt 2006, 903–26). Technology that would only be available in regional medical centers in some countries is available not only in community hospitals but also in clinics and even physicians' offices in the United States. While this means that these technologies are immediately available to Americans, it also means that they are used more often. In 2003 American physicians performed 161 coronary bypass procedures per 100,000 residents, compared to 98 in Canada and 56 in the UK (Organization for Economic Cooperation and Development 2005, 59). New technologies are often more expensive than those they replace. They also often afford new diagnostic or therapeutic capabilities that make it possible to address problems that previously could not be addressed (Jost ed. 2005, 2). In both respects, they bring new costs to the system.

The most important cause of excess health care costs is that, even though we by and large use the same amount of health care products and services per person in the United States, we simply pay higher prices for those products and services than citizens of other countries do. Physicians enjoy much higher incomes in the United States than they do elsewhere, twice the income of physicians in Canada and Germany and almost four times the income of physicians in the UK (Strategic Policy and Research Intergovernmental Affairs 2001). Pharmaceutical expenditures per capita in the United States are 50 percent higher than those in Germany and almost twice those in Japan, even though pharmaceutical expenditures as a percentage of total health expenditures in the United States are lower than they are in most of the reference countries

(Organization for Economic Cooperation and Development 2005, 75). Drugs cost more in the United States even though we use more lower-cost generic drugs in the United States than most other countries do, because we do not regulate drug prices or profits (Danzon and Furukawa 2003).

One study that examined resources used in treating four tracer diseases (diabetes, gallstones, breast cancer, and lung cancer) concluded that in 1990 Americans spent 40 percent more than the Germans in purchasing power parity dollars but received 15 percent fewer health care inputs, while spending 75 percent more than citizens of the UK while receiving only 30 percent more inputs (McKinsey Global Institute 1996, 8-8). Another study showed that Kaiser Permanente provides care more rapidly and effectively to its members than the British National Health Service (NHS), with comparable resource use, but that Kaiser pays over 50 percent more for health care inputs than the NHS does (Feachem, Sekhri, and White 2002, 135–43). In sum, the United States is a great place for health care providers, but it imposes higher costs on health care consumers.

In the end, international experience demonstrates that public health care financing systems are more effective in holding down health care costs than the mixed public-private systems prevailing in the United States (Gerdtham and Jönsson 2000, 12–53). International experience also shows that certain approaches to structuring health care systems, such as using gatekeepers or paying doctors through capitation, may help to hold down costs as well (Gerdtham and Jönsson 2000, 46). Public systems have lower administrative costs, give greater control over the adoption and diffusion of technology, and provide greater control over the prices paid for health care goods and services than our mixed public-private system does. Indeed, even within the United States, public systems cost less than private insurance (Kaiser Commission on Medicaid and the Uninsured 2004).[5]

Other Countries Provide Better (Though Not Perfect) Access to Health Care

A second comparative claim that is often made concerning the American health care system is that the United States is the only developed country that does not provide access to health care for all of its citizens. It is certainly true that many Americans, approximately 46.6 million, or about 16 percent of the population, are not insured at any one time through a private or public insurance program (Denavas-Walt, Proctor, and Lee 2006, 20). The number of Americans insured through employment has been shrinking for years (though it grew briefly in the late 1990s), and enrollment in public programs, though steadily growing, has in many years not been taking up the slack, thus allowing the number of uninsured Americans to continue to grow.[6]

By contrast, all other developed countries assure an approximation of universal access to health care, in most countries by providing a public insurance program that covers most of their population, and in a few countries by mandating and subsidizing the purchase of private insurance.[7] A few of these public insurance programs, such as the German program, do not require participation by the wealthy, while many programs, such as the French and the Dutch, offer additional benefits for the poor and the elderly, such as a waiver of cost sharing or coverage of additional benefits. But all the programs cover at least the poor and the middle class, and most cover the most expensive health care services: hospitalization, physician services, and pharmaceuticals. It is therefore fundamentally true that the American health care system is not only more costly but also less inclusive than those of other countries.

Advocates of market-driven health care challenge this claim, or at least the strength with which the claim is commonly made (Goodman, Musgrave, and Herrick 2004, 27–47, 147–65). They point out that being uninsured in the United States does not mean being denied all access to care, and conversely that being covered by public insurance in other countries does not mean that all have equal access to care.

As discussed in chapter 1, it is true that Americans who are uninsured do not lack all access to health care. We do have an extensive, although inadequate and threatened, safety net in this country, consisting of community and migrant health centers, free and often faith-based clinics, public hospitals, hospital outpatient departments, state mental hospitals, and hospital emergency rooms that provide some level of health care to many of the uninsured (Lewin and Altman eds. 2002). Yet an overwhelming body of evidence shows that the uninsured get less care, get it later when it is of less value, incur greater morbidity, and die younger than the insured (Institute of Medicine 2002b). Uninsurance is also a problem that disproportionately affects minorities, particularly Hispanics and African Americans.[8] One can quibble about how serious a problem lack of health insurance is, but the existence of the problem is undeniable.

How then do other countries fare comparatively? First, no country has achieved complete health equity. Throughout the world, the poor are less healthy than the rich. In England in the late 1980s, four decades after the founding of the National Health Service, the average life expectancy for men in the professional, managerial, and technical occupations was significantly longer than it was for men in unskilled or partly skilled occupations (*Independent Inquiry into Inequalities in Health Report* 1998, 13). Minority groups, and particularly historically subordinated groups like the Maori in New Zealand and aboriginals in Canada, often have worse health statistics than the majority white population (MacMillan, MacMillan, Offord, and Dingle 1996, 1569–78). In a number of countries, moreover, health disparities — for example disparities in mortality rates — are growing, as the health of the affluent and the majority group improves more rapidly than the health of the poor and minorities.[9] Health disparities are a worldwide problem, not simply a problem of the United States.

Variations in access to health care also exist in other countries. Health care resources are often clustered in urban or suburban areas and are less accessible in rural areas (and sometimes inner-city areas) (Barer, Wood, and Schneider 1999; Dunlop, Coyte, and McIssac 2000, 123–33). In some countries health care services are less widely available to the elderly than to younger people (Sutton 1997). In a number of countries deductibles, coinsurance, and co-payments, although usually smaller than those imposed in the United States, are still high enough to deter the poor from seeking health care (Kupor, Liu, Lee, and Yoshikawa 1995; Lexchin and Grootendorst 2004). In all other countries, persons with enough money can buy access to private health care (in the United States if not in their own country), and in virtually all countries the wealthy can also buy private health insurance. For whatever reason, wealthier persons can often get access to better public health care, regardless of the official commitment to equity of access.[10] (van Doorslaer, Masseria, and Koolman 2006).

The simple fact remains, however, that the poor in countries with universal coverage can see a doctor, be hospitalized if necessary, get the medications they need, and in many countries even receive long-term or dental care without having to worry about cost. Though other countries often have user fees for some services, these are usually reasonable in size and are often waived for certain populations — such as pregnant women, children, and people with low incomes — or capped at certain levels to protect the chronically ill.

That the poor receive less medical care in the United States is proven by sophisticated analyses of consumption of medical services conducted by the

OECD Health Equity Research Group.[11] These studies show that in virtually all developed countries, including the United States, poor people see the doctor and are hospitalized more often than wealthier people (though they receive less dental care) (van Doorslaer and Masseria 2004, 14–17). This is simply because the poor are less healthy, and thus need more medical care. If one adjusts for medical condition — comparing persons of equal medical need at different income levels — wealthier persons tend to get more of most medical services than poorer persons do in most countries, though the degree and nature of the disparity varies from country to country. The United States stands out in these comparisons for the starkness of its pro-rich inequalities. Pro-rich inequalities in the likelihood of seeing a doctor for persons of equal medical need are greater in the United States than in any other OECD country, and pro-rich inequalities in the number of doctor visits are greater in the United States than in any other country except for Portugal and Finland (van Doorslaer and Masseria 2004, 69, 70).[12] Also, when the effects of various factors on use of care are further decomposed, it becomes clear that lack of insurance is a significant cause in the United States of shorter hospital stays (although it is less of a factor in discouraging hospital admissions) (van Doorslaer and Masseria 2004, 24). Pro-rich inequalities in the number of dental visits are greater in the United States than in any other country but Portugal. In other words, in most countries the poor do not receive the same amount of medical care as the rich, but in the United States the situation of the poor is clearly worse.

The difficulty that poor Americans face in accessing care is also borne out by a series of six-country comparative studies carried out by the Commonwealth Fund over the past decade. These studies will be discussed in greater depth later in this chapter, as they deal primarily with quality comparisons, but they are also revealing as to access. One study involving adults with health problems in six countries found that patients in the United States were far more likely than patients in other countries to not fill a prescription because of cost, not visit a doctor when sick, or not receive a recommended test or follow-up (Schoen, Osborn, Huynh, Doty, Zapert, Peugh, et al. 2005, W5-519). Another study found that adults of below-average income in the United States ranked last on sixteen of thirty measures of experience with primary care, including access, coordination, and quality-of-care measures. None of the other four countries studied ranked worse on more than six measures (Huynh, Schoen, Osborn, and Holmgren 2006, 22).

Worse access to medical care for poor and uninsured Americans is also confirmed by binational studies. One study found that Canadians had better and more equal access to physicians' services than Americans (Hamilton, Hamilton, and Paarsch 1997). The study also found that this difference was not attributable to race, as both white and nonwhite Americans fared poorly relative to Canadians of similar socio-demographic characteristics. Other studies show that not only do poorer people in the United States receive less health care than poorer people in Canada do, but they also suffer worse health because of it (Lasser, Himmelstein, and Woolhandler 2006; Sanmartin 2006). A series of studies examining cancer survival rates in paired cities in the United States and Canada found them to be significantly better for low-income persons in Canada than in the United States (Gorey, Holowary, Fehringer, Laukkanen, Moskowitz, Webster, et al. 1997; Gorey, Holowary, Fehringer, Laukkanen, Richter, and Meyer 2000, 343–48). Yet another study comparing hospitalization for "avoidable hospital conditions (AHCs)" — conditions that result in hospitalization but could have been avoided through adequate primary care — found that age-adjusted AHC rates were 2.5 times as high in Manhattan as in Paris and varied much more significantly between lower- and higher-income neighborhoods in Manhattan than in Paris, mirroring the results of the studies comparing the United States and Canada (Gusmano, Rodwin, and Weisz 2006, 518–19). Finally, a recent study comparing the health of late-middle-age, non-Hispanic whites in the United States and England, using biologic markers as well as self-reported status, found the English to be significantly healthier than the Americans, across income gradients (Banks, Marmot, Oldfield, and Smith 2006). Worse access to health care in the United States is clearly correlated with worse health.

Other Countries Ration Health Care Resources Differently

Access to health care is not only an issue for the poor. CDHC advocates argue that even if public health insurance systems provide better access for the poor than market-driven health care systems do, they provide worse access for everyone else. If health care resources are not unlimited, and if they are not allocated on the basis of willingness (and thus ability) to pay, they must be allocated on some other basis — they will have to be rationed. The primary and oft-repeated argument against other health care systems, therefore, is that they ration health care, denying health care to some people.

Note that CDHC advocates cannot make this argument — public insurance systems ration or fail to provide "necessary" health care — without contradicting themselves. A basic principle of CDHC is that there is no such thing as "need" for health care, only consumer demand, which is determined by the price faced by the consumer and the value that the individual consumer places on the particular product or service. Nor can CDHC advocates argue that countries with public insurance systems deny their citizens the right to purchase health care. Countries with public insurance programs allow their residents to purchase health care privately if they choose to do so, in another country if necessary but usually in their own, and most countries also allow people who want it to purchase private insurance (Mossialos and Thompson 2004).[13] Rather, the CDHC argument must be that public determinations of insurance coverage, price controls, and budgets distort the patterns of supply and demand that would otherwise exist, and thus make it more difficult for some persons to purchase care they would otherwise demand and for providers to provide goods and services that they would otherwise supply (including technological innovations that they would otherwise create or adopt). CDHC advocates often, however, seem to be arguing instead that rationing denies needed health care outright (Goodman, Musgrave, and Herrick 2004, 17–24).

In no country, including the United States, do all persons receive all the health care that they either want or could benefit from. There is also every indication that in all countries some health care is provided that is of very little benefit to those who receive it. In a few countries, including the United States, health care is primarily allocated on the basis of ability to pay, although even in the United States a great deal of health care is available to persons who have little ability to pay, and some forms of health care, most notably implantable organs, are not primarily distributed on the basis of ability to pay. In most countries health care resources are distributed primarily on the basis of other criteria, though rarely is wealth completely irrelevant.

The primary tool that public insurance systems use to control costs is control of the expenditure of funds. Sometimes, as in the United Kingdom, the budgetary process is explicit and visible. The Department of Health establishes a budget adopted by Parliament for the NHS, which budget is then allocated among the various units of the NHS to provide for health care services. Budgets are more complicated in federal systems. In Canada, for example, the health care system operates at the provincial level, so the budget consists of both federal and provincial allocations for health care goods and services, and is harder to track. Countries that employ the social insurance model are less likely to have a national health care budget, but the level of insurance premiums may be controlled by law, as in Germany, where increases in premiums cannot exceed increases in wages. Social insurers, in turn, negotiate budgets with providers, but these budgets are often specific to one sector or institution. There is no "global" budget, and thus costs are not as carefully controlled. In most public systems costs are ultimately controlled at the level of the provider or local health care purchasing agency. Whether or not this results in shortages or in denial of access to new technologies — in "rationing" — depends a great deal on both the level of expenditures and the organization of the delivery system.

Given that the United States spends far more per capita on health care than other countries do, and that within the United States the distribution of health care expenditures is unequal (with wealthy, fully insured Americans spending more on health care than poor, uninsured Americans in equivalent health), it would be remarkable if wealthy Americans did not receive some additional benefit from their expenditures. One result of our higher level of health care spending is that we enjoy amenities that are rare in other countries. Private rooms are common in American hospitals, and hospital rooms rarely have more than two occupants. In many other countries private rooms are rare, or cost extra, while rooms with more than two occupants are not at all uncommon. Hospitals and clinics in other countries often look worn and frayed, even dirty, compared to the shiny new palaces in which Americans receive health care. Except in the most remote rural areas, Americans rarely have to travel any distance for access to sophisticated diagnostic and treatment technologies that would only be available in regional centers in other countries. We also get the benefit of the most lavishly paid health care professionals and managers in the world. But in what way do our higher expenditures benefit patients?

One benefit is that insured patients in the United States do not have to wait for services in queues to the same extent that citizens of some other countries do. But many Americans have a distorted view of rationing. The two countries with health care systems most visible to Americans, England and Canada, are two of the countries in which, for a variety of reasons, rationing has also been most visible. Quite a number of OECD countries, including Germany, Austria, France, Switzerland, and Japan, do not experience waiting lists as a problem (Siciliani and Hurst 2003). Even within those countries that do experience rationing as a problem, rationing is usually focused on particular procedures and types of providers. Surveys reveal that residents of the UK, Australia, and Canada are more likely than residents of the United States to be able to see a primary-care doctor on the same day that they seek one, although residents of the United States have more prompt access to specialists (Schoen, Osborn, Huynh, Doty, Zapert, Peugh, et al. 2005, W5-519).

Nonetheless it is true that the organization of health care delivery and financing in public insurance programs results in patterns of providing health care goods and services dissimilar from those that would result in a pure market system or in a system designed to respond only to medical need, if either were possible. The Japanese health care system, in which physicians are paid primarily on a fee-for-service basis at very low rates, provides a high volume of very short patient visits (Campbell and Ikegami 1998, 145–66). The German social insurance system, which also pays physicians on a fee-for-service basis, provides on average faster access to primary-care physicians, specialists, and elective surgery than does the American health care system (Schoen, Osborn, Huynh, Doty, Zapert, Peugh, et al. 2005, W5-519). But countries that spend less on health care, have fewer resources for providing health care, and pay based on salary or limited budgets rather than fee for service, do have to struggle with waiting lists (Siciliani and Hurst 2003).

Where they exist, waiting lists are not primarily a manifestation of frustrated consumer demand but rather of unmet need identified by professional judgment. In the UK a gatekeeping general-practitioner must first decide that a patient needs to see a specialist before the patient can get a consultation. A specialist must next decide that the patient needs surgery before the patient progresses to the hospital waiting list. Waiting lists exist, therefore, not necessarily because of a gap between supply and demand but rather because of a gap between supply and need, as professionally determined. It is very possible that similar gaps between need and supply also exist in other countries, including the United States, but that they are simply not measured. One attempt to quantify the shortfall in the United States between need and supply with respect to denial of treatment of the uninsured and underinsured found that implicit waiting lists in the United States were worse than the explicit lists in the UK (Cullis 1993, 23–29). Doctors in the United States are more likely than doctors in the UK to report that their patients have difficulty affording the care they need, while doctors in the UK are more likely to report shortages of resources, such as the latest medical or diagnostic equipment, or hospital beds (Blendon, Schoen, Donelan, Osborn, DesRoches, Scoles, et al. 2001, 233).

In any event, recent initiatives within the UK have significantly reduced waiting times. After half a century of underinvestment in the NHS, the UK has since 2000 dramatically increased NHS funding, increasing real expenditures at a rate of 7 percent to 8 percent per year (Maynard 2005). This increase in funding has led to dramatic reductions in waiting times. When the new program was initiated many patients had to wait over twelve months for elective procedures, but by 2005 inpatient treatment was available to all within nine months, with a further goal of reducing maximum waits to six months. The mean waiting time for elective surgery has been reduced by 30 percent and the median by 21 percent (Maynard 2005). Waiting times for hip replacements, long a critical problem in the NHS, have been dramatically reduced (Aaron, Schwartz, and Cox 2005, 60). Waiting lists are not an inevitable result of public insurance programs but rather result from inadequate health care expenditures and organizational problems. Waiting for medical care is also not unknown in the United States — in a recent survey 39 percent of American adult respondents reported serious problems in getting prompt medical attention when sick without going to an emergency room (Schoen, Doty, Collins, and Holmgren 2006, 5).

Another benefit that Americans enjoy is more rapid and universal access to new medical technologies as they become available. Most public insurance systems (including the Medicare program in the United States) have institutions and procedures for determining which health care technologies they will cover and which they will not. These programs are increasingly based on scientific evaluations of the effectiveness of new technologies (Jost ed. 2005). In a few countries the cost of technologies is also considered, although even in these countries "breakthrough" technologies that treat otherwise untreatable conditions are likely to be covered regardless of their cost. Rarely is coverage denied for effective technologies. More often coverage is approved only for certain medical problems or in certain specific settings (in the hospital rather than in doctor's office), or if certain guidelines are followed. The primary effect of technology assessment programs seems to be to delay the introduction and diffusion of technologies rather than to bar them altogether. Another effect is to privilege existing technologies over new technologies, since existing technologies are rarely evaluated.

New medical procedures tend to be adopted and diffused more quickly in the United States than in other countries. One study examining the adoption of cardiac catheterization, bypass surgery, and angioplasty showed a consistent pattern in the United States of early adoption of the procedures and rapid growth in their use (Technological Change in Health Care Research Network

2001, 25–42). In other countries — Australia, Belgium, Canada, Italy, Singapore, Switzerland, and Taiwan — the procedures were adopted later, but after adoption the growth in use was rapid. In a few cases — England, Scotland, Finland, and Norway — adoption was late and growth in use was slow, never reaching the use rates of other countries. Rapid adoption of new technologies is not an unmixed blessing. There is recent evidence that the United States may have reached the "flat of the curve" on coronary care. Additional expenditures in the past half-decade have produced little in terms of improved care (Skinner, Staiger, and Fisher 2006).

The UK has historically been quite conservative in its adoption of some technologies. Though renal dialysis is no longer rationed by age as it once seems to have been, it is still not as widely used as in the United States (Aaron, Schwartz, and Cox 2005, 30–44). Coronary revascularization, angioplasty, intensive care units, CT scans, and MRIs are all more widely available and used in the United States than in the UK (Aaron, Schwartz, and Cox 2005, 55–58, 64–76, 79–92). These differences are due to differences in health status (more obesity resulting in more diabetes and need for dialysis in the United States) and approaches to treatment (more conservative in the UK), as well as differences in resource availability (Aaron, Schwartz, and Cox 2005, 39–44, 57, 70–75, 108–30). Higher treatment rates, moreover, do not necessarily result in better outcomes in the United States (Aaron, Schwartz, and Cox 2005, 75–76, 89–92). And with respect to rarer conditions that do not require large capital expenditures, such as hemophilia, treatment patterns are quite similar in the United States and the UK (Aaron, Schwartz, and Cox 2005, 44–50).

Here as elsewhere the tendency to emphasize the UK as a reference country is misleading. A number of countries, including Japan, Switzerland, and Austria, have more MRI and CT scanners per million inhabitants than the United States has (Organization for Economic Cooperation and Development 2005, 46–47). Rates of adoption and diffusion differ by technology, with coronary procedures seemingly an outlier in terms of comparative speed of adoption in the United States. Drug therapy for coronary problems, for example, seems fairly similar in the developed countries (Technological Change in Health Care Research Network 2001, 35–56). A recent eight-country study found that at least 90 percent of 249 drug active ingredients (including most of the new chemical entities recently approved in the United States) were available in all but one of the countries (Danzon and Furukawa 2003, W3-524–W3-525). Finally, with respect to some forms of medical care, the United States lags behind other nations. In 2003 the United States had the fourth-worst diphtheria, tetanus, and pertussis (DTP) immunization rates for young children of any OECD nation (Organization for Economic Cooperation and Development 2005, 51). The United States is also lagging far behind European countries in implementing health care information technology (Anderson, Frogner, Johns, and Reinhardt 2006).

The Quality of Health Care in Other Countries Is as Good as Ours

Ultimately, the most important question is whether our higher expenditures on health care in the United States result in better health outcomes. The final question for this chapter, therefore, is this: How does the quality of health care in the United States compare with quality in other countries?

Some commentators point to the infant mortality and life expectancy rates in the United States, which are quite low by international standards, as evidence of relatively poor health care in the United States.[14] Defenders of the American health care system respond to this argument in two ways. First, they point out that life expectancy and infant mortality are determined largely by factors that have little to do with health care: nutrition; the use of alcohol, drugs, and tobacco; exercise; working conditions; age at pregnancy; and living conditions in general. A second argument is that statistics for the United States are skewed by the inclusion of statistics for minorities, and in particular African Americans, whose life expectancy and infant mortality rates are much worse than those of Americans of European and Asian descent (Goodman, Musgrave, and Herrick 2004, 51–54).

These criticisms are fair. They do not, however, exonerate the American health care system from all responsibility for poor mortality and morbidity rates. There is considerable evidence, for example, that stark racial disparities within our health care system contribute significantly to the much worse health of racial minorities, and thus at least some of the fault for racial disparities in vital statistics must be laid at the feet of the health care system (Institute of Medicine 2002c).

In the last half-decade, fortunately, information has finally been collected that allows us to go beyond vital statistics when comparing the quality of different health systems. In particular, the Commonwealth Fund has assembled data comparing patient satisfaction and outcomes of care for five or six countries, including the United States. One of these studies, published in 2005, looked at quality of care as experienced by patients with health problems in six countries (Schoen, Osborn, Huynh, Doty, Zapert, Peugh, et al 2005, W5-509–W5-525). This study found that patients in the United States were more likely than patients in the other countries to have experienced unsatisfactory pain control in the hospital, to have recognized a medical mistake made in their treatment, to have been given an incorrect diagnostic or laboratory test or experienced delay in getting lab results, to have been without a regular doctor, or not with the same doctor, for the past five years, and to have experienced a failure of medical coordination. On the other hand, patients in the United States were more likely than patients in the other countries to have had their doctors explain risks to them before a procedure or hospitalization. By most quality measures, the experiences of patients in the countries covered by the studies were quite similar. A follow–up study using 2005 data yielded similar results (Davis, Schoen, Schoenbaum, Audet, Doty, Holmgren, et al. 2006).

Another recent study compared the performance of the American health care system with those of four other countries using nineteen process and outcome indicators (such as cancer survival rates, transplant survival rates, and vaccination rates). It found that the United States scored best on three indicators (best breast cancer survival rates, lowest measles incidence rate, and highest cervical cancer screening rate), worst on two (worst kidney transplant survival rates, highest incidence of hepatitis B), and somewhere in the middle on the others (Hussey, Anderson, Osborn, Feek, McLaughlin, Millar, et al. 2004, 89–99). In other words, the quality of health care in the United States is much the same as in other developed countries — other countries can provide universal access at a lower cost without sacrificing quality.

Is There an Alternative?

As critical as CDHC advocates are of the current American health care system, they are even more critical of the "solidarity-based" health care systems of other countries. A fundamental belief of CDHC advocates is that government is incapable of competently governing a health care system. As other developed countries have public insurance systems, by definition they must be inferior to our own system, which, for all of its faults, is still generally private.

As this chapter has demonstrated, however, the health care systems of other countries generally function better than our own. They cost less, and provide better access to health care for the poor, similar access for everyone else, and health care of comparable quality. None of them rely on a consumer-driven approach. Rather, all rely on government to control costs and assure access. They offer, therefore, an alternative — perhaps a superior alternative — to CDHC. We now turn to the most important question: how we should fix our broken American health care system.

CHAPTER 11

How to Fix Our Broken Health Care System: Where Do We Start?

The primary message of this book is that the uncomplicated world of CDHC advocates is not our world. The reality of the American health care system, as revealed through historical, economic, ethical, and empirical inquiry, cannot be comprehended by the simple stories that they tell. The problems that afflict our health care system are not all attributable to moral hazard. They will not be solved by simply shifting costs to consumers. International experience amply confirms this. Other nations have achieved universal access to health care of high quality, at lower costs, without relying extensively on cost sharing. This is not to say that CDHC advocates lack useful insights, and it certainly does not argue against empowering consumers to play a more significant role in our health care system. It does mean that on the whole we will need to look elsewhere to solve the problems of our health care system.

In the Preface I described the basic issues that must be addressed in designing a health care financing system. The first is the skewed distribution of health care costs — in any given year a small minority of the population consumes a large proportion of all health care. Conversely, most of the population uses virtually no health care. The cost of health care consumed by the most expensive portion of the population, moreover, is unaffordable by all but a very small minority of the wealthiest Americans. Health insurance is therefore necessary to assure access to health care. This fact is uncontroversial: every developed nation has some form of health insurance, and even the most ardent CDHC advocates recognize the necessity of at least catastrophic insurance.

The most important problem that must be confronted in designing a health care system is not skewed health care costs. Rather it is the problem of unaffordability. It is not simply that health care is unaffordable for the few who experience catastrophic costs — insurance can take care of that. It is rather that health insurance is unaffordable for many. Not only are health care costs skewed, but income and wealth are skewed as well. In 2004 the average employment-related family health insurance policy cost $9,950 (Kaiser Family Foundation / Health Research and Educational Trust 2004, 2). In 2004 the median household income in the United States was $44,684 (Fronczek 2005, 2). The earnings of 48.5 percent of Americans were at or below 300 percent of the poverty level ($14,974 for a family of three), while 31.2 percent of American families earned less than 200 percent of the poverty level (U.S. Bureau of the Census 2005). In 2006 the cost of the average employment-related family health insurance policy increased to $11,480, 7.7 percent greater than the cost a year earlier, while workers' earnings rose only 3.8 percent (Kaiser Family Foundation / Health Research and Educational Trust 2006, 1). Health insurance is increasingly becoming unaffordable to many Americans.

Nongroup insurance policies are less expensive than employment-related group policies, particularly for young and healthy families (Kaiser Family Foundation / eHealthInsurance 2004, 5). They impose higher cost-sharing obligations, however, and offer fewer benefits. Low-income Americans already pay a much higher proportion of their income for health care cost sharing than wealthier Americans do, and shifting more costs to poorer Americans will result, as previous chapters have demonstrated, in greater financial distress and worse health outcomes (Merlis, Gould, and Mahato 2006, 5–6).

All other developed countries address the problem of skewed income distribution by shifting health care costs from those less able to pay to those more able to pay. This would certainly be possible in the United States. In 2003 the top fifth of American households had average incomes of $138,500 (Shapiro and Friedman 2006, 2). The top 1 percent had average incomes of $701,500. In 2004 the top 1 percent of the population garnered 19.5 percent of the nation's pretax income.[1]

These resources are largely ignored when it comes to paying for health care. Health care in the United States is financed by employers' contributions toward premiums (which result in commensurate reductions in wages), by direct employee contributions (or direct payment of premiums in the nongroup market), and by regressive payroll taxes (which pay for Medicare Part A). We have one of the most regressive approaches to financing of any country in the world (Wagstaff and van Doorslaer 2000). This system has resulted in a steady decline in the number of Americans covered by employment-based insurance; individual and family financial crises among the uninsured and underinsured; massive cost shifting by health care institutions as they try to cover the costs of the uninsured; and continual fiscal crises at the federal and state level as government attempts to cover those who cannot be covered by the private market (Institute of Medicine 2003b).

CDHC advocates identify the central problem of our health care system as moral hazard: the excessive consumption of health care products and services because of excessive insurance. There is substantial evidence of waste and overuse of products and services in the American health care system. There is also some evidence that people with CDHC coverage spend less on health care and are more selective in their purchasing decisions. On the other hand, there is also evidence that HDHPs cause low-income families to forgo necessary health care and to suffer financial distress, and that many who have HDHPs do not also have funded HSAs to cushion the burden of increased cost sharing. Most developed health care systems do include some element of cost sharing, but most also recognize that cost sharing must be limited if it is not to result in denying access to health care for persons with limited resources.

The final major issue identified in the Preface in designing a health care system is the organization of a system of providers and the means to pay them. There are many possible approaches, and the approach chosen will to a considerable extent depend on how health care is financed. The issue of health care organization and payment will therefore be discussed simultaneously with the design of a health care finance system.

Different Solutions for Different Problems

There is little point in discussing alternative health care systems that do not have any chance of political success in the United States. Any health care system that will be politically acceptable in the United States will have to include a primary role for private enterprise. The health care systems of all developed nations rely on private provision of health care to at least some extent. But in the United States not only private provision but also some role for private health insurance seems to be a political necessity. This is unfortunate, as government administration of health care finance seems to be an important factor in controlling costs in other countries, and our most successful health care system—the Veterans Health Administration—is a government-run system (Mahar 2006, 257–64). But Americans have a strong preference for private markets and are particularly unlikely to accept government provision of health care (Blendon, Benson, and DesRoches 2003, W3-405, W3-408–W3-409).[2] As a practical matter, the private health insurance lobby is very powerful in the United States, and elimination of private health insurance is a political impossibility.

Yet government must play a major role in any system of health care finance. Government is the largest and most efficient risk spreader, and thus has the greatest capacity to spread the most expensive health care risks. More importantly, only government is capable of redistributing income: markets simply cannot do this. Government must therefore take responsibility for assuring that health care is affordable to those who cannot otherwise afford it.

Market competition should be used to bring down costs and improve quality where competition is feasible. But as demonstrated in chapter 10, public budgets have been shown to be very effective in other countries for controlling health care costs and should be used where they can be, particularly for government programs. While public regulation is needed to assure quality, professional oversight should also be encouraged to assist with quality improvement. What we need, that is to say, is a mix of public and private solutions.

Fortunately, we have a number of models for achieving a mix of governmental and private risk bearing. The recently adopted Medicare prescription drug program offers one such model.[3] The recent attempt by the state of Massachusetts to reduce the number of uninsured also provides a mixed public-private solution. The experience of other health care systems that mix public and private insurance, such as the Dutch, German, and Australian systems, can also assist us (Jost 2001, 450–63). The Dutch system is of particular interest, because it divides responsibility between public and private insurance in part based on the nature of the risk borne (Jost 2001, 460–63).[4]

First, in a reformed health care system, as with the Dutch system and the new Medicare drug benefit, catastrophic risk should be assumed by the government. This can be done in at least two ways. The approach taken in the Netherlands is to designate for government financing those extraordinarily expensive products and services that are least affordable by the population generally and that constitute a high proportion of the costs borne by those whose health care is most expensive: long-term skilled nursing facility care, hospitalizations that last more than a specified period, inpatient mental health care, and certain specific very expensive medical procedures, drugs, and devices (such as organ transplants and chemotherapy agents).[5] An alternative that has recently received increased attention is government reinsurance of the highest-cost individuals, the approach taken by the Medicare Part D drug program.[6] Once the costs of a particular individual passed a given threshold—for example $50,000—a government reinsurance program would take over (Swartz 2006; Jacobi 2005) Either approach would shift the highest risks—those risks least likely to be bearable by particularly vulnerable groups—to the risk bearer with the greatest financial resources and the greatest ability to spread risk most broadly. The government already insures bank accounts and home loans and provides insurance against natural catastrophes, and providing catastrophic coverage to health care seems like a natural extension.

Second, at the other end of the spectrum, cosmetic procedures and "lifestyle care"[7] should be financed privately, either out of pocket or through a private insurance market, should one develop. Most public and private insurance programs, not only in the United States but also in other countries, already take this approach. Market competition seems to have been quite successful in bringing down the cost of cosmetic procedures—which can be priced much more easily as discrete procedures than diagnostic and therapeutic interventions can, and are usually sought by a clientele with the money to afford them. Insurers seem able to distinguish between reconstructive surgery to correct cleft palates or other abnormal disfiguring conditions, which they cover, and cosmetic breast enlargement or wrinkle removal to improve normal appearance, which they do not.

Third, low-cost payment for predictable items and services could also remain the private responsibility of persons who have adequate means to cover these costs. Expenditures for eyeglasses, routine dental checkups and care, and most over-the-counter drugs, for example, are relatively predictable and affordable.[8] It would probably also make sense to pay for a limited number of visits to physicians for routine primary care—say the first three or four per year. This could alternatively be handled through a modest deductible, in the range of $300 to $500, for all but low-income families. These low-cost events are where the RAND HIE found the greatest savings to be had from cost sharing.

There is also little reason to incur the additional costs of billing and claims processing when routine, low-cost products and procedures are involved.[9]

Optometrists, opticians, and purveyors of over-the-counter drugs already advertise their prices, and dentists and primary care physicians should follow suit. All professionals and providers should be required to list their prices on a publicly provided internet site for a set list of routine services, to allow easy comparison shopping.[10] As insurers would pay no more than these published prices for professional services,[11] direct competition by providers for patients might bring down insurance prices as well (though it is likely that insurers would continue to get better prices from providers than private individuals can, because insurers purchase in volume). Competition among health care professionals would begin to look more like the competition that now exists among lawyers for providing routine services, such as bankruptcies, divorces, and real estate closings.

An exception should be made for the obligation to cover routine, low-cost services for persons with very low incomes, for whom even these expenses should be covered. For those under 135 percent of the poverty level, a government program should cover these costs.[12] The program should also cover these costs for those with incomes between 135 percent and 200 percent of poverty, although these beneficiaries could bear nominal cost-sharing obligations.[13] People with this little income would be unduly burdened by the cost of these basic services, and there is little to be gained by causing them to forgo basic primary dental or medical care, which might cause them to require more expensive care later or make it difficult for them to participate in the workforce.[14] The byzantine eligibility requirements of the Medicaid program, which make eligibility turn on characteristics wholly unrelated to need, should be removed.

Fourth, a basic set of preventive services should be available to all, financed by a public program, regardless of ability to pay. This should include immunizations, preventive screenings, well-baby physicals, prenatal care, and periodic physicals for older people. Preventive services are already covered by Medicare and for low-income children through the Medicaid Early Periodic Screening, Diagnosis and Treatment (EPSDT) program. Preventive services already need not be subject to the HDHP deductible under the federal law.[15] They are also covered by many tax-subsidized employment-related health insurance plans. This provision would merely spread government assistance for preventive care to the rest of the population.

Fifth, there is everything else — most acute care, most care for the management of chronic conditions that does not result in long-term care or hospitalization (including outpatient mental health care), most prescription drugs and durable medical equipment, and various therapies. These products and services should be covered by insurance. Everyone should be required by law to carry this insurance, just as all but three states now require everyone who owns a car to carry liability insurance. Just as car owners cannot shift the cost of accidents to their victims by refusing to carry liability insurance, persons who can afford health insurance should not be able to shift the cost of the medical care they might need to society by refusing to carry health insurance.

Employers should be encouraged to continue to provide health insurance as an employment benefit, either by self-insuring or by purchasing insurance for their employees. As the administrators of the Blue Cross plans discovered in the 1930s, considerable savings in marketing, underwriting, and administrative costs can be achieved by providing insurance to groups that form for reasons unrelated to health care needs, and employee groups are well suited to this end.

Individuals and families could also buy insurance in the nongroup insurance market. Insurers should be required to accept all applicants and to price their plans by using community rating, which should save underwriting costs. Because insurance would no longer cover catastrophic costs, and because it would also not have to cover low-cost but widely used routine services, it should be much more affordable than it is now. The risks that it covers should also be much more predictable, greatly reducing the threat to insurers posed by adverse selection (and reducing the cost of the insurance). Nongroup insurance could continue to be regulated by the states or could be regulated under federal solvency, capitalization, and claims practices standards that would meet current guidelines of the National Association of Insurance Commissioners (NAIC).

The federal government should offer its own insurance plan (as could perhaps state governments), which would compete with employer-provided and individual insurance. The plan should be run by an independent federal corporation and should be self-financing from premiums.[16] If the government could not compete against private insurers, the government program would cease to exist. But if it had lower administrative costs than private insurers, it could introduce real efficiency-based competition into insurance markets.

Each plan should be required to cover all necessary and non-experimental health care that did not fall into the four other categories of care discussed above. Plans should be allowed to use drug formularies as long as all categories and classes of necessary drugs were covered. New products and services, as well as questionable existing products and services, should be subject to rigorous technology assessment.[17] Products and services found to be ineffective or not effective enough in relation to their cost should not be covered by the public program. Private programs could cover them, but probably at higher premiums. Noncoverage determinations should be explicit, transparent, and not subject to change unless all insureds in a plan were given ninety days' notice and the opportunity to change to another plan. Plans could also engage in utilization review, but subject (as is usually the case now) to internal and external appeal procedures (Berman-Sandler 2004, 237–75).

Private plans could form provider networks, and plans with leaner networks could presumably offer lower prices. The plans would need to fully disclose, however, the limits of their networks, as well as cover specialists competent to provide all necessary services. Private plans could offer additional coverage — for example lifestyle treatments, or coverage of low-cost and predictable services with an additional premium.

Data should be collected on the risk distribution among various plans. If, as is likely, the government plan ended up with a significantly worse risk distribution than the other plans, it could be subsidized from tax revenues as necessary to compensate for this adverse risk selection. People who wanted a richer benefit package could pay more for a more generous private plan, while those willing to live with more constrained provider networks could also choose cheaper private plans, if any were offered.

Finally, cost sharing should be used to ensure that consumers are made sensitive to health care costs where this makes sense. For example, tiered pharmaceutical plans, which make the insured pay more for non-generic drugs and for therapeutically equivalent brand-name drugs whose manufacturers refuse to offer discounts to insurers, have shown success in controlling health care costs without adverse health consequences, and could continue under the new plan (Motheral and Fairman 2001, 1299). Reasonable co-payments for physician visits might be appropriate to discourage excessive use. Higher co-payments might be useful for emergency room visits to discourage the use of the emergency room for primary care. Plans would have to have reasonable out-of-pocket maximums, however, based on household income. Deductibles should not be permitted, since the exclusion of coverage for low-cost services effectively serves as a deductible.

Cost sharing should not be imposed in situations where it is inappropriate to create an economic disincentive for the use of care. The patient is rarely the decision maker with respect to hospitalization, for example, and therefore a financial disincentive for hospitalization is inappropriate.[18] Where a patient is receiving a generic pharmaceutical or a preferred brand-name pharmaceutical to manage a chronic disease, a financial disincentive is inappropriate, because care should not be discouraged where lack of that care might seriously threaten health or increase costs later. It may make sense, therefore, to exclude certain maintenance drugs from cost sharing.

While this approach to insurance would guarantee that everyone was insured, steps would still need to be taken to make this insurance affordable to all. Everyone whose income fell below 135 percent of the poverty level (including most Medicaid recipients) should receive a voucher from the federal government equal to the cost of the government insurance plan. Those whose incomes were between 135 percent and 300 percent of the poverty level should receive a voucher of diminishing value designed to make sure that no one would need to pay more than 10 percent of his or her income for health care.[19] Finally, those persons who would have otherwise been eligible for Medicare should be covered by the government program (unless they opted for a private plan), but would need to pay what they would otherwise have paid for Part B and D premiums. Tax subsidies for health insurance for the wealthy should end, as CDHP advocates have long contended.

The approach described above would extend health insurance to all Americans. It would accomplish this by addressing the problems of both risk and affordability, while still preserving a role for private initiative and consumer responsibility. It would also have great promise for controlling costs.

The payment of providers should be handled differently, depending on the kind of services they provided. The government catastrophic care program would deal primarily with institutional providers, which it could pay on an administered price basis, as they are paid now by Medicare and Medicaid. Alternatively, the government could negotiate budgets with providers (as payers do in the German system) or purchase blocks of services from providers who provide care most efficiently or care of the highest quality (Jost 2001, 243–48). The government preventive care program could also negotiate prices, perhaps through a competitive bidding process. Vaccines and screening tests, for example, could be bought in quantity from the lowest bidder who could provide services of acceptable quality, or from the provider who provided services of the highest quality. The government acute care insurance company would probably pay for services on an administered price basis. Private providers would not be required to participate in the public program, and prices would have to be set high enough that they would participate voluntarily. Private insurance programs would negotiate fees, as they do now. Low-cost, high-frequency services would mostly be paid out of pocket, based on advertised prices.

Government payment policies, as well as government technology assessment programs, must be to the greatest extent possible be freed from political pressure. One of the greatest weaknesses of the current Medicare system is the extent to which payment and coverage decisions are driven by interest group politics (Vladeck 1999). This tendency dramatically increases the cost of the program to the disadvantage of taxpayers. Some other countries have achieved more success in controlling costs and in controlling the introduction of technologies that are not cost-effective by using processes based more on expertise or on direct negotiations with interest groups and less on political influence (Jost ed. 2005).

This proposal takes advantage of the government's ability to control costs, proven throughout the world, but also of both managed competition and consumer-driven market strategies. The government program would be competing for business with private insurers, and if it set the prices that it paid providers too high, or was unable to control fraud and abuse, it would have to raise premiums and would lose members to the private plans. Alternatively, if the government program set the prices that it paid providers too low, and was unable to attract providers of high quality, it would also lose market share to private insurers. But if, as would be most likely, it was able to underprice private insurers without sacrificing quality (as Medicare now is), it would set an example for the private sector to follow. Competition between public and private insurance programs would keep both in check.

If cost control succeeded, a number of powerful interests would be very unhappy. One person's cost is another's income or profit (Evans 1990, 117). If health care cost containment were ever successfully implemented in the United States, doctors, hospitals, health insurers, and drug companies could be counted on to whine about their loss of income, and about the threat that this would pose to the nation's health. One need not be too cynical to be suspicious of the support that these providers offer for CDHC. Do they really believe that it will cut into their incomes?

In other countries, health care professionals earn far less than they do in the United States when their income is compared to the income of the average worker, and somehow they manage to get by. Intelligent and competent women and men continue to be attracted to the health care professions, which still offer above-average compensation as well as interesting, challenging, and rewarding work. There is no reason why health care providers, as opposed to other providers of goods and services, should be entitled to income protection not extended to others in the economy.

Actually, limiting the growth in health care costs would likely have an impact on the nation's economy. Health care is one of the few things that are still predominantly produced domestically in the United States, and growth in the health care sector has been one of the primary engines of job creation in our country.[20] Imposing serious constraints on the growth of health care costs would likely take a toll on job growth. But to the extent that we pay excessively high prices for health care, decreasing those prices could allow us to move investment to sectors of the economy where that money could be used more productively. And cutting the costs paid by employers for health insurance benefits (and thus the cost of compensation for workers) would be likely to promote job growth, at least in the short run. In any event, we should not allow health care to consume an ever-greater share of our national income unless we actually prefer to spend money on it rather than on other goods and services. The plan proposed here would allow us to make both political decisions as to how much we want to spend as a nation and personal decisions as to how much we want to spend as individuals on health care.

To facilitate that political choice, and also to assure that the costs of health care are borne broadly and progressively, the cost of the government programs should be financed through a broad-based tax such as the income tax, rather than by a narrow and regressive payroll tax. The tax should be earmarked for health care (as the Medicare payroll tax is now) — either through a percentage surcharge on the income tax or through the creation of an independent tax — to make the health care spending visible and transparent. Alternatively, a value-added consumption tax could be used to finance health care if one could be designed that was not wholly regressive. Polls show that a substantial majority of Americans prefer increased government spending that would make health care available to all over further tax cuts, and a significant minority (43 percent) would even support substantial tax increases for this purpose (Blendon, Benson, and DesRoches 2003, W3-410). It should therefore be possible to raise enough money in this way to fund the program, as long as the additional funds in fact went to purchase health care.

The proposed program could also be structured to address our problems of quality of care and medical error. Current licensing, accreditation, certification, institutional regulation, and drug and device approval and monitoring programs should continue in place, and be continually improved, until better means of assuring institutional competence are discovered. Both public and private insurers should be encouraged to experiment with pay-for-performance approaches to paying providers. Maintaining a diversity of payers for most services should facilitate experimentation in this area. The creation of databases that might permit competition on the basis of quality should also be encouraged to allow comparative shopping for services, and reliable comparative information on quality, as it emerges, should be made available on the internet sites where providers would post price information. This competition should encourage providers to specialize and to become better at doing what they do best. This proposal would also be compatible with the formation of multi-specialty groups, which have been widely identified since the days of the Costs of Medical Care study as a means to improve the quality of health care. Further, a national and uniform system of health insurance should be used to facilitate the adoption of electronic patient records and reminder systems. Most importantly, the federal government should devote significant funding to identifying the best clinical practices, and should publish the resulting information on internet sites to which the public and all providers would have access. What is needed, in sum, is to pursue a variety of potential approaches, including but by no means limited to providing comparative information to consumers — the CDHC strategy.

Getting It Done

Now comes the hard part — getting the proposal adopted into law. It is difficult to interpret the presidential election of 2004 (or even the congressional elections of 2006) as a ringing endorsement of a national health insurance program. In fact, it is likely that over the next few years our health care system will continue to deteriorate in all respects. The well-funded chorus of CDHC advocates may continue to drown out the voices of CDHC skeptics. We are likely to see an expansion of CDHPs, as employers, ever more frustrated with their inability to control increases in health insurance premiums, try to shift more of the cost to employees (Gabel, Whitmore, Rice, and Lo Sasso 2004, W4-215–W4-217). These plans may well include HSAs, HRAS, or some yet-to-be-designed mechanism for providing tax subsidies for health benefit plans with high cost-sharing obligations. Additional tax credit schemes will probably make it through Congress, possibly aimed at relatively low-income uninsureds. The amount of these credits will probably be too low to offer much help to those who are really poor, but their existence may well induce even more employers to drop coverage. Congress may, by adopting partial solutions, do serious damage to our employment-based health insurance system, which has made our lack of a universal public health insurance system at least tolerable.

As this is taking place, our public insurance system may also deteriorate. The president is likely to try cutting back further on Medicaid entitlements, as was done in the Deficit Reduction Act of 2005 (Kaiser Commission on Medicaid and the Uninsured 2006). If the states cut back on their increasingly unaffordable Medicaid benefits, which is particularly likely if we slide back into recession, the number of uninsured will continue to increase. Hospitals may for a time be able to continue caring for the uninsured through their uncompensated care programs, but this cannot go on forever. Pressure will mount on Congress to repeal EMTALA, pressure to which it may at some point succumb.

In the meantime, health care costs will continue to soar, as the Medicare drug program continues to be implemented, as billions of dollars are dumped into the Medicare Advantage program to subsidize uncompetitive private plans (Biles, Nicholas, Cooper, Adrion, and Guterman 2006), as employers continue to abandon the business of controlling costs, and as some consumers, because of CDHPs, pay retail rather than wholesale prices for provider services. By the next presidential election, we will in all likelihood have several million more Americans uninsured and health care costs that consume far more of the gross domestic product than they do now.[21]

When all else fails, we might try the obvious: learning from the experience of other nations. Of course that experience is mixed, but it tends to show that in this one particular corner of the economy, government often outperforms the private sector. We could, and should, join the rest of the world in making public health insurance available to all. To move in that direction, several things need to happen. First, a way must be found to get the news media to pay attention to reasoned voices on health policy. For years, right-wing advocacy centers have steadily and loudly beat the drum for their market-oriented solutions to our health care problems. The media have been hearing this drum beat for so long that they have begun to march to it — either accepting the positions of the right as truth or at least seeing them as valid positions that must be presented in every debate and at most need to be balanced occasionally with differing perspectives. Some media sources can be counted on to present negative and misleading caricatures of the health care systems of other nations. Few Americans realize, for example, that other nations offer quicker access to primary care than the United States does, or have more sophisticated health information systems. Supporters of a national health policy need to be loud and insistent. They need to get out accurate information on how health care systems actually function in other nations and why market-based solutions are not the entire answer to all of our problems.

When the time comes, perhaps in 2008, perhaps in 2012, to again move forward on health reform, progress may need to be made incrementally. The Medicare drug bill demonstrates that America still has a commitment to insuring the elderly, just as the State Children's Health Insurance Program (SCHIP), established in 1997, showed that we have a commitment to covering poor children. Public coverage still continues to expand as private coverage contracts (Cohen and Martinez 2006, 10). Perhaps catastrophic coverage for all or comprehensive coverage for children can come next. Alternatively, there may come a point when so many middle-class Americans (or their adult children) are uninsured that the "path dependency" responsible for deterring us from national health insurance will lose its grip.

One barrier that will certainly have to be overcome is the opposition of interest groups that profit from the current system — insurers, small businesses, the pharmaceutical companies, and organized medicine. It is these interests that were largely responsible for killing President Clinton's plan and all attempts before it to bring about universal coverage (Laham 1996, 205–11; Quadagno 2005). As the situation of the health care system becomes more dire, however, some of these interests may conclude that they have more to gain than to lose by supporting a national health program. Accommodating these interests within the program, as Medicare did in using insurers to process claims, might make the reform more palatable to them. But if interest groups continue to oppose reform, members of Congress may ultimately have to listen to their constituents rather than to these obstructionist interest groups.

One of the biggest problems that we will face when the time comes to adopt a new program will be the problem of cost. The program proposed in this book will certainly require billions of additional public dollars. How many is difficult to say, although the catastrophic coverage program proposed here would have covered the $45.9 billion that the private sector spent on nursing home care in 2005, and much of the $264.5 billion spent by the private sector on hospital care in that year (Catlin, Cowan, Heffler, Washington, and National

Health Accounts Team 2007, 150). It is important to understand, however, that government money spent on the program would not all be new money. The government currently spends over $208 billion dollars a year in tax subsidies for private insurance (Selden and Gray 2006), and the president seems eager to spend more by creating new tax subsidies. The Medicaid program spends over $300 billion on caring for the poor, much of which already goes for nursing home care and care of the chronically ill.[22] The Medicare and Medicaid programs already spend billions of dollars to cover the costs of the uninsured through disproportionate-share hospital payments and medical education cost subsidies (Institute of Medicine 2003a, 54). Bankruptcies shift yet more of the cost of caring for the poor to uncompensated providers, who ultimately try to shift those costs to their patients and insurers. All these subsidies and cost-shifting efforts would be eliminated by universal coverage. Moreover, the cost to government of the new program would not even all be tax money. Much of the cost of the acute care government insurance program would be financed by premiums collected from persons who chose to participate in the program.

The plan could also result in some savings. A recent report by the Institute of Medicine on the cost of uninsurance in America concluded that "the aggregate, annualized cost of the diminished health and shorter life spans of Americans who lack health insurance is between $65 and $130 billion for each year of health insurance foregone" (Institute of Medicine 2004, 58). The cost-control provisions of the proposed plan should also reduce its additional cost. A recent study estimated that the implementation of fully standardized health care information exchange and interoperability could save our health care system $77.8 billion a year (Walker, Pan, Johnston, Adler-Milstein, Bates, and Middleton 2005, w5–w10). It would be much easier to implement such a system with the rationalization of our health insurance system that this book proposes.

But it cannot be denied that the total cost of health care will continue to rise for the foreseeable future, and under this proposal, the proportion of that cost borne by Americans as taxpayers rather than by Americans as private citizens would grow as well. Still, this is a cost we can bear. Assuming that our national productivity continues to increase as it has over much of the past century, we are essentially looking at devoting to health care a growing share of an ever-expanding pie. Between 1970 and 2005 the proportion of the GDP spent on health care grew from 7.2 percent to 16 percent (Catlin, Cowan, Heffler,

Washington, and National Health Accounts Team 2007). But over that same period, the real GDP grew from $3.77 trillion to $11.05 trillion in constant (2000) dollars. Even if the proportion of GDP that we spend on health care keeps growing, and more of this money is tax money, we will still have on average far more private money two or three decades from now than we do now to spend on the future equivalent of SUVs, exotic coffees, video games, or whatever happens to be in fashion at the time, and still be able to pay for health care.[23]

The question is ultimately not whether we can afford to provide health care for all. The question is not even, as I hope this book has demonstrated, whether it is possible to find a way to do this. The question is rather whether we want to do it. If we want to, we can.

Preface

1. CDHC advocates also support other approaches to reforming health care finance, such as tiered networks, tiered pharmacy benefits, and providing more information to consumers. Since these reforms are also consistent with other approaches, including managed competition and even a universal public insurance program (reference drug pricing is commonly used in European systems), they are not the focus of this book.

2. Internal Revenue Code 223.

3. Early in the twentieth century when medical costs were still very low by contemporary standards, attempts were made to finance health care through borrowing, but even at that time they were largely unsuccessful. See chapter 4.

Chapter 1: Our Broken American Health Care System

1. The Centers for Disease Control provides an alternative count of the number of uninsured based on the National Health Interview Survey. In 2005 the CDC determined that 41.2 million Americans were uninsured at any one time while 51.3 million had been uninsured at one point during the preceding year. The CDC count indicates that the number of uninsured has decreased over the past two years, because even though private insurance coverage has declined, public insurance coverage, particularly of children, has grown more rapidly (Cohen and Martinez 2006, 1, 3).

2. The most important factors causing the decline in employer-sponsored coverage are loss of employment and declining "job quality," i.e. the shift of employment to lower-wage jobs or jobs in smaller firms or in sectors of the economy less likely to offer insurance (Reschovsky, Strunk, and Ginsburg 2006).

3. For a more thorough analysis of the period from 1996 to 1999 see Short and Graefe 2003.

4. This is because many unemployed Americans—the elderly, the disabled, and children—are covered by public insurance programs.

5. During 2005 only 80 percent of employees who worked for employers that offered coverage were eligible for coverage, and only 83 percent of those who were eligible took up coverage; therefore over a third of workers employed by firms that offered coverage were not actually covered (Kaiser Family Foundation 2005a).

6. Employee's contributions averaged $226 a month for family coverage in 2005 (Fronstin 2006b, 4, 6).

7. 32.7 percent of Hispanics are uninsured, as are 30.6 percent of Americans aged 18–24 (DeNavas-Walt, Proctor, and Lee 2006, 22).

8. Families with incomes above 400 percent of the poverty line who are uninsured at some point over a four-year period are most likely to have a single gap of coverage and are rarely uninsured for the entire period (Short and Graefe 2003, 250).

9. See www.Tonik.us.

10. The study by the Institute of Medicine estimated the cost to the United States due to forgone health at between $65 billion and $130 billion a year (Wolman and Miller 2004, 402).

11. There is also evidence, however, that in recent years survival gains with respect to heart disease have stagnated while costs have continued to increase. Expenditure increases do not always result in better health (Skinner, Staiger, and Fisher 2006).

12. The decline in post-retirement health coverage is also attributable to changes in accounting conventions that require employers to recognize liabilities for retirement benefits in their financial statements (Fronstin 2005).

13. The largest proportion of these expenditures, 43 percent, goes for prescription drugs, followed by expenditures for physician services at 26 percent (Kaiser Family Foundation 2006b).

14. See "President Bush Discusses Quality, Affordable Health Care," at http://usinfo.state .gov/usa/s012804.htm (28 January 2004).

15. There is considerable support for "pay for performance" in health care (Berenson 2003; Hyman and Silver 2001). Others believe, however, that pay for performance would be difficult to do well, and may not be a good idea (Vladeck 2003).

16. At best, they may be able to assure that care is of minimal quality (Jost 1995, 858–64).

17. As of 2005, 61 percent of covered workers were enrolled in PPOs, with 21 percent in HMOs and 15 percent in POS plans, compared to 35 percent in PPOs, 31 percent in HMOs, and 24 percent in POS plans a decade earlier in 1996 (Kaiser Family Foundation 2005b).

18. Indeed, Medicaid recipients are more likely to use emergency rooms for care than the uninsured are, a fact only partially explained by health status (Cunningham 2006, 242).

19. Though physicians are the largest source of uncompensated charity care, the proportion of doctors who provide charity care has declined from 76.3 percent in 1996–97 to 68.2 percent in 2004–5 (Cunningham and May 2006, 1).

20. A recent five-country study found that 60 percent of Americans with above-average incomes and 70 percent of Americans with below-average incomes found it very or somewhat difficult to get medical care on nights, weekends, or holidays without going to an emergency room (Huynh, Schoen, Osborn, and Holmgren 2006, x).

21. By contrast, private pharmaceutical companies invested $10.2 billion in research and development in 2001 (National Science Board 2004, 4-16, 4-30).

22. In 2003 pharmaceutical companies spent $25 billion on product promotion, twice the amount they had spent five years earlier (Blue Cross Blue Shield Association 2005, 40).

Chapter 2: The Consumer-Driven Prescription

1. They will also, it is hoped, charge lower prices because they save on administrative costs by not having to deal with insurers (Goodman, Musgrave, and Herrick 2004, 110–11).

2. According to one recent estimate, heart transplants cost from $50,000 to $287,000, averaging $148,000, while liver transplants cost from $66,000 to $367,000, averaging $235,000 ("Transplant" 2004).

3. Health care providers already provided nearly $36 billion in unreimbursed care to the uninsured in 2001 (Institute of Medicine 2003b, 52–53).

4. Health Insurance Portability and Accountability Act, Pub. L. No. 104-191, 301, 110 Stat. 1936, 2037 (1996), codified at I.R.C. 220.

5. Pub. L. No. 105-33, 4006, 111 Stat. 251, 331–34.

6. Too few people signed up for the HIPAA demonstration project to allow the GAO to conduct an evaluation (General Accounting Office 1998, 1).

7. Pub. L. No. 108-173, 1201, codified at I.R.C. 223.

8. I.R.C. 62(a)(19), 106(d)(1), 223(a), 3231(e)(11), 3306(b)(18), 3401(a)(22). An excellent account of the law that governs HSAs and the policy issues that they raise is found in Kaplan 2005.

9. I.R.C. 223(c)(2)(A)(i)(I) & (II). See also 2007 HSA Indexed Amounts, http://www .treas.gov/offices/public-affairs/hsa/07IndexedAmounts.shtml. The insurer may, however, cover preventive medical expenses, such as screenings or vaccinations, before the deductible is met. I.R.C. 223(c)(2)(C), I.R.S. Notice 2004-23, 2004-15 I.R.B. 725.

10. I.R.C. 223(c)(2)(A)(ii)(I) & (II). See also 2007 HSA Indexed Amounts, http://www .treas.gov/offices/public-affairs/hsa/07IndexedAmounts.shtml.

11. Under the original legislation creating HSAs, tax-subsidized contributions were also limited to the amount of the HDHP deductible. This requirement was eliminated by Congress in the waning hours of the 109th Congress, increasing dramatically the potential for shielding money from taxes in an HSA. H.R. 6408, sec. 303. Persons aged fifty-five to sixty-five may also make an additional "catch-up" contribution. I.R.C. 223(b)(3)(A).

12. I.R.C. 223(f)(1).

13. I.R.C. 223(f)(2) & (f)(4)(A).

14. I.R.C. 213(d), Rev. Rul. 2003-102, 2003-38, I.R.B. 559; Notice 2004-2, 2004-2 I.R.B. 269, 272.

15. I.R.C. 223(f)(4).

16. I.R.C. 223(f)(4)(C).

17. I.R.C. 223(f)(8).

18. Revenue Rulings 2002-41, 2002-45.

19. See Consumer Directed Health Care Inc., Investment Scenario, http://www.cdhcinc .com/Excel/HSA%20Value%20Projector.xls.

20. I thank James Knight for this insight.

21. See Davis, Doty, and Ho 2005 on the financial implications of CDHC for consumers.

22. In 2004, according to one estimate, 144 million Americans paid no income tax. This estimate was based on there being 58 million households that did not pay tax, including 14 million households that did not earn sufficient income to require filing taxes and 44 million households that filed a tax return but did not owe taxes. Over 90 percent of these Americans earned under $20,000 a year (Moody and Hodge 2004).

23. See chapter 8.

1. Epstein posits at one point, for example, a hypothetical in which a choice must be made between (1) apportioning limited health care assets equally among ten wealthy and ten poor critically ill patients, resulting in a 50 percent chance of survival for each person (meaning that half of the wealthy and half of the poor survive) and (2) allowing the wealthy to spend all of their assets on themselves, increasing their chance of survival to 80 percent (eight survive), since they have access to greater health resources, but giving no health resources to the poor patients and letting all ten of them die. Epstein asserts that society is better off with the second choice, because it will allow eight productive people to survive rather than five productive and five unproductive people (Epstein 1997, 114–15).

2. While researching this book I received an email from a prominent CDHC advocate stating, "In all of social science — whether economics, politics, sociology, history, etc. — there is only one model that (a) is internally consistent and (b) can explain and predict. That is the social science model developed by economists. All the rest is gobbledygook. And more often than not, it is highly opinionated, value-laden gobbledygook."

3. European Economic and Social Committee 2004, 3.

4. Goodman seems particularly skeptical as to the value of substance abuse and mental health treatments (Goodman and Musgrave 1992, 105).

5. They do not emphasize the vital role that public funding plays in promoting this research, but rather the importance of private investment, particularly by the drug industry.

6. Regina Herzlinger's extended "Breakfast Insurance" fable seeks to capture everything that is wrong with our current health care system, as well as her solution to its problems, in one extended metaphor (Herzlinger ed. 2004, 61–73). Her choice of the insured breakfast for her metaphor is particularly interesting because in fact breakfast buffets, presenting essentially the same moral hazard problems as conventional insurance, are common. My unfortunately extensive experience with breakfast buffets demonstrates that (1) most people are reasonable in their selection of dishes from breakfast buffets and do not keep on eating everything in sight simply because the dishes have no marginal cost, and (2) the price and quality of breakfast buffets vary significantly, but are usually reasonable in relation to alternative à la carte dishes on the menu. There must be a literature on consumer behavior in the face of breakfast buffets, but neither I nor seemingly Regina Herzlinger has studied it. A web search linking the terms "breakfast buffet" and "consumer behavior" brings up a host of seminars or conferences on consumer behavior that begin the day with a breakfast buffet.

7. This is the conclusion of public choice economics, which is embraced explicitly or implicitly by the supporters of CDHC (Goodman, Musgrave, and Herrick 2004, 187–89). See chapter 7.

8. More moderate CDHC advocates recognize the legitimate role of regulation to assure the safety and efficacy of drugs (Herzlinger 1997, 233).

9. The deaths arise because Americans spend money on overregulated health care that

they could otherwise spend on safer automobiles and other products that protect lives. By this logic, of course, any reduction in expenditures anywhere in the economy could save lives.

10. Though CDHC advocates repeatedly attack Medicaid, EMTALA, and other programs for the poor, when they are comparing the American health care system to the systems of other countries they can speak quite favorably of these programs, noting that Medicaid recipients "use services at rates comparable to those with private insurance" and that "the poor often have access to the most advanced technology and therapies" (Goodman, Musgrave, and Herrick 2004, 35).

11. The authors also assert that extending to all medical expenses the income tax deductions and exclusions currently offered for employment-based insurance would dramatically reduce the incidence of low cost-sharing, employment-based insurance and increase the incidence of high-cost-sharing individual policies. This would increase total cost sharing, which would in turn reduce the demand for health care and total health care expenditures (Cogan, Hubbard, and Kessler 2005, 36–37, 66–68).

12. Welfare used to be the exclusive function of local government, but we abandoned that approach because it was humiliating, intrusive, and often politically corrupt (Jost 2003, 67–69).

13. Paradoxically, some CDHC advocates recognize that nongroup health insurance is often unavailable to the uninsured because of medical underwriting, or provides poor value for money because it offers very limited coverage (Herzlinger ed. 2004, 37).

14. See e.g. Cogan, Hubbard, and Kessler 2005, 18: "Most of the new uninsured come from the most affluent group [households earning more than $50,000 a year], many of whom are relatively healthy young adults." The authors also state: "Providing health insurance to the 14 million people who are already eligible for public programs but do not accept it is a difficult challenge. Approximately half of this group was offered but declined public coverage" (Cogan, Hubbard, and Kessler 2005, 19). Among the reasons they offer for the poor take-up of public benefits are "the inferiority of program benefits, inconvenience, cultural attitudes and stigma, and poor information" (Cogan, Hubbard, and Kessler 2005, 19), implying that enrolling in public programs is just too much trouble for eligible low-income persons. By contrast, public program advocates attribute poor take-up primarily to barriers imposed by the Medicaid bureaucracy, and point to higher take-up in states where barriers are reduced and active outreach efforts are made.

15. They do admit, however, that price information is currently not available for many services (Goodman and Musgrave 1992, 53).

16. Herzlinger believes that entrepreneurs will produce information but sees a vital role for government as well (Herzlinger ed. 2004, 183).

17. Herzlinger also sees a role for a government agency like the Securities and Exchange Commission (Herzlinger ed. 2004, 148, 797–810; Herzlinger 1997, 268).

18. Another strategy that some advocate is long-term insurance contracts allowing insureds to stay with an insurer as long as they like regardless of changes in their health, with initial premiums based on the risk of the insured at the time of application, with subsequent increases in risk shifted to the insurer (Cannon and Tanner 2005, 87–88).

Chapter 4: The First Time Around

1. Indeed many hospitals began as charity institutions, and expected the doctors who practiced to offer their services for free as well (Starr 1982).
2. About two-thirds of hospitals in the United States in 1931 were governmental, though two-thirds of the governmental hospitals were mental hospitals (Committee on Costs of Medical Care 1932, 5).
3. This was encouraged by doctors who realized how dangerous and unsanitary hospitals were (Cathell 1922, 220–21).
4. Tonsillectomies and adenoidectomies accounted for 27.5 percent of admissions in 1929–31 (Stevens 1989, 106–7).
5. The justification for this position was the inability of consumers to evaluate the claims of advertising physicians, and the fear that advertising would be resorted to primarily by the least competent physicians.
6. The classic statement of this thesis is found in articles by Reuben Kessel (1970).
7. By 1914 only 1 percent of medical care benefits were covered in this way (Starr 1982, 209).
8. State governments also provided hospitals for the mentally ill and persons with tuberculosis (Committee on Costs of Medical Care 1932, 52–53).
9. Davis (1941) notes this as a factor in the failure of medical service bureaus (55).
10. In one survey of over five hundred African Americans with syphilis cited by the study, only 14 percent had received any professional medical care, and only 3 percent were receiving the standard medication for syphilis (Committee on Costs of Medical Care 1932, 10).
11. This notion of medical need as independent of economic demand was common at the time. Michael Davis argued a decade later that physiological need exists first, which then translates to recognized need, which finally translates into demand, constrained by "expense, ignorance, prejudice, or indifference" (Davis 1941, 42).

Chapter 5: The Nonaccidental System

1. Indemnity products became more common in Blue Cross in the 1950s under cost pressure (Somers and Somers 1961, 304; Harris 1964, 408).
2. Some plans did impose coinsurance and deductibles for ancillaries (Somers and Somers 1961, 304, 305–6; Dickerson 1963, 302).
3. These deductibles were often from $500 to $750 for individual policies, as high as the levels found today (Somers and Somers 1961, 282, 312, 332).
4. The disadvantage of indemnity insurance, of course, is that it imposes all the marginal costs of health care above indemnity limits on the consumer, and that these costs can be crippling with catastrophic diseases (Frech and Ginsburg 1978, 30–31).
5. American Medical Association v. United States, 317 U.S. 519 (1943).
6. Though most insurance was sold to groups, both commercial insurers and the Blues also offered nongroup insurance. Blue Cross plans would sign up individuals through well-advertised drives during open-enrollment periods that would last from a week to a month (Reed 1947, 61–62, 67). This method resulted in a better risk pool than could be obtained by merely allowing enrollment at any time. The commercial in-

surers, and to a lesser degree the Blues, underwrote these policies rather carefully, rejecting many who applied for them. Although Blue Cross initially community-rated its individual insurance, it eventually also moved to experience rating, which was commonly used by the commercial insurers (Stevens 1989, 261).

7. Pub. L. 729, 56 Stat. 765, sec. 10 (1942).

8. Internal Revenue Service Special Ruling, CCH 6587 (Oct. 26, 1943).

9. At the time 15 percent of the population had only hospital insurance, while 14 percent had comprehensive insurance or insurance for medical as well as surgical and hospital costs. In 1949 health insurance covered 26 percent of hospital costs, 10 percent of physicians' fees, and less than 1 percent of other medical costs (U.S. Senate 1951, 3).

10. In the same year 145 million Americans had surgical insurance and 52 million major medical coverage.

11. Private insurance coverage peaked in the late 1970s and 1980s and has declined since. In 1979 almost 90 percent of Americans under the age of sixty-five had some form of private health insurance (Gabel 1999, 65).

12. Between 1954 and 1958 the proportion of total major medical enrollment under comprehensive policies grew from 3 percent to 32 percent (Somers and Somers 1961, 383).

13. By 1998, 97 percent were covered for prescription drugs and 96 percent for outpatient mental health services. In addition, 84 percent of employees were covered for routine physicals, while only 6 percent had had such coverage in 1977 (Gabel 1999, 68).

14. Employers paid 30 percent of gross cost and 20 percent of net cost for dependent coverage.

15. Virtually all employees in multi-employer plans also fully paid for dependent coverage, but only 18 percent of employees in single-employer plans subject to collective bargaining had dependent insurance fully covered by their employer; 9 percent of employees in such plans fully funded dependent coverage themselves (U.S. Department of Labor 1960b). Employer contributions varied by coverage as well. In 1959 only one out of three collectively bargained major medical plans covering individual employees (as opposed to hospital plans) were financed solely by the employer, and one in nine were financed solely by the employee (U.S. Department of Labor 1961, 6–7). (On labor policy see also Somers and Somers 1961, 228–46.)

16. Inland Steel Co. v. NLRB, 170 F.2d 247 (7th Cir.), cert. denied, 336 U.S. 960 (1949).

17. The Taft-Hartley Act, passed in 1947, prohibited exclusively union-run plans (Klein 2004, 49; Munts 1967, 11).

18. The unions also favored comprehensive insurance rather than more limited surgical or medical policies (Harris 1964, 409).

19. They were also concerned that it might encourage malingering and absenteeism, and that it might discriminate against healthy workers who would not benefit from it (Baker and Dahl 1945, 26).

20. Other sources put the level of employer self-insurance in the late 1980s somewhat lower, though still above 50 percent. See Health Insurance Association of America, Source Book of Health Insurance Data (1990), table 2.8 [p. 27].

21. Later rulings left the issue unclear until the code change of 1954 (Steuerle and Hoffman 1979; Thomasson 2002, 240–41).

22. Before the Second World War only the richest Americans paid income tax. Because of increases in both wages and taxes during the war, however, most Americans paid income tax by the time the war ended.

23. See U.S. Department of Labor 1961, 3–4, listing among the advantages of cost sharing under major medical plans that it discourages overutilization, gives patients an incentive to police medical fees, and eliminates administrative costs of payments for small claims. Major medical cost sharing was criticized at the time by union leaders, who saw it as benefiting few workers and leaving most small bills uncovered. Union leaders also saw it as discouraging prompt treatment and preventive care.

24. A Senate report in 1951 noted that "independent" health plans covered more than 80 percent of their subscribers' services, including occasionally dental and nursing care (U.S. Senate 1951, 4).

Chapter 6: The Origins of Consumer-Driven Health Care

1. This concern was recognized in the minority report of the Committee on the Costs of Medical Care (Committee on Costs of Medical Care 1932, 166).

2. This was also true of surgery, which was often the only physician service covered by insurance (U.S. Senate 1951, 10).

3. There was a widespread belief that this had been the experience of the National Health Service when it was established in Britain after the war, especially with respect to dental work and eyeglasses (Somers and Somers 1961, 294–96).

4. Named after Milton Roemer, a well-known mid-twentieth-century health policy scholar. Roemer's law did not in fact precisely reflect the views of Roemer, who had observed only that under conditions of full insurance available beds would be filled, not that controlling construction would control costs (Payton and Powsner 1980, 253, 268–77).

5. This idea has been developed further by John Nyman. See chapter 7.

6. Pauly expressed skepticism about the use of deductibles to control moral hazard, recognizing that once an insured exceeded the deductible, further spending was unrestrained (Pauly 1968, 536).

7. 23 March 1978, 650–58; 30 March 1978, 709–20.

8. 421 U.S. 773 (1975).

9. At conferences sponsored by the American Enterprise Institute to develop and advocate market-based proposals for reforming the American health care system, the approach emphasizing the consumer's choice at point of purchase through cost sharing was also represented by Laurence S. Seidman (Seidman 1981, 450; Seidman 1980, 307).

10. Telephone interview with John Goodman, 12 September 2005. See also http://www.sourcewatch.org/index.php?title=National _ Center _ for _ Policy _ Analysis.

11. Telephone interview with John Goodman, 12 September 2005.

12. Pub. L. 104-191, 110 Stat. 1936.

13. Individuals could claim tax deductibility for contributions of up to 65 percent of the deductible amount and families for up to 75 percent. Deductibles for individuals had to be between $1,500 and $2,250, for families between $3,000 and $4,500 (Bunce 2001, 12).

14. IRS Revenue Ruling 2001-41 and Notice 2002-45, published in Internal Revenue Bulletin 2002-28, 15 July 2002.

1. CDHC skeptics, of course (including myself), also have their own political agenda. Mine, as I announced in the Preface, is based on a belief that all Americans should have access to health care, regardless of their ability to purchase it.

2. The resemblance between neoclassical economics and physics, the most mathematical of the sciences, is striking. In particular, however, the resemblance is to nineteenth-century physics. More modern developments in physics, which could also have relevance to economics, have not been incorporated (Mirowski 1989).

3. Similarly, McCloskey points out that much economic literature is understandable only to those who already understand it and that its incomprehensibility "merely terrifies the onlookers" (1990, 60). McCloskey is particularly insightful in describing the use of statistics by economists. McCloskey notes that noneconomists tend to use statistics "essay style, the way quotations are used" and that the statistics "do not carry much of the argument" (1990, 62). By contrast, economists use statistics as proof: "statistics are deployed monographically, the thing to be established, the output of the argument, the way the story is told" (1990, 62). "The point is that economists favor the figure of argument making-a-set-of-accounts. Accounting is in fact the master metaphor of economics, the source of most of its quantitative bite. The metaphor alarms noneconomists, puzzled by the cavalier way in which bits of numbers are flung into the calculation" (1990, 63).

4. Mirowski notes that most economists have in fact always held psychology in contempt, and have always been more interested in their own models of behavior than in actual behavior (1989, 236).

5. Becker (1976) defines the stable preferences at the foundation of economics as referring not to preferences for specific market goods or services but rather to the "fundamental aspects of life, such as health, prestige, sensual pleasure, benevolence, or envy," in short, to all human desiderata (5). He also suggests that economic analysis can deal with 'shadow' imputed prices" as well as real prices, and with transactions involving incomplete information, high transaction costs, and emotional as well as rational decisions (6). He concludes: "[A]ll human behavior can be viewed as involving participants who maximize their utility from a stable set of preferences and accumulate an optimal amount of information and other inputs in a variety of markets" (14). In sum, if all the assumptions fundamental to economics are sufficiently relaxed and expanded, economics encompasses all human motivations and all of human behavior.

6. The most comprehensive description of the limitations of the neoclassical model for describing health care is found in Rice 2002. Uwe Reinhardt, also an economist, has written several articles noting the limited usefulness of traditional welfare economics for directing health policy (Reinhardt 1998; Reinhardt 2002). Robert Evans, a Canadian health economist, has written a number of articles challenging the health policy prescriptions of American health economists, as well as their politics (Evans 1997; Evans 1990). See also critiques of the prescriptions of economics for health care in Frankford 1992 and Kuttner 1997.

7. Once comparative information is published in a magazine or posted on the internet, it is available to anyone who can find a copy of the magazine (at a library, for example)

or gain access to the web site on which the information is found, or onto which the information has been copied.

8. In fairness, Becker and Stigler are not talking about preferences for particular products as such, but rather about broader tastes. Unless preferences are defined in the most global terms (almost all of us prefer pleasure to pain), the assumption that preferences are innate and immutable is heroic.

9. Indeed, many people feel overwhelmed by the multitude of choices that face them every day (Schwartz 2004, 9–44). Experimental evidence suggests that persons faced with more choices among products may be less willing to purchase any product at all (Schwartz 2004, 126–31).

10. Indeed, some experimental evidence shows that when people are forced to give reasons for decisions their decisions change, and they tend to make decisions with which they are ultimately less satisfied (Schwartz 2004, 137–42).

11. People also tend to weigh sunk costs in their decisions, contrary to the counsel of economists. Having purchased a $50 ticket to the theater, a consumer is likely to go to the performance, even if she would have been unlikely to do so had she not bought the ticket already. One explanation of this behavior is the desire to avoid regret (Schwartz 2004, 72–73, 160–62).

12. Indeed, psychological research shows that motivation to do some tasks decreases if financial rewards are offered for the work (Stone 2002, 73).

13. There is also considerable evidence for "hedonic adaptation"—people get used to pleasure or pain—so that in the long run, happiness or satisfaction has less to do with the choices we make, including purchases, than it does with our underlying nature (Schwartz 2004, 167–79).

14. California Dental Association v. Federal Trade Commission, 526 U.S. 726 (1999).

15. One survey found that 84 percent of health economists and 93 percent of economic theorists who expressed an opinion agreed with the statement that "third-party payment results in patients using services whose costs exceed their benefits, and this excess of costs over benefits amounts to at least 5% of total health care expenditures" (Fuchs 1996, 8).

16. Initially this insurance was only hospital insurance, but the policies were often service-benefit policies without deductibles. By the time the tax status of employer contributions was clarified, medical and surgical benefits were common as well.

17. Nyman notes further that purchasing insurance does not eliminate uncertainty. It simply changes the nature of the uncertainty from whether one will incur the risk of illness to whether one will remain healthy and thus lose the premium paid (Nyman 2003, 54).

18. Nyman observes that the difference between a standard gamble and an insurance policy explains why society creates associations such as Gamblers Anonymous for habitual gamblers but has not, as of yet, found it useful to create associations to discourage the purchase of insurance (Nyman 2003, 135) (although CDHC advocates may see the value in such associations).

19. Nyman acknowledges that for employees, the cost of this "load" is offset by tax subsidies, but notes that many people, including until recently the self-employed, buy health insurance that is not tax subsidized, and thus must find health insurance to be of real value (Nyman 2003, 27).

20. Nyman also notes that some of the behavior described by economists as moral hazard is in fact better described as adverse selection. People with pre-existing conditions, that is, purchase insurance to gain access to goods and services that are in fact useful for their conditions, but that they would not purchase in the absence of insurance (Nyman 2003, 45).

21. They are also misleading to the extent that they use demand by the uninsured as a baseline for calculating insurance-based demand. The uninsured tend to be poor, and thus unable to purchase health care that is in fact of very high value (Nyman 2003, 107).

22. Nyman also notes that separate insurance is rarely purchased (at least not without tax subsidies) for dental care or for alternative or complementary health care (such as massage therapy), where usage by the healthy is the norm and the possibility of the opportunistic use of insurance is high, suggesting that consumers are quite capable of determining when insurance is efficient and when it is not (Nyman 2003, 138).

23. Nyman also points out that the purchase of high-cost, life-saving procedures is possible because of income transfers through insurance, not because of reduced prices, and thus welfare loss is not a problem (Nyman 2003, 70).

24. Nyman favors cost sharing imposed on care that is likely to be inefficient and the use of HSAs for covering routine or preventive care for healthy people (Nyman 2003, 154–55).

25. Even CDHC advocates recognize that catastrophic insurance plays an important role in providing security against major health care shocks.

26. Uwe Reinhardt states, "The distribution of benefits in kind inevitably feeds the horses to feed the birds, so to speak," but he recognizes that the "horses" may be more effective in lobbying for feed than the "birds" are (Reinhardt 1998, 38). Though public choice does not explain everything, it does explain a lot.

27. This was not true of the theories of earlier economists like Marx, Mill, Ricardo, and Smith, who focused more on the economics of the production of wealth and less on consumers' decision making (Dobb 1973). As Dobb notes, one characteristic of the "Jevonian Revolution" was that "[Q]uestions of property-ownership or class-relations and conflicts were regarded as falling outside the economist's domain, not directly affecting, in major respects at least, the phenomena and relations with which economic analysis was property concerned" (Dobb 1973, 172). See also Dobb 1973, 242–45, describing the dependence of Pareto optimality on the original distribution of wealth.

28. There is always the risk, however, that in treating love as scarce and in organizing our lives to get along without it, we may discourage its growth (McCloskey 1990, 143).

29. Market ideology, for example, has been used to perpetuate racial disparities in health care. Racial segregation in health care, a continuing problem, has long been justified as simply reflecting the consumer preferences of whites and of blacks for separate facilities (Stone 2005, 72–75). Cost sharing also imposes greater burdens on blacks than on whites, both because their income tends to be lower and because their health status tends to be worse (Stone 2005, 78–79). Market ideology thus provides a neutral explanation (economic motivation or necessity) to justify behavior that is in fact racist (Stone 2005, 79–80).

Chapter 8: But Does It Work?

1. The experiment also included another plan involving individual deductibles of $150 and family deductibles of $450, with 95 percent coinsurance for outpatient services and free inpatient care (Newhouse and Insurance Experiment Group 1993, 9).

2. The poor used more inpatient services, however, where the cap was likely to be exceeded and thus cost sharing less influential (Newhouse and Insurance Experiment Group 1993, 45–46).

3. Personal communication, Naoki Ikegami, 3 July 2006. Japan does have fairly low out-of-pocket expenditure limits, which undoubtedly influence the effectiveness of cost sharing.

4. See Gaynor, Li, and Vogt 2006, finding that reductions in pharmaceutical spending related to cost sharing are largely offset by increases in outpatient and inpatient care. See also Gibson, Ozminkowski, and Goetzel 2005, concluding that high levels of cost sharing for pharmaceuticals can result in disruptions in treatment and reduced use of essential medications.

5. The study defined "underinsured" as having medical expenses amounting to 10 percent or more of income (for poor families 5 percent or more) or deductibles of 5 percent or more of income (Schoen, Doty, Collins, and Holmgren 2005, W5-291–W5-292).

6. A fourth form of tax-subsidized spending account, the flexible spending account or FSA, is not discussed in the text because there was never any requirement that an FSA be coupled with an HDHP, and other features of FSAs — most notably the "use it or lose it" requirement that prohibits funds in the accounts from accumulating from year to year — keep them from having the demand-constraining feature of consumer-driven savings accounts.

7. That CDHC increases the financial burden on the sick while conferring financial benefits directly on the wealthy is a powerful argument against MSAs in a publicly funded system, such as that of Canada (Forget, Deber, and Roos 2002).

8. The HIE supports this argument to some extent, as it found little evidence of increased expenditures in anticipation of exceeding the deductible, at least until participants came very close to meeting the deductible (Newhouse and Insurance Experiment Group 1993, 82–83).

9. Of course, if the HSA holder subsequently has real medical expenses up to the deductible, the HSA owners will have to convince the HDHP insurer that the money was really spent on covered charges, or HDHP coverage will not be available.

10. See Park and Greenstein, 2006, critiquing the methodology of the Blue Cross survey, which lumped together enrollees in the individual and employer-based coverage markets and failed to distinguish between those who chose an HDHP and those offered no choice by their employer.

11. Experience with 401(k) plans has shown that many eligible employees do not participate, that only 8.4 percent of eligible employees make the maximum employee contributions allowed by law (including only 0.5 percent of those earning from $20,000 to $39,999 and 2.5 percent of those earning $40,000 to $59,999), that participants often make poor investment decisions, and that many cash out their accounts when they change jobs (Munnell and Sundén 2004, 53–94).

12. The amount spent by employers was $4,148 for individuals and $10,844 for families, compared to $4,385 for individuals and $11,765 for families for PPO products (Kaiser Family Foundation / Health Research and Educational Trust 2006, 7).

13. Amendments adopted at the end of 2006 to the MMA provisions allow employers to make larger contributions to the HSAs of non-highly compensated employees than of "highly compensated" employees (roughly, owners or employees who earn in excess of $100,000 a year or are in the top 20 percent of employees based on compensation), but require all contributions for non-highly compensated employees to be comparable. Whether this will result in increased HSA contributions for lower-income employees remains to be seen. H.R. 6111, sec. 306.

14. Out-of-pocket spending accounted for 58 percent of health care spending in China in 2002 (Blumenthal and Hsiao 2005, 1165–70).

Chapter 9: Legal, Ethical, and Regulatory Issues

1. The issues raised by the first half of this chapter are currently the subject of an empirical study being conducted by Professors Mark Hall and Carl Schneider and funded by a Robert Wood Johnson Investigator Award. The legal issues have been extensively reviewed by Professor Haavi Morreim, who shared with me a prepublication draft of her recently published article in the *Vanderbilt Law Review* on this topic.

2. On the other hand, as noted in chapter 5, the typical major medical policy in the 1970s — contrary to what is commonly believed today — had comparatively high deductibles and coinsurance obligations, and pharmaceutical coverage was still not the norm. The major difference between the 1970s and today, indeed, might be that today's expensive and effective tests and drugs were not available in the 1970s, and a day in the hospital cost only $150 (National Center for Health Statistics 2000, table 122).

3. 530 U.S. 211 (2000).

4. Magan Medical Clinic v. California State Board of Medical Examiners, 57 Cal. Rptr. 256, 263 (Cal. App. 1967).

5. 793 P.2d 479, 483–84 (Cal. 1990).

6. See Broemmer v. Abortion Serv., 840 P.2d 1013 (Ariz. 1992).

7. Stauss v. Biggs, 525 A.2d 992, 1000 (Del. 1987).

8. See 45 C.F.R. 164.506, 164.512 (the HIPAA Privacy Regulations).

9. See D.A.B. v. Brown, 570 N.W.2d 168 (Minn. App. 1997); Neade v. Portes, 739 N.E.2d 496 (Ill. 2000).

10. American Bar Association Model Rules of Professional Conduct, Rule 1.16.

11. By analogy, several cases have recognized obligations on the part of health care providers to assist their patients in nonmedical matters, such as filling out forms excusing an absence from work, Chew v. Meyer, 527 A.2d 828 (Md. Ct. Spec. App. 187), or forms supporting an insurance application, Murphy v. Godwin, 303 A.2d 668 (Del. Super. 1973).

12. See Canterbury v. Spence, 464 F.2d 772 (D.C. 1972).

13. Arato v. Avedon, 858 P.2d 598, 608 (Cal. 1993), citing Moore v. Regents of University of California, 793 P.2d 479, 485 at note 10 (Cal. 1990).

14. At least one court has held that a patient has the right to be fully informed of the relative risks and benefits of treatments that might be alternatives to a recommended

treatment, even if the patient cannot afford more expensive alternatives (Bernard v. Char, 903 P.2d 667 (Haw. 1995)). Other courts have recognized a more general right of "informed refusal": the right to be informed as to the availability of additional diagnostic tests or alternative treatments and the risks of failing to have them (Gates v. Jensen, 595 P.2d 919 (Wash. 1979); Truman v. Thomas, 611 P.2d 902 (Cal. 1980); Smith v. Reisig, 686 P.2d 285 (Okla. 1984)). These cases have not been widely followed, though a number of state informed consent statutes require the disclosure of "reasonable," "possible," or "practical" alternatives to proposed tests or treatments (Krause 1999, 323–38). One barrier to cases raising this issue will be the nature of the patient's injury. If the only injury that the patient suffers in not being told of a treatment alternative is having to pay for a more expensive procedure, the difference in cost is unlikely to be sufficient to justify tort litigation, though the patient may have a case in small claims court (Morreim 2006, 1224).

15. This obligation to inform patients as to the cost implications of decisions is largely unfulfilled today. According to a recent study, although 79 percent of doctors surveyed believed that their patients wanted to discuss out-of-pocket costs with them, only 35 percent of physicians and 15 percent of patients reported ever having discussed out-of-pocket costs in an encounter between physician and patient. Only 16 percent of patients reported believing that their physicians were aware of the magnitude of their out-of-pocket costs, and only 21 percent of physicians reported that they knew in general how much their patients spent out of pocket (Alexander, Casalino, and Meltzer 2003, 955–56).

16. 42 U.S.C. 1395dd.

17. The Hill-Burton program provided grants and loans for the construction of hospitals but required recipient hospitals to provide "a reasonable volume of services to persons unable to pay therefor" and service to their communities (42 U.S.C. 291c(e)(2)).

18. 42 U.S.C. 1396o(e). But see 42 U.S.C. 1396o-1(d)(2), allowing providers in some circumstances to refuse treatment to recipients who cannot afford co-payments.

19. Wilson v. Chesapeake Health Plan, Inc., No. 88019032/CL76201 (Baltimore City Cir. Ct. 1988), discussed in Furrow, Greaney, Johnson, Jost, and Schwartz 2004, 239–40, but see Mraz v. Taft, 619 N.E.2d 483 (1993) (no obligation on the part of hospital or nursing home to advise patient that he qualified for Medicaid).

20. 64 P.2d 208 (Utah 1937).

21. The "respectable minority" or "two schools of thought" doctrine, for example, has long recognized that doctors often disagree on the best course of treatment for particular conditions (Furrow, Greaney, Johnson, Jost, and Schwartz 2000, 288–90).

22. See Baxley v. Rosenblum, 400 S.E.2d 502, 507 (S.C. Ct. App. 1991) (allowing assumption of risk instruction where the patient, who was a physician, refused the treatment option recommended by his doctor). Assumption of risk has also been applied in cases involving Jehovah's Witnesses who refuse blood transfusions. See Kurtis A. Kemper, "Annotation, Contributory Negligence, Comparative Negligence, or Assumption of Risk, Other than Failing to Reveal Medical History or Follow Instructions, as Defense in Action against Physician or Surgeon for Medical Malpractice," 108 A.L.R. 5th 385 (2005).

23. Schneider v. Revici, 817 F.2d 987 (2d Cir. 1987); Boyle v. Revici, 961 F.2d 1060 (2d Cir. 1992); Morreim 2006, 1226–29.

24. Under the classic contributory negligence doctrine, a defendant was completely excused from liability if the plaintiff was also negligent and the plaintiff's negligence contributed to the injury. Many jurisdictions have abandoned the contributory negligence doctrine in favor of comparative negligence, under which the damages due to the plaintiff for the defendant's negligence are merely reduced to recognize the comparative contribution of the plaintiff's negligence to the injury (Murphy 1991, 159–61).

25. Grippe v. Momtazee, 705 S.W.2d 551 (Mo. App. 1986); Chudson v. Ratra, 548 A.2d 172 (Md. App. 1988); Ferro v. Boswell, 530 S.E.2d 533 (2000); Wisker v. Hart, 766 P.2d 168 (Kan. 1988); Morreim 2006, 1229–32. There are limits to the patient's obligation, however: Stager v. Schneider, 494 A.2d 1307 (1985), held that a patient had no obligation to call a radiologist to inquire about the results of an x-ray where the doctor had failed to inform the patient of the results.

26. Foreman v. Pillsbury, 753 F.Supp. 14 (D.C.C. 1990).

27. Kirklus v. Stanley, 833 N.E.2d 952 (2005).

28. Heartland Health Systems v. Chamberlin, 871 S.W.2d 8 (Mo. App. 1993).

29. Galloway v. Methodist Hospital, 658 N.E.2d 611 (1995).

30. Victory Memorial Hospital v. Rice 1986, 493 N.E.2d 117 (Ill. App.2 Dist. 1986); Mercy Hospital, Inc. v. Carr 1974, 297 So.2d 598 (Fla. App. 1974); Payne v. Humana Hospital Orange Park, 661 So.2d 1239 (Fla. App. 1995); Doe v. HCA Health Services of Tennessee 2001, 46 S.W.3d 191 (Tenn. 2001). See also Majid v. Stubblerfield, 589 N.E.2d 1045 (Ill.App. 1992) (physician entitled to reasonable fee measured by comparable charges in the community). See also Morreim 2006, 1251–58, discussing the problem of defining "reasonableness" of charges in the absence of functioning markets, and the problem of assembling and presenting evidence of reasonableness.

31. Hall v. Humana Hospital Daytona Beach, 686 So.2d 653 (Fla. App. 1996); Galloway v. Methodist Hospital 1995, 658 N.E.2d 611 (1995).

32. See also Greenfield v. Manor Care, Inc., 705 So.2d 926 (Fla. App. 1997), finding that the wife of a patient stated a claim to recover for unjust enrichment where the facility had collected an allegedly unreasonable fee.

33. 29 U.S.C. 1011, 1015.

34. Our findings were published in "The Role of State Regulation in Consumer-Driven Health Care," 31 *American Journal of Law and Medicine* 395–418 (2005). See also Geisel 2005; Butler 2006.

35. 26 U.S.C. 223(c)(2)(A)(i) (2004).

36. I.R.S. Notice 2004-43, 2004-27 I.R.B. 10.

37. 26 U.S.C.S. 223(d)(1)(B).

38. This may well be because most insurers with which we spoke have decided to avoid these concerns altogether by using banks to administer HSAs, and the one insurer with which we spoke that is administering its own accounts has considerable experience with consumer-driven health care. But it was surprisingly difficult to locate anyone who had thought through this problem.

39. At least forty-two states have such laws (Rich and Erb 2005, 269).

40. Alternatively, a physician whose competency is incorrectly questioned by an insurer report card might also sue for defamation.

Chapter 10: Are Consumers Our Only Hope?

1. Two of the best sources for up-to-date information are the web sites of the European Observatory on Health Systems and Policies, http://www.euro.who.int/observatory, and the Health Policy Monitor web site of the Bertelsmann Stiftung, www.health policymonitor.org. As of this writing, one of the most current sources is a special issue of the journal *Health Economics*, "Analyzing the Impact of Health System Changes in the EU Member States," vol. 14, no. 51 (September 2005).

2. In a few countries, however, primary-care doctors are public employees and in some nonprofit hospitals they are common (Grosse-Tebbe and Figueras 2004).

3. The only wealthier OECD country measured in terms of GDP per capita is tiny Luxembourg, which spends far less than the United States on health care per capita.

4. The issue of defensive medicine is complex and well beyond the scope of this book. Some sources claim that malpractice accounts for as much as 10 percent of health care costs, most of which is attributable to defensive medicine. See Price Waterhouse Coopers, *The Factors Fueling Rising Healthcare Costs, 2006,* 7. These claims are largely based on a widely publicized study by Kessler and McClellan which found evidence of defensive medicine with respect to heart attacks and ischemic heart disease based on a review of Medicare data, and then projected these costs to all other medical procedures (Kessler and McClellan 1996). Subsequent attempts to verify these projections have failed to substantiate them. Clearly doctors believe that they engage in defensive medicine, but this does not mean that they do. In fact many factors encourage the provision of care, including fee-for-service financing, professional training, and most importantly, the desire to do everything that can be done to help and protect patients (Baker 2005).

5. In 2004 it was estimated that per capita spending for a Medicaid recipient in poor health would increase from $9,615 to $14,785 if the person were insured privately and services were provided at private utilization levels and at private costs (Kaiser Commission on Medicaid and the Uninsured 2004, 7).

6. Between 2000 and 2004 employer-sponsored coverage fell 4.6 percentage points, while Medicaid and state-sponsored insurance increased by 2.4 percentage points, supplemented by small increases in Medicare and other government programs (Holahan and Cook 2005, W5-499). Overall there was an increase of six million in the number of uninsured.

7. As of 2006 the Netherlands was pursuing this approach.

8. In 2004 13.2 percent of whites were uninsured, compared to 21.2 percent of blacks, 34.3 percent of Hispanics, and 18.8 percent of others (Holahan and Cook 2005, W5-506).

9. In England in the 1970s and the 1980s, for example, the life expectancy of higher-class men grew by two years while that of lower-class men grew by only 1.4 years, widening the gap (Independent Inquiry into Inequalities in Health Report 1998, 13).

10. This seems to be particularly true of specialist care.

11. The problem of equity has been studied extensively by Eddy van Doorslaer, Adam Wagstaff, and Christina Masseria, who have produced a number of papers for the OECD. See e.g. van Doorslaer and Masseria 2004; van Doorslaer, Wagstaff, van der

Burg, Christiansen, De Graeve, Duchesne, et al. 2000; and van Doorslaer, Masseria, and Koolman 2006.

12. There is, however, a pro-poor tilt in hospital admissions in the United States, probably reflecting the greater generosity of Medicaid and Medicare coverage for hospital care than for other forms of care, as well as the effect of the Emergency Medical Treatment and Active Labor Act (van Doorslaer and Masseria 2004, 17).

13. A number of Canadian provinces prohibit the purchase of private insurance to cover publicly funded services, but these laws are of questionable enforceability after the Canadian Supreme Court's recent decision in Chaoulli v. Quebec (Attorney General), striking down Quebec's prohibition under the Quebec Charter (Flood, Roach, and Sossin 2005).

14. The United States ranks twenty-sixth in the OECD in infant and neonatal mortality and twenty-third in life expectancy at birth (Organization for Economic Cooperation and Development 2005, 19, 31).

Chapter 11: How to Fix Our Broken Health Care System

1. This was up from 17.5 percent the previous year, with the highest growth among those whose earnings placed them in the top one-tenth of 1 percent (Aron-Dine and Shapiro 2006, 2).

2. In fact, although there has been a dramatic shift toward support for market approaches to health care among policy élites in recent years, public support for a government role in the financing of health care remains robust (Schlesinger 2004, 974–80).

3. This program is administered by private risk-bearing prescription drug plans which are paid based on bid premiums, but the plans only bear full risk within specified risk corridors. The government shares the risk for costs above these risk corridors, and the government bears most of the risk of catastrophic payments (Kaiser Family Foundation 2004, 7).

4. The Dutch health care system has been restructured as of 2006 so that most acute care is now covered through a privately insured managed competition system, but the basic structure of the system remains as described here (Netherlands Ministry of Health, Welfare and Sport 2005).

5. This list is obviously somewhat arbitrary, but it is intended to capture events that are both high in cost and likely to be imposed on patients particularly unable to bear the cost.

6. Under the Part D program, the government pays 80 percent of the amount paid by prescription drug or Medicare advantage plans for drugs of beneficiaries whose expenses exceed the out-of-pocket limit (42 U.S.C. 1395w-115(a)(2) & (b)).

7. Lifestyle drugs might include drugs for erectile dysfunction or toenail fungus.

8. Where over-the-counter drugs can be readily substituted for more expensive brand-name drugs, it might well make sense to cover OTCs and offer them with a lower co-payment.

9. There is of course the risk that consumers will fail to purchase medically necessary services, necessitating higher costs later if conditions deteriorate. This risk is considerably lessened under this proposal, however, because preventive services are covered by a separate program.

10. Since laboratory tests and diagnostic imaging would be covered by insurance, professionals would only need to set and publish prices for their consultation services.

11. They could of course negotiate lower prices.

12. This would equal (as of 2006) $12,920 for a single individual and $17,321 for a couple (Kaiser Family Foundation 2006b). The Medicare prescription drug legislation does not require premium payments for individuals whose incomes fall below this level (Kaiser Family Foundation 2006b).

13. For most state children's health insurance programs the income eligibility level is 200 percent of the poverty level (U.S. Department of Agriculture 2001). States that chose to provide coverage at higher levels would be allowed to do so.

14. It would be necessary to develop some simple means of determining who was eligible for these subsidies, for example by using income tax filings. Also, a creative and aggressive outreach program would be needed to assure that those eligible for the program would actually be signed up for it.

15. I.R.C. 223(c)(2)(C) (2000). See I.R.S. Notice 2004-23, 2004-1 C.B. 725.

16. Until recently the largest "private insurer" in Australia—Medibank Private—was a government-sponsored insurer, created to make certain that a private insurer was available in markets otherwise not served by private insurance (Jost 2001, 454).

17. See Jost ed. 2005, discussing international experience with the use of technology assessment for coverage determinations.

18. A possible exception here would be where a procedure could be performed just as safely and effectively on an outpatient or inpatient basis, in which case financial incentives might be appropriate to encourage the patient to use the less expensive approach. The RAND study did find that cost sharing reduced hospitalization, but also that it reduced appropriate hospitalizations to the same extent as inappropriate ones, suggesting that a better tool needs to be found to encourage the appropriate use of hospital care (Newhouse and Insurance Experiment Group 1993, 172–76).

19. Note that since catastrophic costs were excluded, policies would cost much less than they do now; 10 percent of income is usually considered an upper limit for out-of-pocket medical spending for insured persons before they are considered "underinsured." See Schoen, Doty, Collins, and Holmgren 2005, W5-291–W5-292. This figure is also a good benchmark for defining the maximum that a family should have to spend on cost sharing and insurance premiums.

20. The Bureau of Labor Statistics, for example, identifies the "education and health services industry" as the industry sector that will experience the fastest growth in employment from 2004 to 2014, while six of the "ten fastest growing occupations" that it identifies for 2004–14 are health care occupations (U.S. Bureau of Labor Statistics 2005, tables 1 [p. 5], 3c [p. 7]).

21. It is projected that by 2010 health care costs will grow to over $2.8 billion and consume 18 percent of GDP (Borger, Smith, Truffer, Keehan, Sisko, Poisal, et al. 2006, w-61–w-62). It is difficult to find recent projections of the growth in the number of uninsured, but older sources project growth to between forty-eight and sixty-one million people by 2009 (Custer and Ketsche 2000, 18–19).

22. In 2004 Medicaid spent $292.7 billion, including $99.1 billion on hospital care and $64.8 billion on long-term care (Smith, Cowan, Heffler, Catlin, and National Health Accounts Team 2006, 191).

23. If we simply project the future rate of increase in worker productivity at 1.1 percent a year, as compared to 1.5 percent a year over the past fifty years, productivity per worker will expand from $67,473 in 2000 to $105,982 in 2035, in constant 2002 dollars (Moon, Storeyguard, and Urban Institute 2002). Even if American health care costs double during that time in constant dollars, Americans will still have a great deal of discretionary money left over.

BIBLIOGRAPHY

Aaron, H. J. 1994. "Distinguished Lecture on Economics in Government: Public Policy, Values and Consciousness." *Journal of Economic Perspectives* 8, no. 2, 3–21.

Aaron, H. J., Schwartz, W. B., and Cox, M. 2005. *Can We Say No? The Challenge of Rationing Health Care.* Washington: Brookings Institution.

Adam Smith Institute. 2002. "Around the World in 80 Ideas: Saving Your Health," ed. E. Butler and K. Boyfield, http://www.adamsmith.org/80ideas/ idea/17.htm.

Agency for Healthcare Research and Quality. 2005. *2005 National Healthcare Quality Report.* Washington: Agency for Healthcare Research and Quality.

Agrawal, V., Ehrbeck, T., Packard, K. O., and Mango, P. 2005. *Consumer-Directed Health Plan Report: Early Evidence Is Promising.* Pittsburgh: McKinsey and Company.

Alexander, G. C., Casalino, L. P., and Meltzer, D. O. 2003. "Patient-Physician Communication about Out-of-Pocket Costs." *Journal of the American Medical Association* 290, 953–58.

Alexander, G. C., Hall, M. A., and Lantos, J. 2006. "Rethinking Professional Ethics in the Cost-Sharing Era." *American Journal of Bioethics* 6, no. 4, W17–W22.

AMA Health Policy Group. 2004. *Health Savings Accounts at a Glance.* Chicago: American Medical Association.

American Medical Association. 2006. *Competition in Health Insurance: A Comprehensive Study of U.S. Markets, 2005 Update.* Chicago: American Medical Association.

America's Health Insurance Plans. 2005a. *Individual Health Insurance: A Comprehensive Survey of Affordability, Access, and Benefits.* Washington: America's Health Insurance Plans.

——. 2005b. *State Laws Affecting HSAs: Impediments and Tax Treatments as of August 12, 2005.* Washington: America's Health Insurance Plans.

——. 2006. *Census Shows 3.2 Million People Covered by HSA Plans.* Washington: America's Health Insurance Plans.

Anderson, G. F., Frogner, B. K., Johns, R. A., and Reinhardt, U. E. 2006. "Health Care Spending and Use of Information Technology in OECD Countries." *Health Affairs* 25, no. 3, 819–31.

Anderson, G. F., Hussey, P. S., Frogner, B. K., and Waters, H. R. 2005. "Health Spending in the United States and the Rest of the Industrialized World." *Health Affairs* 24, no. 4, 903–26.

Anderson, G. F., Reinhardt, U. E., Hussey, P. S., and Petrosyan, V. 2003. "It's the Prices,

Stupid: Why the United States Is So Different from Other Countries." *Health Affairs* 22, no. 3, 89–105.

Anis, A. H., Guh, D. P., Lacaille, D., Marra, C. A., Rashidi, A. A., Li, X., et al. 2005. "When Patients Have to Pay a Share of Drug Costs: Effects on Frequency of Physician Visits, Hospital Admissions and Filling of Prescriptions." *Canadian Medical Association Journal* 173, 1335–40.

Aron-Dine, A., and Shapiro, I. 2006. *New Data Show Extraordinary Jump in Income Concentration in 2004.* Washington: Center for Budget and Policy Priorities.

Arrow, K. 1963. "Uncertainty and the Welfare Economics of Medical Care." *American Economic Review* 53, 941–73.

———. 1968. "The Economics of Moral Hazard: Further Comment." *American Economic Review* 58, no. 3, 537–39.

Artiga, S., and O'Malley, M. 2005. *Increasing Premiums and Cost Sharing in Medicaid and SCHIP: Recent State Experience.* Washington: Kaiser Commission on Medicaid and the Uninsured.

Atella, V., Peracchi, F., Depalo, D., and Rossetti, C. 2005. *Drug Compliance, Co-payment and Health Outcomes: Evidence from a Panel of Italian Patients.* Rome: Centre for International Studies on Economic Growth.

Augurzky, B., Bauer, T., and Schaffner, S. 2006. *Copayments in the German Health System: Do They Work?* Essen: RWI.

Bacon, A. S. 1928. "Hospital Budget-Savings Plan for Prospective Mothers." *American Hospital Association Bulletin* 2, no. 1, 68–70.

Baicker, K., Chandra, A., Skinner, J. S., and Wennberg, J. E. 2004. "Who You Are and Where You Live: How Race and Geography Affect the Treatment of Medicare Beneficiaries." Health Affairs Web Exclusive, 7 October, VAR-33–VAR-44.

Baker, H., and Dahl, D. 1945. *Group Health Insurance and Sickness Benefit Plans in Collective Bargaining.* Princeton: Princeton University Press.

Baker, T. 2005. *The Medical Malpractice Myth.* Chicago: University of Chicago Press.

"Bankers Form Health Savings Account Council." 2005. http://www.aba.com/Press+Room/122005HealthSavingscouncil.htm.

Banks, J., Marmot, M., Oldfield, Z., and Smith, J. P. 2006. "Disease and Disadvantage in the United States and England." *Journal of the American Medical Association* 295, 2037–45.

Barer, M. L., Wood, L., and Schneider, D. G. 1999. *Toward Improved Access to Medical Services for Relatively Underserved Populations: Canadian Approaches, Foreign Lessons.* Vancouver: Centre for Health Services and Policy Research.

Barr, M. D. 2001. "Medical Savings Accounts in Singapore: A Critical Inquiry." *Journal of Health Politics, Policy and Law* 26, 709–26.

Becker, G. 1976. *The Economic Approach to Human Behavior.* Chicago: University of Chicago Press.

Bellanger, M. M., and Mossé, P. R. 2005. "The Search for the Holy Grail: Combining Decentralised Planning and Contracting Methods in the French Health Care System." *Health Economics* 14, no. S1, S119–S132.

Berenson, R. 2003. "Paying for Quality and Doing It Right." *Washington & Lee Law Review* 60, 1315–44.

———. 2007. "Doctoring Health Care, II." *American Prospect* 18, no. 1, 13–16.

Berk, M. L., and Monheit, A. C. 2001. "The Concentration of Health Care Expenditures Revisited." *Health Affairs* 20, no. 2, 9–18.

Berman-Sandler, L. 2004. "Independent Medical Review: Expanding Legal Remedies to Achieve Managed Care Accountability." *Annals of Health Law* 13, 237–75.

Biles, B., Nicholas, L. H., Cooper, B. S., Adrion, E., and Guterman, S. 2006. *The Cost of Privatization: Extra Payments to Medicare Advantage Plans*. Rev. edn. New York: Commonwealth Fund.

Bilyk, J. 2006. "Growing Discomfort: Farmers Eye Health Savings Accounts as Alternative to Mounting Health Insurance Costs," http://www.MyWebTimes.com, 21 February.

Birch, S. 2004. "Charging the Patient to Save the System? Like Bailing Water with a Sieve." *Canadian Medical Association Journal* 170, 1812–13.

Blendon, R. J., Benson, J. M., and DesRoches, C. M. 2003. "Americans' Views of the Uninsured: An Era for Hybrid Proposals." Health Affairs Web Exclusive, 27 August, w3-405–w3-414.

Blendon, R. J., Schoen, C., DesRoches, C. M., Osborn, R., Scoles, K. L., and Zapert, K. 2002. "Inequities in Health Care: A Five-Country Survey." *Health Affairs* 21, no. 3, 182–91.

Blendon, R. J., Schoen, C., DesRoches, C., Osborn, R., and Zapert, K. 2003. "Common Concerns amid Diverse Systems: Health Care Experiences in Five Countries." *Health Affairs* 22, no. 3, 106–21.

Blendon, R., Schoen, C., Donelan, K., Osborn, R., DesRoches, C. M., Scoles, K., et al. 2001. "Physicians' Views on Quality of Care: A Five Country Comparison." *Health Affairs* 20, no. 3, 233.

Bloche, M. G. 1999. "Clinical Loyalties and the Social Purposes of Medicine." *Journal of the American Medical Association* 281, 268–74.

Blue Cross Blue Shield Association. 2005. *Medical Cost Reference Guide: Facts and Trends to Support Knowledge-Driven Solutions*. Chicago: Blue Cross Blue Shield Association.

———. 2006. *Medical Cost Reference Guide: Facts and Trends to Support Knowledge-Driven Solutions*. Chicago: Blue Cross Blue Shield Association.

Blumenthal, D., and Hsiao, W. 2005. "Privatization and Its Discontents: The Evolving Chinese Health Care System." *New England Journal of Medicine* 353, 1165–70.

Board of Trustees, Federal Hospital Insurance and Federal Supplementary Medical Insurance Trust Funds. 2006. *2006 Annual Report*. Washington: Board of Trustees, Federal Hospital Insurance and Federal Supplementary Medical Insurance Trust Funds.

Bohan, C. 2006. "Bush Spars with Democrats over Health Agenda." Reuters News, 15 February.

Borger, C., Smith, S., Truffer, C., Keehan, S., Sisko, A., Poisal, J., et al. 2006. "Health Spending Projections through 2015: Changes on the Horizon." Health Affairs Web Exclusive, 22 February, w61–w73.

Boulding, K. 1969. "Economics as a Moral Science." *American Economic Review* 59, no. 1, 1–12.

Bowen, W. R. 2005. "Policy Innovation and Health Insurance Reform in the American States: An Event History Analysis of State Medical Savings Account Adoptions (1993–1996)." Diss., Florida State University.

Brennan, T. A., Leape, L. L., Laird, N. M., Hebert, L., Localio, A. R., Lawthers, A. G., et

al. 1991. "Incidence of Adverse Events and Negligence in Hospitalized Patients: Results of the Harvard Medical Practice Study I." *New England Journal of Medicine* 324,
370–76.

Brink, S., Modaff, J., and Sherman, S. 1993. *Variation by Duration in Small Group
Medical Insurance Claims, Society of Actuaries Transactions, 1991–1992.* Chicago:
University of Chicago.

Brown, L. D. 1993. "Competition and the New Accountability: Do Market Incentives and
Market Outcomes Conflict or Cohere?" *Competitive Approaches to Health Care Re-
form*, ed. R. J. Arnould, R. F. Rich, and W. White, 223–44. Washington: Urban
Institute Press.

Brown, M. K. 1997–98. "Bargaining for Social Rights: Unions and the Reemergence of
Welfare Capitalism, 1945–1952." *Political Science Quarterly* 112, no. 4, 645–74.

Bunce, V. C. 2001. "Medical Savings Accounts: Progress and Problems under HIPAA."
Policy Analysis, no. 411. Washington: Cato Institute.

Buntin, M. B. 2005. *"Consumer-Driven" Health Plans: Implications for Health Care
Quality and Cost.* Santa Monica: Rand.

Buntin, M. B., Damberg, C., Haviland, A., Kapur, K., Lurie, N., McDevitt, R., and
Marquis, M. S. "Consumer-Directed Health Care: Early Evidence about Effects on
Cost and Quality." Health Affairs Web Exclusive, 24 October, w516–w530.

Business Week Online. 2002. "Does the New Health Care Shape Up?," http://www.busi
nessweek.com/print/bwdaily/dnflash/may2002/nf20020520 _ 1296.htm?db.

Busse, R. 2004. "Disease Management in Germany's Statutory Health Insurance System."
Health Affairs 23, no. 3, 56–67.

Busse, R., and Riesberg, A. 2004. *Health Care Systems in Transition: Germany.* London:
European Observatory on Health Systems and Policies.

Busse, R., Saltman, R. B., and Dubois, H. F. W. 2004. "Organization and Financing of
Social Health Insurance Systems: Current Status and Recent Policy Developments."
Social Health Insurance Systems in Western Europe, ed. R. Saltman, R. Busse, and
J. Figueras, 33–80. Maidenhead: Open University Press.

Butler, P. A. 2006. *Protecting Consumers in an Evolving Health Insurance Market.* Washington: National Committee for Quality Assurance.

California Health Care Foundation. 2003. "Insurance Markets: Ready or Not: Consumers Face New Health Insurance Choices," http://www.chcf.org/documents/insur
ance/TAReadyOrNot.pdf.

Campbell, J. C., and Ikegami, N. 1998. *The Art of Balance in Health Policy: Maintaining
Japan's Low-Cost, Egalitarian System.* Cambridge: Cambridge University Press.

Cannon, M. F. 2006. *Health Savings Accounts: Do the Critics Have a Point?* Washington:
Cato Institute.

Cannon, M. F., and Tanner, M. D. 2005. *Healthy Competition: What's Holding Back
Health Care and How to Free It.* Washington: Cato Institute.

Cassell, E. J., Leon, A. C., and Kaufman, S. G. 2001. "Preliminary Evidence of Impaired
Thinking in Sick Patients." *Annals of Internal Medicine* 134, no. 12, 1120–23.

Cathell, D. W. 1922. *Book on the Physician Himself from Graduation to Old Age.* Baltimore: D. W. Cathell.

Catlin, C., Cowan, C., Heffler, S., Washington, B., and National Health Expenditure

Account Team. 2007. "National Health Spending in 2005: The Slowdown Continues." *Health Affairs* 26, no. 1, 142–53.

Center for Medicare and Medicaid Services, Office of Public Affairs. 2006. "CMS Announces Steps to Improve Access to Consumer Directed Health Care in Medicare," http://www.cms.hhs.gov/apps/media/press/release.asp?Counter=1894.

Chalkey, M., and Robinson, R. 1997. *Theory and Evidence on Cost Sharing in Health Care: An Economic Perspective.* London: Office of Health Economics.

Chinitz, D., Wismar, M., and LePen, C. 2004. "Governance and (Self)-Regulation in Social Insurance Systems." *Social Health Insurance Systems in Western Europe,* ed. R. Saltman, R. Busse, and J. Figueras, 155–69. Maidenhead: Open University Press.

Christianson, J., Parente, S., and Feldman, R. 2004. "Consumer Experiences in a Consumer-Driven Health Plan." *Health Services Research* 39, no. 4, 1123–40.

Cigna Health Care. 2006. "Cigna Choice Fund (SM) Study Provides New Insights on Consumer Decision-making in Consumer-Driven Health Plans," http://www.prnews wire.com/cgi-bin/stories.pl?ACCT=104&STORY=/www/story/02-02-2006/000427 3524&EDATE=.

Coase, R. 1960. "The Problem of Social Cost." *Journal of Law and Economics* 3, 1–44.

Cogan, J. F., Hubbard, R. G., and Kessler, D. P. 2005. *Healthy, Wealthy, and Wise: Five Steps to a Better Health Care System.* Jackson, Tenn.: American Enterprise Institute.

Cohen, B. 2006. "The Controversy over Hospital Charges to the Uninsured: No Villains, No Heroes." *Villanova Law Review* 51, 95–148.

Cohen, R. A., and Martinez, M. E. 2006. *Health Insurance Coverage: Estimates from the National Health Interview Survey, 2005.* Atlanta: Centers for Disease Control.

Cohn, J. 2005. "Crash Course." *New Republic,* 7 November, 18.

Collins, S. R., Davis, K., Doty, M. M., Kriss, J. L., and Holmgren, A. L. 2006. *Gaps in Health Insurance: An All-American Problem.* New York: Commonwealth Fund.

Collins, S., Davis, K., Schoen, C., Doty, M. M., and Kriss, J. L. 2006. *Health Coverage for Aging Baby Boomers: Findings from the Commonwealth Fund Survey of Older Adults.* New York: Commonwealth Fund.

Collins, S. R., Schoen, C., Kriss, J. L., Doty, M. M., and Mahato, B. 2006. *Rite of Passage? Why Young Adults Become Uninsured and How New Policies Can Help.* New York: Commonwealth Fund.

Committee on the Costs of Medical Care. 1932. *Medical Care for the American People.* Chicago: University of Chicago Press.

Coughlin, T. A., Long, S. K., and Shen, Y. 2005. "Assessing Access to Care under Medicaid: Evidence for the Nation and Thirteen States." *Health Affairs* 24, no. 4, 1073–83.

Cover the Uninsured Week. 2006. "Income and Poverty Status," http://covertheuninsured week.org/factsheets/display.php? FactSheetID=108, retrieved 4 February 2005.

Creese, A. 1997. "User Fees." *British Medical Journal* 315, 202–3.

Croley, S. P. 1998. "Theories of Regulation Incorporating the Administrative Process." *Columbia Law Review* 98, 1–168.

Cross, M. A. 2004. "Will Providers Seek New Contracts as Consumer-Directed Plans Grow?" *Managed Care,* May, 42–44.

Cullis, J. 1993. "Waiting Lists and Health Policy." *Rationing and Rationality in the National Health Services,* ed. S. Frankel and R. West, 15–41. London: Macmillan.

Culyer, A. J., and Evans, R. G. 1996. "Normative Rabbits from Positive Hats: Mark Pauly on Welfare Economics." *Journal of Health Economics* 1, no. 2, 243–51.

Cunningham, P. J. 2006. "Medicaid/SCHIP Cuts and Hospital Emergency Department Use." *Health Affairs* 25, no. 1, 237–47.

Cunningham, P. J., and May, J. H. 2006. *A Growing Hole in the Safety Net: Physician Charity Care Declines Again*. Washington: Center for Studying Health Systems Change.

Cunningham, P., Staiti, A., and Ginsburg, P. B. 2006. *Physician Acceptance of New Patients Stabilizes in 2004–5*. Washington: Center for Studying Health Systems Change.

Custer, W. S., and Ketsche, P. 2000. *The Changing Sources of Health Insurance*. Washington: Health Insurance Association of America.

Cutler, D. M. 2004. *Your Money or Your Life: Strong Medicine for America's Health Care System*. New York: Oxford University Press.

Danzon, P. M., and Furukawa, M. F. 2003. "Prices and Availability of Pharmaceuticals: Evidence from Nine Countries." Health Affairs Web Exclusive, 29 October, W3-521–W3-536.

Dash, E. 2006. "Health Savings Promise a Windfall for U.S. Banks." Red Orbit, 29 January, http://www.redorbit.com/news/display/?id=373206.

Davis, K., Doty, M. M., and Ho, A. 2005. *How High Is Too High? Implications of High-Deductible Health Plans*. New York: Commonwealth Fund.

Davis, K., Schoen, C., Schoenbaum, S. C., Audet, A. J., Doty, M. M., Holmgren, A. L., et al. 2006. *Mirror, Mirror on the Wall: An Update on the Quality of American Health Care through the Patient's Lens*. New York: Commonwealth Fund.

Davis, M. 1941. *America Organizes Medicine*. New York: Harper and Bros.

Davis, M. M., and Rorem, C. R. 1932. *The Crisis in Hospital Finance*. Chicago: University of Chicago Press.

Dawes, R. M., Faust, D., and Meehl, P. E. 2002. "Clinical Versus Actuarial Judgment." *Heuristics and Biases: The Psychology of Intuitive Judgment*, ed. T. Gilovich, D. Griffin, and D. Kahneman, 716–29. Cambridge: Cambridge University Press.

Deloitte Center for Health Solutions. 2006. *Survey: Consumer-Driven Health Plan Cost Growth Significantly Slower Than Other Plans*. Washington: Deloitte Center for Health Solutions.

de Meza, D. 1983. "Health Insurance and the Demand for Medical Care." *Journal of Health Economics* 2, 47–54.

Demsetz, H. 1972. "When Does the Rule of Liability Matter?" *Journal of Legal Studies* 1, no. 1, 13–28.

DeNavas-Walt, C., Proctor, B. D., and Lee, C. H. 2006. *Income, Poverty, and Health Insurance Coverage in the United States, 2005*. Washington: U.S. Government Printing Office.

Deyo, R. A., and Patrick, D. L. 2005. *Hope or Hype: The Obsession with Medical Advances and the High Cost of False Promises*. New York: American Management Association.

Diamond Cluster International. 2006. "President's Vision for Healthcare Reform Could Define Winners and Losers among Insurers, Financial Services Firms." Press Release, 22 February.

Dickerson, O. D. 1959. "The Problem of Overutilization in Health Insurance." *Journal of Insurance* 26, no. 1, 65–72.

———. 1963. *Health Insurance*. Rev. edn. Homewood, Ill.: Richard D. Irwin.

Dobb, M. 1973. *Theories of Value and Distribution since Adam Smith: Ideology and Economic Theory*. Cambridge: Cambridge University Press.

Dobbin, F. R. 1992. "The Origins of Private Social Insurance: Public Policy and Fringe Benefits in America, 1920–1950." *American Journal of Sociology* 97, no. 5, 1416–50.

Donaldson, C., and Gerard, K. 1989. "Countering Moral Hazard in Public and Private Health Care Systems." *Journal of Social Policy* 18, 235–51.

Dorschner, J. 2006. "Pain in the Premium." *Miami Herald*, 9 April, E, 1.

Doty, M., Edwards, J., and Holmgren, A. 2005. *Seeing Red: Americans Driven into Debt by Medical Bills*. New York: Commonwealth Fund.

Dreyfuss, R., and Stone, P. H. 1996. "MediKill." *Mother Jones*, January–February, 22–27.

Druss, B. G., Marcus, S. C., Olfson, M., and Pincus, H. A. 2002. "The Most Expensive Medical Conditions in America." *Health Affairs* 21, no. 4, 105–11.

Dunlop, S., Coyte, P. C., and McIssac, W. 2000. "Socio-economic Status and the Utilization of Physicians' Services: Results from the Canadian National Population Health Survey." *Social Science and Medicine* 51, no. 1, 123–33.

Easterlin, R. 1974. "Does Economic Growth Improve the Human Lot? Some Empirical Evidence." *Nations and Households in Economic Growth: Essays in Honor of Moses Abramovitz*, ed. P. A. David and M. W. Reder. New York: Academic Press.

———. 2004. *The Reluctant Economist: Perspectives on Economics, Economic History, and Demography*. Cambridge: Cambridge University Press.

eHealthInsurance. 2006. "Health Savings Accounts, January 2005–December 2005," 10 May.

Eichner, M. J., McClellan, M. B., and Wise, D. A. 1996. "Insurance or Self Insurance? Variation, Persistence, and Individual Health Accounts." Cambridge, Mass.: National Bureau of Economic Research.

Elhauge, E. 1994. "Allocating Health Care Morally." *California Law Review* 82, 1449–1544.

Enthoven, A. 1980. *Health Plan: The Only Practical Solution to the Soaring Cost of Medical Care*. Reading, Mass.: Addison-Wesley.

Enthoven, A., and Kronick, R. A. 1989. "A Consumer-Choice Health Plan for the 1990s: Universal Health Insurance in a System Designed to Promote Quality and Economy." *New England Journal of Medicine* 320, 29–37.

Epstein, R. 1997. *Mortal Peril: Our Inalienable Right to Health Care?* Reading, Mass.: Addison-Wesley.

Ehrenreich, B., and Ehrenreich, J. 1970. *The American Health Empire: Power, Profits and Politics*. New York: Random House.

European Economic and Social Committee and the Committee on the Regions. 2004. *Modernizing Social Protection for the Development of High-Quality, Accessible and Sustainable Health Care and Long-Term Care: Support for the National Strategies Using the "Open Method of Coordination."* Brussels: European Parliament.

Evans, R. 1990. "Tension, Compression and Shear: Directions, Stresses, and Outcomes of Health Care Cost Control." *Journal of Health Politics, Policy and Law* 15, 101–28.

———. 1997. "Going for the Gold: The Redistributive Agenda behind Market-Based Health Care Reform." *Journal of Health Politics, Policy and Law* 22, 427–65.

———. 1998. "Toward a Healthier Economics, Reflections on Ken Bassett's Problem." *Health, Healthcare, and Health Economics: Perspectives on Distribution*, ed. M. L. Barer, T. E. Getzen, and G. L. Stoddart, 465–500. New York: John Wiley and Sons.

Evans, R. G., and Barer, M. L. 1995. "User Fees for Health Care: Why a Bad Idea Keeps Coming Back (or, What's Health Got to Do with It?)." *Canadian Journal on Aging* 14, no. 2, 360–90.

Evans, R. G., Barer, M. L., Stoddart, G. L., and Bhatia, V. 1993. *Who Are the Zombie Masters, and What Do They Want?* Vancouver: Centre for Health Services and Policy Research.

Eversley, J., and Webster, C. 1997. "Light on the Charge Brigade." *Health Service Journal* 107, 26–28.

Families USA. 2004. *One in Three Non-Elderly Americans without Health Insurance, 2002–2003.* New York: Families USA.

Farina, C. R., and Rachlinski, J. J. 2002. "Foreword: Post-Public Choice?" *Cornell Law Review* 87, 267–79.

Farnsworth, Douglass. 2006. "Moral Hazard in Health Insurance: Are Consumer-Directed Plans the Answer?" *Annals of Health Law* 15, 251–73.

Feachem, R. G. A., Sekhri, N. K., and White, K. L. 2002. "Getting More for Their Dollar: A Comparison of the NHS with California's Kaiser Permanente." *British Medical Journal* 324, 135–43.

Federal Trade Commission / Department of Justice. 2004. *Improving Health Care: A Dose of Competition.* Washington: Federal Trade Commission.

Feldman, R., and Christianson, J. 2004. "Evaluation of the Effect of a Consumer-Driven Health Plan on Medical Care Expenditures and Utilization." *Health Services Research* 39, no. 4, 1189–1210.

Feldman, R., and Dowd, B. 1991. "A New Estimate of the Welfare Loss of Excess Health Insurance." *American Economic Review* 81, no. 1, 297–301.

———. 1993. "What Does the Demand Curve for Medical Care Measure?" *Journal of Health Economics* 12, 193–200.

Feldstein, M. 1971. "A New Approach to National Health Insurance." *Public Interest* 23, 93–120.

Fisher, E. S., and Welch, H. G. 1999. "Avoiding the Unintended Consequences of Growth in Medical Care." *Journal of the American Medical Association* 281, 446–53.

Flood, C. M., Roach, K., and Sossin, L. 2005. *Access to Care, Access to Justice: The Legal Debate over Private Health Insurance in Canada.* Toronto: University of Toronto Press.

Forget, E. L., Deber, R., and Roos, L. L. 2002. "Medical Savings Accounts: Will They Reduce Costs?" *Canadian Medical Association Journal* 167, 143–47.

Fotaki, M., and Boyd, A. 2005. "From Plan to Market: A Comparison of Health and Old Age Care Policies in the UK and Sweden." *Public Money and Management* 25, no. 4, 237–43.

Fowles, J. E., Kind, E. A., Braun, B. L., and Bertko, J. 2004. "Early Experience with Employee Choice of Consumer-Directed Health Plans and Satisfaction with Enrollment." *Health Services Research* 39, no. 4, part II, 1141–58.

Fox, D. 1979. "From Reform to Relativism: A History of Economists and Health Care." *Milbank Quarterly* 57, no. 3, 297–336.

Frank, R. 1985. *Choosing the Right Pond: Human Behavior and the Quest for Status*. Oxford: Oxford University Press.

Frankford, D. M. 1992. "Privatizing Health Care: Economic Magic to Cure Legal Medicine." *Southern California Law Review* 66, no. 1, 1–98.

Frech, H. E., III, and Ginsburg, P. B. 1978. *Public Insurance in Private Medical Markets: Some Problems of National Health Insurance*. Washington: American Enterprise Institute.

Frederick, S., Loewenstein, G., and O'Donoghue, T. 2004. "Time Discounting and Time Preference: A Critical Review." *Advances in Behavioral Economics*, ed. C. F. Camerer, G. Loewenstein, and M. Rabin, 162–222. Princeton: Princeton University Press.

Friedman, M. 1962. *Capitalism and Freedom*. Chicago: University of Chicago Press.

Fronczek, P. 2005. *Income, Earnings, and Poverty from the 2004 American Community Survey*. Washington: U.S. Bureau of the Census.

Fronstin, P. 2005. The *Impact of the Erosion of Retiree Health Benefits on Workers and Retirees*. Washington: Employee Benefit Research Institute.

——. 2006a. *The Tax Treatment of Health Insurance and Employment-Based Health Benefits*. Washington: Employee Benefit Research Institute.

——. 2006b. *Workers' Health Insurance: Trends, Issues, and Options to Expand Coverage*. New York: Commonwealth Fund.

Fronstin, P., and Collins, S. R. 2005. *Early Experience with High-Deductible and Consumer-Driven Health Plans: Findings from the EBRI / Commonwealth Fund Consumerism in Health Care Survey*. Washington: Employee Benefit Research Institute.

——. 2006. "Early Experience with High-Deductible and Consumer-Driven Health Plans." EBRI Issue Brief 300.

Fuchs, B., and James, J. 2005. *Health Savings Accounts: The Fundamentals*. Washington: National Health Policy Forum.

Fuchs, V. R. 1996. "Economics, Values, and Health Care Reform." *American Economic Review* 86, no. 1, 1–24.

Furrow, B. R., Greaney, T. L., Johnson, S. H., Jost, T. S., and Schwartz, R. L. 2000. *Hornbook on Health Law*. 2nd edn. St. Paul: West Group.

——. 2004. *Health Law: Cases, Materials and Problems*. 5th edn. St. Paul: West.

Gabel, J. R. 1999. "Job-Based Health Insurance, 1977–1998: The Accidental System under Scrutiny." *Health Affairs* 18, no. 6, 62–74.

Gabel, J., DiCarlo, S., Fink, S., and de Lissovoy, G. 1989. "Employer-Sponsored Health Insurance in America." *Health Affairs* 8, no. 2, 116–28.

Gabel, J. R., Ginsburg, P. B., Pickreign, J. D., and Reschovsky, J. D. 2001. "Trends in Out-of-Pocket Spending by Insured American Workers, 1990–1997." *Health Affairs* 20, no. 2, 47–57.

Gabel, J., Jajick-Toth, C., de Lissovoy, G., Rice, T., and Cohen, H. 1988. "The Changing World of Group Health Insurance." *Health Affairs* 7, no. 3, 48–65.

Gabel, J., Pickreign, J., and Whitmore, H. 2006. "Behind the Slow Enrollment Growth of Employer-Based Consumer-Directed Health Plans." *Issue Brief, Findings from HSC* 107, December.

Gabel, J. R., Whitmore, H., Rice, T., and Lo Sasso, A. T. 2004. Employers' Contradictory Views about Consumer-Driven Health Care: Results from a National Survey. Health Affairs Web Exclusive, 21 April, W4-210–W4-218.

Garber, A. M., Jones, C. I., and Romer, P. M. 2006. *Insurance and Incentives for Medical Innovation.* Cambridge, Mass.: National Bureau of Economic Research.

Gaynor, M., and Vogt, W. B. 1997. "What Does Economics Have to Say about Health Policy Anyway? A Comment and Correction on Evans and Rice." *Journal of Health Politics, Policy and Law* 22, 475–96.

Gayor, M., Li, J., and Vogt, W. B. 2006. "Is Drug Coverage a Free Lunch? Cross-Price Elasticities and the Design of Prescription Drug Benefits." National Bureau of Economic Research Working Paper.

Geisel, J. 2005. "State Laws May Stymie HSA Development." *Business Insurance*, 30 May, 11.

General Accounting Office. 1998. *Medical Savings Accounts: Results from Surveys of Insurers.* Washington: General Accounting Office.

Gerdtham, U., and Jönsson, B. 2000. "International Comparisons of Health Expenditure: Theory, Data, and Econometric Analysis." *Handbook of Health Economics*, vol. 1A, ed. A. J. Culyer and J. P. Newhouse, 12–53. Amsterdam: Elsevier.

Giaimo, S. 2002. *Markets and Medicine: The Politics of Health Care Reform in Britain, Germany and the United States.* Ann Arbor: University of Michigan Press.

Gibson, T. B., Ozminkowski, R. J., and Goetzel, R. Z. 2005. "The Effects of Prescription Drug Cost Sharing: A Review of the Evidence." *American Journal of Managed Care* 11, 730–40.

Gilmer, T., and Kronick, R. 2005. "It's the Premiums, Stupid: Projections of the Uninsured through 2013." Health Affairs Web Exclusive, 5 April, W5-143–W5-149.

Gilovich, T., Griffin, D., and Kahneman, D., eds. 2002. *Heuristics and Biases: The Psychology of Intuitive Judgment.* Cambridge: Cambridge University Press.

Ginsburg, P. B., and Mannheim, L. M. 1973. "Insurance, Copayment, and Health Services Utilization: A Critical Review." *Journal of Economics and Business* 25, no. 3, 142–53.

Gladwell, M. 2005. *Blink: The Power of Thinking without Thinking.* New York: Little, Brown.

Glied, S. A. 2001. "Challenges and Options for Increasing the Number of Americans with Health Insurance." *Inquiry* 38, no. 2, 90–105.

———. 2002. "Health Insurance Expansions and the Content of Coverage: Is Something Better than Nothing?" Unpublished.

———. 2005. "The Employer-Based Health Insurance System: Mistake or Cornerstone?" *Policy Challenges in Modern Health Care*, ed. D. Mechanic, L. Rogut, and D. Colby, 37–52. New Brunswick: Rutgers University Press.

Goodman, J. C. 1980a. *National Health Care in Great Britain: Lessons for the U.S.A.* Dallas: Fisher Institute.

———. 1980b. *The Regulation of Medical Care: Is the Price Too High?* San Francisco: Cato Institute.

Goodman, J. C., and Musgrave, G. L. 1992. *Patient Power: Solving America's Health Care Crisis.* Washington: Cato Institute.

———. 1994. *Patient Power: The Free Enterprise Alternative to Clinton's Health Plan.* Washington: Cato Institute.

Goodman, J. C., Musgrave, G. L., and Herrick, D. M. 2004. *Lives at Risk: Single Payer National Health Insurance around the World.* Lanham, Md.: Rowman and Littlefield.

Goodman, J., and Rahn, R. 1984. "Salvaging Medicare with an IRA." *Wall Street Journal,* 20 March, 1.

Gorey, K. M., Holowary, E. J., Fehringer, G., Laukkanen, E., Moskowitz, A., Webster, D. J., et al. 1997. "An International Comparison of Cancer Survival: Toronto, Ontario and Detroit, Michigan, Metropolitan Areas." *American Journal of Public Health* 87, no. 7, 1156–63.

Gorey, K. M., Holowary, E. J., Fehringer, G., Laukkanen, E., Richter, N. L., and Meyer, C. M. 2000. "An International Comparison of Cancer Survival: Relatively Poor Areas of Toronto, Ontario and Three Metropolitan Areas." *Journal of Public Health* 22, no. 3, 343–48.

Government Accountability Office. 2005. *Federal Employees Health Benefits Program: Early Experience with a Consumer-Directed Plan.* Washington: Government Accountability Office.

———. 2006. *Consumer-Directed Health Plans: Small but Growing Enrollment Fueled by Rising Cost of Health Care Coverage.* Washington: Government Accountability Office.

Grabowski, H. G., and Wang, Y. R. 2006. "The Quantity and Quality of Worldwide New Drug Introductions, 1982–2003." *Health Affairs* 25, no. 2, 452–60.

Graves, J. A., and Long, S. K. 2006. *Why Do People Lack Health Insurance?* Washington: Urban Institute.

Grosse-Tebbe, S., and Figueras, J. 2004. *Snapshots of Health Systems: The State of Affairs in 16 Countries in Summer 2004.* London: European Observatory on Health Systems and Policies.

Gruber, L. R., Shadle, M., and Polich, C. L. 1988. "From Movement to Industry: The Growth of HMOs." *Health Affairs* 7, no. 3, 197–208.

Gusmano, M., Rodwin, V. G., and Weisz, D. 2006. "A New Way to Compare Health Systems: Avoidable Hospital Conditions in Manhattan and Paris." *Health Affairs* 25, no. 2, 510–20.

Hacker, J. S. 2006. *The Great Risk Shift.* New York: Oxford University Press.

Hadley, J., and Cunningham, P. J. 2005. *Perception, Reality and Health Insurance: Uninsured Are as Likely as Insured to Perceive Need for Care but Half as Likely to Get Care.* Washington: Center for Studying Health System Change.

Häkkinen, U. 2005. "The Impact of Changes in Finland's Health Care System." *Health Economics* 14 (S1), S101–S118.

Hall, M. A. 1993. "Informed Consent to Rationing Decisions." *Milbank Quarterly* 71, no. 4, 645–68.

———. 1997. *Making Medical Spending Decisions.* Oxford: Oxford University Press.

———. 2001. "The Structure and Enforcement of Health Insurance Rating Reforms." *Inquiry* 37, no. 4, 376–88.

———. 2002. "Law, Medicine, and Trust." *Stanford Law Review* 55, 463–527.

———. 2005. "The Death of Managed Care: A Regulatory Autopsy." *Journal of Health Politics, Policy and Law* 30, 427–52.

———. 2006. "Paying for What You Get and Getting What You Pay For: Legal Responses to Consumer-Driven Health Care." *Law and Contemporary Problems* 2006, 69.

Hall, M. A., Dugan, E., Zheng, B., and Mishra, A. K. 2001. "Trust in Physicians and Medical Institutions: What Is It, Can It Be Measured, and Does It Matter?" *Milbank Quarterly* 79, no. 4, 613–39.

Hall, M. A., and Havighurst, C. C. 2005. "Reviving Managed Health Care with Health Savings Accounts." *Health Affairs* 24, 1490–1500.

Halvorson, G. C. 2004. "Commentary: Current MSA Theory: Well-Meaning but Futile." *Health Services Research* 39, no. 4, 1119–22.

Hamilton, B. H., Hamilton, V. H., and Paarsch, H. J. 1997. "The Distribution of Outpatient Services in Canada and the U.S.: An Empirical Model of Physician Visits." Working paper, on file with author.

Hammer, P., Haas-Wilson, D., and Sage, W. M. 2001. "Kenneth Arrow and the Changing Economics of Health Care: 'Why Arrow? Why Now?'" *Journal of Health Politics, Policy and Law* 26, 835–50.

Hanvoravongchai, P. 2002. *Medical Savings Accounts: Lessons Learned from Limited International Experience*. Geneva: World Health Organization.

Harris, S. E. 1964. *The Economics of American Medicine*. New York: Macmillan.

Havighurst, C. 1973. "Controlling Health Care Costs: Strengthening the Private Sector's Hand." *Journal of Health Politics, Policy and Law* 1, 471–98.

Havighurst, C. C., and Goodman, J. C. 1980. *The Regulation of Medical Care: Is the Price Too High?* San Francisco: Cato Institute.

Hayek, F. A. 1960. *The Constitution of Liberty*. Chicago: University of Chicago Press.

Health Insurance Association of America. 1991. *Source Book for Health Insurance Data, 1991*. Washington: Health Insurance Association of America.

———. 1998. *Source Book for Health Insurance Data, 1998*. Washington: Health Insurance Association of America.

Health Insurance Institute. 1966. *1966 Source Book of Health Insurance Data*. New York: Health Insurance Institute.

Heffler, S., Smith, S., Keehan, S., Clemens, M. K., Zezza, M., and Truffer, C. 2004. "Health Spending Projections through 2013." Health Affairs Web Exclusive, 11 February, W4-79–W4-93.

Helman, R., Mathew Greenwald & Associates, and Fronstin, P. 2006. "2006 Health Confidence Survey: Dissatisfaction with Health Care System Doubles since 1998." *EBRI Notes* 27, no. 11, 2–10.

Hervey, T. K., and McHale, J. V. 2004. *Health Law and the European Union*. Cambridge: Cambridge University Press.

Herzlinger, R. E. 1991. "Health Competition: A Third Approach to the Medical Insurance Crisis." *Atlantic*, August, 69–81.

———. 1994. "The Fundamental Forces Reshaping U.S. Health Care and How to Respond to Them." *Managed Care Quarterly* 2, no. 1, 27–30.

———. 1997. *Market-Driven Health Care*. Reading, Mass.: Addison-Wesley.

———, ed. 2004. *Consumer-Driven Health Care: Implications for Providers, Payers, and Policymakers*. San Francisco: Jossey-Bass.

Hibbard, J. 2003. *Decision Making in Consumer-Directed Health Plans*. Washington: American Association of Retired Persons.

Himmelstein, D. U., Warren, E., Thorne, D., and Woolhandler, S. 2005. "Illness and In-

jury as Contributors to Bankruptcy." Health Affairs Web Exclusive, February, W5-63–
W5-73.

Holahan, J., and Cook, A. 2005. "Changes in Economic Conditions and Health Insurance
Coverage, 2000–2004." Health Affairs Web Exclusive, 1 November, W5-498–W5-508.

Hsu, J., Price, M., Huang, J., Brand, R., Fung, V., Hui, R., et al. 2006. "Unintended
Consequences of Caps on Medicare Drug Benefits." *New England Journal of Medicine*
354, 2349–59.

Hunt, K. A., Weber, E. J., Showstack, J. A., Colby, D. C., and Callaham, M. L. 2006.
"Characteristics of Frequent Users of Emergency Departments." *Annals of Emergency
Medicine* 48, 1–8.

Hurley, J. 1998. "Welfarism, Extra-welfarism and Evaluative Economic Analysis in the
Health Sector." *Health, Health Care and Health Economics: Perspectives on Distribution*, ed. M. L. Barer, T. E. Getzen, and G. L. Stoddart, 373–96. New York: John Wiley
and Sons.

Hurley, R. E., Pham, H. H., and Claxton, G. 2005. "A Widening Rift in Access and
Quality: Growing Evidence of Economic Disparities." Health Affairs Web Exclusive,
December, w5-566–w25-576.

Hussey, P. S., Anderson, G. F., Osborn, R., Feek, C., McLaughlin, V., Millar, J., et al. 2004.
"How Does the Quality of Care Compare in Five Countries?" *Health Affairs* 23, no. 3,
89–99.

Huynh, P. T., Schoen, C., Osborn, R., and Holmgren, A. 2006. *The U.S. Health Care
Divide: Disparities in Primary Care Experiences by Income.* New York: Commonwealth Fund.

Hyman, D., and Hall, M. 2001. "Two Cheers for Employment-Based Health Insurance."
Yale Journal of Health Policy 2, 23–43.

Hyman, D. A., and Silver, C. 2001. "You Get What You Pay For: Result-Based Compensation in Health Care." *Washington & Lee Law Review* 58, 1427–92.

Ilse, L. W. 1953. *Group Insurance and Employee Retirement Plans.* New York: Prentice-
Hall.

Independent Inquiry into Inequalities in Health Report [Acheson Report]. 1998. London:
Her Majesty's Stationery Office.

Institute of Medicine. 2000. *To Err Is Human: Building a Safer Health Care System.*
Washington: National Academy Press.

——. 2001a. *Coverage Matters: Insurance and Health Care.* Washington: National
Academy Press.

——. 2001b. *Crossing the Quality Chasm: A New Health System for the Twenty-First
Century.* Washington: National Academy Press.

——. 2002a. *Care without Coverage: Too Little, Too Late.* Washington: National Academy Press.

——. 2002b. *Health Insurance Is a Family Matter.* Washington: National Academy
Press.

——. 2002c. *Unequal Treatment: Confronting Racial and Ethnic Disparities in Health
Care.* Washington: National Academy Press.

——. 2003a. *Hidden Costs, Value Lost: Uninsurance in America.* Washington: National
Academy Press.

------. 2003b. *A Shared Destiny: Community Effects of Uninsurance*. Washington: National Academy Press.

------. 2004. *Insuring America's Health: Principles and Recommendations*. Washington: National Academy Press.

------. 2006. *Preventing Medication Errors*. Washington: National Academy Press.

Jacobi, J. 2005. "Government Reinsurance Programs and Consumer-Driven Care." *Buffalo Law Review* 53, 537–75.

Jacobson, P. D. 2002. *Strangers in the Night: Law and Medicine in the Managed Care Era*. New York: Oxford University Press.

Jones, C. 1988–89. "Class Tax to Mass Tax." *Buffalo Law Review* 37, 685–737.

Jost, T. 1988. "The Necessary and Proper Role of Regulation to Assure the Quality of Health Care." *Houston Law Review* 25, 525–98.

------. 1995. "Oversight of the Quality of Medical Care: Regulation, Management, or the Market." *Arizona Law Review* 37, 825–69.

------. 2001. "Public and Private Approaches to Insuring the Uninsured." *New York University Law Review* 76, 419–92.

------. 2003. *Disentitlement? The Threats Facing Our Public Health Care Programs and a Rights-Based Response*. New York: Oxford University Press.

------. 2004. "Why Can't We Do What They Do? National Health Reform Abroad." *Journal of Law, Medicine and Ethics* 32, 433–41.

------. 2005. "Consumer-Driven Health Care in South Africa." *Journal of Health and Biomedical Law* 1, no. 2, 83–109.

------, ed. 2005. *Health Care Coverage Determinations: An International Comparative Study*. Maidenhead: Open University Press.

Jost, T. S., and Hall, M. 2005. "The Role of State Regulation in Consumer-Driven Health Care." *American Journal of Law and Medicine* 31, 395–418.

Kahneman, D., and Tversky, A. 1979. "Prospect Theory: An Analysis of Decision under Risk." *Econometrica* 47, no. 2, 263–92.

Kaiser Commission on Medicaid and the Uninsured. 2004. *Medicaid: A Lower-Cost Approach to Serving a High-Cost Population*. Washington: Kaiser Family Foundation.

------. 2006. *Deficit Reduction Act of 2005: Implications for Medicaid*. Washington: Kaiser Family Foundation.

Kaiser Family Foundation. 2004. *Prescription Drug Coverage for Medicare Beneficiaries: An Overview of the Medicare Prescription Drug, Improvement, and Modernization Act of 2003*. Washington: Kaiser Family Foundation.

------. 2005a. *Income Eligibility for Parents Applying for Medicaid by Annual Income as a Percent of Federal Poverty Level (FPL)*. Washington: Kaiser Family Foundation.

------. 2005b. *Trends and Indicators in the Changing Health Care Marketplace*. Washington: Kaiser Family Foundation.

------. 2006a. *Health Poll Report Survey: Selected Findings on the 2006 State of the Union Address and Health Care*. Washington: Kaiser Family Foundation.

------. 2006b. "Snapshots: Health Care Costs," http://www.kff.org/insurance/snapshot/index.cfm.

------. 2006c. "National Survey of Enrollees in Consumer-Directed Health Plans," http://www.kff.org/kaiserpolls/pomr112906pkg.cfm.

Kaiser Family Foundation / eHealthInsurance. 2004. *Update on Individual Health Insurance*. Washington: Kaiser Family Foundation.

Kaiser Family Foundation / Health Research and Educational Trust. 2004. *Employer Health Benefits: 2004 Annual Survey*. Washington: Kaiser Family Foundation.

———. 2006. *Employer Health Benefits: 2005 Annual Survey*. Washington: Kaiser Family Foundation.

Kaplan, R. L. 2005. "Who's Afraid of Personal Responsibility? Health Savings Accounts and the Future of American Health Care." *McGeorge Law Review* 36, 535–68.

Kapp, M. 2006. "Patient Autonomy in the Age of Consumer-Driven Health Care: Informed Consent and Informed Choice." *Journal of Health and Biomedical Law* 2, no. 1, 1–31.

Kawachi, I. 2005. "Why the United States Is Not Number One in Health." *Healthy, Wealthy, and Fair: Health Care and the Good Society*, ed. J. A. Marone and L. R. Jacobs, 19–36. Oxford: Oxford University Press.

Kelman, M. 1988. "On Democracy-Bashing: A Skeptical Look at the Theoretical and 'Empirical' Practice of the Public Choice Movement." *Virginia Law Review* 74, 199–273.

Kessel, R. A. 1958. "Price Discrimination in Medicine." *Journal of Law and Economics* 1, 20–53.

———. 1970. "The A.M.A. and the Supply of Physicians." *Law and Contemporary Problems* 35, no. 2, 267–83.

Kessler, D., and McClellan, M. 1996. "Do Doctors Practice Defensive Medicine?" *Quarterly Journal of Economics* 111, 353–90.

Klarman, H. E. 1957. "Medical Care Costs and Voluntary Health Insurance." *Journal of Insurance* 24, no. 1, 23–41.

Klein, J. 2003. *For All These Rights*. Princeton: Princeton University Press.

———. 2004. "The Politics of Economic Security: Employee Benefits and the Privatization of New Deal Liberalism." *Journal of Policy History* 16, no. 1, 34–65.

Knight, J. G. 2005. "What HSAs Mean for Banks." *American Banker*, 29 April, 11.

Korobkin, R. 1999. "The Efficiency of Managed Care 'Patient Protection' Laws: Incomplete Contracts, Bounded Rationality and Market Failure." *Cornell Law Review* 85, 1–88.

Krause, J. H. 1999. "Reconceptualizing Informed Consent in an Era of Health Care Cost Containment." *Iowa Law Review* 85, 281–305.

———. 2003. "Foreword: Federal-State Conflicts in Health Care, Federalism in Health Care Symposium." *Houston Journal of Health Law and Policy* 3, 151–60.

Ku, L., and Broaddus, M. 2005. *Out-of-Pocket Medical Expenses for Medicaid Beneficiaries Are Substantial and Growing*. Washington: Center on Budget and Policy Priorities.

Ku, L., and Wachino, V. 2005. *The Effect of Increased Cost-Sharing in Medicaid: A Summary of Research Findings*. Washington: Center on Budget and Policy Priorities.

Kupor, S. A., Liu, Y., Lee, J., and Yoshikawa, A. 1995. "The Effect of Co-payments and Income on the Utilization of Medical Care by Subscribers to Japan's National Health Service." *International Journal of Health Services* 25, no. 2, 295–312.

Kuttner, R. 1997. *Everything for Sale: The Virtues and Limits of Markets*. New York: Alfred A. Knopf.

LaDou, J., and Kikens, J. D. 1977. *Medicine and Money*. Cambridge: Ballinger.

Laham, N. 1996. *A Lost Cause: Bill Clinton's Campaign for National Health Insurance*. Westport, Conn.: Praeger.

Lambrew, J. M. 2005. *"Choice" in Health Care: What Do People Really Want?* New York: Commonwealth Fund.

Lasser, K. E., Himmelstein, D. U., and Woolhandler, S. 2006. "Access to Care, Health Status, and Health Disparities in the United States and Canada: Results of a Cross-National Population-Based Survey." *American Journal of Public Health* 96, no. 7, 1300–1307.

Lave, J. R., and Lave, L. B. 1970. "Medical Care and Its Delivery: An Economic Appraisal." *Law and Contemporary Problems* 35, no. 2, 252–66.

Leape, L. L., Brennan, T. A., Laird, N., Lawthers, A. G., Localio, A. R., Barnes, B. A., et al. 1991. "The Nature of Adverse Events in Hospitalized Patients: Results of the Harvard Medical Practice Study II." *New England Journal of Medicine* 324, 377–84.

Lee, R. I., and Jones, L. W. 1933. *The Fundamentals of Good Medical Care*. Chicago: University of Chicago Press.

Lee, T. H., and Zapert, K. 2005. "Do High-Deductible Health Plans Threaten Quality of Care?" *New England Journal of Medicine* 353, 1202–4.

Levine, M. E., and Forrence, J. L. 1990. "Regulatory Capture, Public Interest, and the Public Agenda: Toward a Synthesis." *Journal of Law, Economics and Organization* 6, 167–98.

Lewin, M. E., and Altman, S., eds. 2002. *America's Health Care Safety Net: Intact but Endangered*. Washington: Institute of Medicine.

Lexchin, J., and Grootendorst, P. 2004. "Effects of Prescription Drug User Fees on Drug and Health Services Use and on Health Status in Vulnerable Populations: A Systematic Review of the Evidence." *International Journal of Health Services* 34, no. 1, 101–22.

Lim, M. 2004. "Shifting the Burden of Health Care Finance: A Case Study of Public-Private Partnership in Singapore." *Health Policy* 69, no. 1, 83–92.

Lindert, P. 2004. *Growing Public*. Cambridge: Cambridge University Press.

Liu, Y. 2002. "Reforming China's Urban Health Insurance System." *Health Policy* 60, no. 2, 133–50.

Lo Sasso, A. T., Rice, T., Gabel, J. R., and Whitmore, H. 2004. "Tales from the Frontier: Pioneers' Experience with Consumer-Driven Health Care." *Health Services Research* 39, no. 4, part 2, 1071–90.

Luft, H. S. 1978. "How Do Health Maintenance Organizations Achieve Their Savings?" *New England Journal of Medicine* 298, 1336–43.

Lyke, B. 2006. *Health Savings Accounts: Overview of Rules for 2006*. Washington: Congressional Research Service.

Maciosek, M. V., Coffield, A. B., Edwards, N. M., Flottemesch, T. J., Goodman, M. J., and Solberg, L. I. 2006. "Priorities among Effective Clinical Preventive Services: Results of a Systematic Review and Analysis." *American Journal of Preventive Medicine* 31, no. 1, 52–61.

MacMillan, H. L., MacMillan, A. B., Offord, D. R., and Dingle, J. L. 1996. "Aboriginal Health." *Canadian Medical Association Journal* 155, 1569–78.

Mahar, M. 2006. *Money-Driven Medicine*. New York: Collins.

Mann, C. C., and Plummer, M. L. 1991. *The Aspirin Wars, Money, Medicine, and 100 Years of Rampant Competition*. New York: Alfred A. Knopf.

Mann, C., and Westmoreland, T. 2004. "Attending to Medicaid." *Journal of Law, Medicine and Ethics* 32, 416–25.

Marchildon, G. P. 2005. *Health Systems in Transition: Canada*. London: European Observatory on Health Systems and Policies.

Mariner, W. K. 2004. "Can Consumer-Choice Plans Satisfy Patients? Problems with Theory and Practice in Health Insurance Contracts." *Brooklyn Law Review* 69, 485–542.

Marmor, T. R. 2001. "Comparing Global Health Care Systems: Lessons and Caveats." *Global Health Care Markets*, ed. W. W. Wieners, 7–23. San Francisco: Jossey-Bass.

———. 2007. *F-Cubed: Fads, Fallacies and Foolishness in Medical Care Management and Policy*. Singapore: World Scientific.

Marmor, T. R., and Boyum, D. A. 1993. "The Political Considerations of Procompetitive Reform." *Competitive Approaches to Health Care Reform*, ed. R. J. Arnould, R. F. Rich, and W. White, 245–56. Washington: Urban Institute Press.

Marmor, T., and Mashaw, J. L. 2006. "Understanding Social Insurance: Fairness, Affordability, and the 'Modernization' of Social Security and Medicare." Health Affairs Web Exclusive, 21 March, w114–w134.

Maxwell, J., Temin, P., Zaman, S., and Petigara, T. 2005. "Are California's Large Employers Moving to Catastrophic Health Insurance Coverage?" Health Affairs Web Exclusive, 17 May, w5-233–w5-239.

Maynard, A. 2005. "Increasing Investment in the UK-NHS: Some Policy Challenges." *Reforming Health Social Security: Proceedings of an International Seminar*. Washington: World Bank.

Maynard, A., ed. 2005. *The Public-Private Mix for Health*. Abingdon, Oxon: Radcliffe Medical.

McCloskey, D. N. 1990. *If You're So Smart: The Narrative of Economic Expertise*. Chicago: University of Chicago Press.

McGuire, T. G. 2000. "Physician Agency." *Handbook of Health Economics*, ed. A. J. Culyer and J. P. Newhouse, vol. 1A, 462–536. Amsterdam: Elsevier.

McKinsey Global Institute. 1996. *Health Care Productivity*. Los Angeles: McKinsey and Company.

Mechanic, D. 1998. "The Functions and Limitations of Trust in the Provision of Medical Care." *Journal of Health Politics, Policy and Law* 23, 661–86.

Medicare Payment Advisory Commission. 2006. *Report to Congress: Medicare Payment Policy*. Washington: Medicare Payment Advisory Commission.

Mehlman, M. J. 1990. "Fiduciary Contracting: Limitations on Bargaining between Patients and Health Care Providers." *University of Pittsburgh Law Review* 51, 365–418.

Melhado, E. M. 1988. "Competition versus Regulation in American Health Policy." *Money, Power, and Health Care*, ed. E. M. Melhado, W. Feinberg, and H. M. Swartz, 15–102. Ann Arbor: Health Administration Press.

———. 1998. "Economists, Public Provision, and the Market: Changing Values in Policy Debate." *Journal of Health Politics, Policy and Law* 23, 215–63.

Merenstein, D., Daumit, G. L., and Powe, N. R. 2006. "Use and Costs of Nonrecommended Tests during Routine Preventive Health Exams." *American Journal of Preventive Medicine* 30, no. 6, 521–27.

Merlis, M., Gould, D., and Mahato, B. 2006. *Rising Out-of-Pocket Spending for Medical Care: A Growing Strain on Family Budgets.* Washington: Commonwealth Fund.

Minicozzi, A. 2006. "Medical Savings Accounts: What Story Do the Data Tell?" *Health Affairs* 25, no. 1, 256–67.

Mirowski, P. 1989. *More Heat Than Light: Economics as Social Physics, Physics as Nature's Economics.* Cambridge: Cambridge University Press.

Mitchell, W. C., and Munger, M. C. 1991. "Economic Models of Interest Groups: An Introductory Survey." *American Journal of Political Science* 35, 512–46.

Moffit, R. E. 1999. "High Anxiety: Working Families Need Market-Based Health Care Reform." *Empowering Health Care Consumers through Tax Reform,* ed. G. Arnett, 35–53. Ann Arbor: University of Michigan Press.

Monheit, A. C. 2003. "Persistence in Health Expenditures in the Short Run: Prevalence and Consequences." *Medical Care* 41, no. 7, suppl., 53–64.

Moody, J. S., and Hodge, S. A. 2004. "The Growing Class of Americans Who Pay No Federal Income Taxes," www.taxfoundation.org/news/show/206.html.

Moon, M., Storeyguard, M., and the Urban Institute. 2002. *Solvency or Affordability? Ways to Measure Medicare's Financial Health.* Washington: Kaiser Family Foundation.

Morone, J. A. 1993. "The Ironic Flaw in Health Care Competition: The Politics of Markets." *Competitive Approaches to Health Care Reform,* ed. R. J. Arnould, R. F. Rich, and W. White, 207–22. Washington: Urban Institute Press.

Morreim, E. H. 2001. *Holding Health Care Accountable.* New York: Oxford University Press.

———. 2006. "High-Deductible Health Plans: New Twists on Old Challenges from Tort to Contract." *Vanderbilt Law Review* 59, 1207–61.

Morrisey, M. A. 2005. *Price Sensitivity in Health Care: Implications for Health Care Policy.* Washington: National Federation of Independent Business Research Foundation.

Mossialos, E., and Dixon, A. 2002. "Funding Health Care: An Introduction." *Funding Health Care: Options for Europe,* ed. E. Mossialos, A. Dixon, J. Figueras, and J. Kutzin, 1–30. Buckingham: Open University Press.

Mossialos, E., and Mrazek, M. 2002. "Entrepreneurial Behaviour in Pharmaceutical Markets and the Effects of Regulation." *Regulating Entrepreneurial Behaviour in European Health Care Systems,* ed. R. B. Saltman, R. Busse, and E. Mossialos, 146–62. Buckingham: Open University Press.

Mossialos, E., and Thompson, S. 2004. *Voluntary Health Insurance in the European Union.* London: European Observatory on Health Systems and Policies.

Motheral, B., and Fairman, K. A. 2001. "Effect of a Three-Tier Prescription Copay on Pharmaceutical and Other Medical Utilization." *Medical Care* 39, 1293–1304.

Munnell, A. H., and Sundén, A. 2004. *Coming Up Short: The Challenge of 401(k) Plans.* Washington: Brookings Institution Press.

Munts, R. 1967. *Bargaining and Health: Labor Unions, Health Insurance And Medical Care.* Madison: University of Wisconsin Press.

Murphy, S. W. 1991. "Contributory Negligence in Medical Malpractice: Are the Standards Changing to Reflect Society's Growing Health Care Consumerism." *University of Dayton Law Review* 17, 151–80.

National Association of Health Underwriters. 2006. *2006 Benefit Buying Trends Study Chartpack*. Lisle, Ill.: Chapter House.

National Center for Health Statistics. 2000. *Health, United States, 2000*. Hyattsville, Md.: National Center for Health Statistics.

———. 2005. *Health, United States, 2005*. Hyattsville, Md.: National Center for Health Statistics.

National Center for Policy Analysis. 1990. *An Agenda for Solving America's Health Care*. Dallas: National Center for Policy Analysis.

National Conference of State Legislatures. 2004–6. *State Legislation on Health Savings Accounts and Consumer-Directed Health Plans*. Washington: National Conference of State Legislatures.

National Science Board. 2004. "Science and Engineering Indicators," http://www.nsf.gov/statistics/seind04/.

Netherlands, Kingdom of. Ministry of Health, Welfare and Sport. 2005. *Health Insurance in the Netherlands: The New Health Insurance System from 2006*. The Hague: Ministry of Health, Welfare and Sport.

Newhouse, J. 1974. "A Design for a Health Insurance Experiment." *Inquiry* 11, 5–24.

———. 2004. "Consumer-Directed Health Plans and the Rand Health Insurance Experiment." *Health Affairs* 23, no. 6, 107–13.

Newhouse, J. P., and the Insurance Experiment Group. 1993. *Free for All? Lessons from the Rand Health Insurance Experiment*. Cambridge: Harvard University Press.

Normand, C., and Busse, R. 2002. "Social Health Insurance Financing." *Funding Health Care: Options for Europe*, ed. E. Mossialos, A. Dixon, J. Figueras, and J. Kutzin, 59–79. Buckingham: Open University Press.

Nozick, R. 1974. *Anarchy, State, and Utopia*. New York: Basic Books.

Nyman, J. A. 2003. *The Theory of Demand for Health Insurance*. Stanford: Stanford University Press.

Oberlander, J. 2006. "The Political Economy of Unfairness in U.S. Health Policy." *Law and Contemporary Problems* (forthcoming).

Oliver, A., Mossialos, E., and Wilsford, D., eds. 2005. "Legacies and Latitude in European Health Policy." *Journal of Health Politics, Policy and Law* 30, no. 1.

Oliver, T. R. 2004. "Policy Entrepreneurship in the Social Transformation of American Medicine: The Rise of Managed Care and Managed Competition." *Journal of Health Politics, Policy and Law* 29, 701–34.

Olson, L., Tang, S. S., and Newacheck, P. W. 2005. "Children in the United States with Discontinuous Health Insurance Coverage." *New England Journal of Medicine* 353, 382–91.

Organization for Economic Cooperation and Development. 2005. *Health at a Glance: OECD Indicators, 2005*. Paris: Organization for Economic Cooperation and Development.

Parente, S. T., Feldman, R., and Christianson, J. B. 2004a. "Employee Choice of Consumer-Driven Health Insurance in a Multiplan, Multiproduct Setting." *Health Services Research* 39, no. 4, 1091–1111.

———. 2004b. "Evaluation of the Effects of a Consumer Choice Health Plan on Medical Expenditures and Utilization." *Health Services Research* 39, no. 4, 1189–1209.

Park, E., and Greenstein, R. 2006. "Latest Enrollment Data Still Fail to Dispel Concerns about Health Savings Accounts." Washington: Center on Budget and Policy Priorities.

Park, E., and Solomon, J. 2005. *Health Opportunity Accounts for Low-Income Medicaid Beneficiaries: A Risky Approach.* Washington: Center on Budget and Policy Priorities.

Pauly, M. V. 1968. "The Economics of Moral Hazard: Comment." *American Economic Review* 58, no. 3, 531–37.

———. 1971. *An Analysis of National Health Insurance Proposals.* Washington: American Enterprise Institute.

———. 1980. "Overinsurance: The Conceptual Issues." *National Health Insurance: What Now, What Later, What Never?*, 201–19. Washington: American Enterprise Institute for Public Policy Research.

———.1992. "The Public Policy Implications of Using Outcome Statistics." *Brooklyn Law Review* 58, 35–53.

———. 1994. *An Analysis of Medical Savings Accounts: Do Two Wrongs Make a Right?* Washington: American Enterprise Institute.

———. 1997. *Health Benefits at Work.* Ann Arbor: University of Michigan Press.

Pauly, M. V., and Goodman, J. C. 1995. "Tax Credits for Health Insurance and Medical Savings Accounts." *Health Affairs* 14, no. 1, 125–39.

Payton, S., and Powsner, R. M. 1980. "Regulation through the Looking Glass: Hospitals, Blue Cross and Certificate of Need." *Michigan Law Review* 79, 203–77.

Peele, P. B. 1993. "Evaluating Welfare Losses in the Health Care Market." *Journal of Health Economics* 12, 205–8.

Porter, M., and Teisberg, E. 2006. *Redefining Health Care: Creating Value-Based Competition on Results.* Boston: Harvard Business School Press.

Posner, R. A. 1969. "The Federal Trade Commission." *University of Chicago Law Review* 37, 47–89.

———. 2002. *Economic Analysis of Law.* New York: Aspen.

Price Waterhouse Coopers. *The Factors Fueling Rising Healthcare Costs, 2006,* 7.

Quadagno, J. 2005. *One Nation Uninsured.* New York: Oxford University Press.

Reden and Anders Ltd. 2005. *Consumer Directed Insurance Products: Survey Results.* Minneapolis: Reden and Anders.

Reed, L. S. 1947. *Blue Cross and Medical Service Plans.* Washington: Federal Security Agency.

Regopoulos, L., Christianson, J. B., Claxton, G., and Trude, S. 2006. "Consumer-Directed Health Insurance Products: Local-Market Perspectives." *Health Affairs* 25, no. 3, 766–73.

Reinhardt, U. 1998. "Abstracting from Distributional Effects: This Policy Is Efficient." *Health, Health Care, and Health Economics: Perspectives on Distribution,* ed. M. L. Barer, T. E. Getzen, and G. L. Stoddert, 1–52. New York: John Wiley and Sons.

———. 2002. Foreword. *The Economics of Health Reconsidered,* 2nd edn, ed. T. E. Rice, xi–xxii. Chicago: Health Administration.

Remler, D., and Glied, S. 2006. "How Much More Cost Sharing Will Medical Savings Accounts Bring?" *Health Affairs* 25, no. 4, 1070–78.

Reschovsky, J. D., Strunk, B. C., and Ginsburg, P. 2006. "Why Employer-Sponsored Insurance Coverage Changed, 1997–2003." *Health Affairs* 25, no. 3, 774–91.

Rhoads, S. E. 1985. *The Economist's View of the World: Government, Markets, and Public Policy*. Cambridge: Cambridge University Press.

Rice, T. 1992. "An Alternative Framework for Evaluating Welfare Losses in the Health Care Market." *Journal of Health Economics* 11, no. 1, 85–92.

———. 1997. "Can Markets Give Us the Health Care System We Want?" *Journal of Health Politics, Policy and Law* 22, 383–425.

———. 2002. *The Economics of Health Reconsidered*, 2nd edn. Chicago: Health Administration.

Rice, T., de Lissovoy, G., Gabel, J., and Ermann, D. 1985. "The State of PPOs: Results from a National Survey." *Health Affairs* 4, no. 4, 25–40.

Rice, T., and Morrison, K. R. 1994. "Patient Cost Sharing for Medical Services: A Review of the Literature and Implications for Health Care Reform." *Medical Care Review* 51, no. 3, 235–87.

Rich, R. F., and Erb, C. T. 2005. "The Two Faces of Managed Care Regulation and Policymaking." *Stanford Law and Policy Review* 16, 233–76.

Ringel, J. S., Hosek, S. D., Vollaard, B. A., and Mahnovski, S. 2002. *The Elasticity of Demand for Health Care: A Review of the Literature and Its Application to the Military Health System*. Santa Monica: Rand Health.

Robinson, J. C. 2002. "Reinvention of Health Insurance in the Consumer Era." *Journal of the American Medical Association* 291, 1880–86.

Robinson, R. 2002. "User Charges in Health Care." *Funding Health Care: Options for Europe*, ed. E. Mosiallos, A. Dixon, J. Figueras, and J. Kutzin, 161–83. Buckingham: Open University Press.

Rodwin, M. A. 1995. "Strains in the Fiduciary Metaphor: Divided Physician Loyalties and Obligations in a Changing Health Care System." *American Journal of Law and Medicine*, 21, 241–58.

Roemer, M. I. 1970. "Controlling and Promoting the Quality of Medical Care." *Law and Contemporary Problems* 35, 284–304.

Roos, N. P., Shapiro, E., and Tate, R. 1989. "Does a Small Minority of Elderly Account for a Majority of Health Care Expenditures? A Sixteen Year Perspective." *Milbank Quarterly* 67, nos. 3–4, 347–69.

Rosen, G. 1946. *Fees and Fee Bills: Some Economic Aspects of Medical Practice in Nineteenth Century America*. Baltimore: Johns Hopkins University Press.

Ross, J. S., Bradley, E. H., and Busch, S. H. 2006. "Use of Health Care Services by Lower-Income and Higher-Income Uninsured Adults." *Journal of the American Medical Association* 295, 2027–36.

Rowe, E. K. 1955. "Health, Insurance and Pension Plans in Union Contracts." U.S. Department of Labor Bulletin no. 1187. Washington: U.S. Government Printing Office.

Rubin, E. L. 2002. "Public Choice, Phenomenology, and the Meaning of the Modern State: Keep the Bathwater, but Throw Out That Baby." *Cornell Law Review* 87, 309–61.

Rubin, R. J., and Mendelson, D. N. 1995. "A Framework for Cost Sharing Policy Analysis." *Sharing the Costs of Health: A Multi-Country Perspective*, ed. N. Mattison, 2-1–2-164. Basel: Pharmaceutical Partners for Better Healthcare.

Sage, W. 1999. "Regulating through Information: Disclosure Laws and American Health Care." *Columbia Law Review* 99, 1701–1829.

Sagoff, M. 1986. "Values and Preferences." *Ethics* 96, 301–16.

Saltman, R. B., and Dubois, H. F. W. 2004. "The Historical and Social Base of Social Health Insurance Systems." *Social Health Insurance Systems in Western Europe*, ed. R. B. Saltman, R. Busse, and J. Figueras, 21–32. Maidenhead: Open University Press.

Sanmartin, C. 2006. "Comparing Health and Health Care Use in Canada and the United States." *Health Affairs* 25, no. 4, 1133–42.

Scherer, M. 2004. "Medicare's Hidden Bonanza." *Mother Jones*, March–April, 22.

Schlesinger, M. 2004. "Reprivatizing the Public Household: Medical Care in the Context of American Public Values." *Journal of Health Politics, Policy and Law* 29, 969–1004.

———. 2005. "The Dangers of the Market Panacea." *Healthy, Wealthy, and Fair: Health Care and the Good Society*, ed. J. A. Marone and L.R. Jacobs, 91–136. Oxford: Oxford University Press.

Schneider, C. E. 1998. *The Practice of Autonomy: Patients, Doctors, and Medical Decisions*. Oxford: Oxford University Press.

Schoen, C., Doty, M. M., Collins, S. R., and Holmgren, A. L. 2005. "Insured but Not Protected: How Many Adults Are Underinsured?" Health Affairs Web Exclusive, 14 June, W5-289–W5-302.

Schoen, C., How, S. K., Weinbaum, I., Craig, J. E., and Davis, K. 2006. *Public Views on Shaping the Future of the U.S. Health System*. New York: Commonwealth Fund.

Schoen, C., Osborn, R., Huynh, P. T., Doty, M., Zapert, K., Peugh, J., et al. 2005. "Taking the Pulse of Health Care Systems: Experiences of Patients with Health Problems in Six Countries." Health Affairs Web Exclusive, 3 November, W5-509–W5-525.

Schor, E. 2006. "Dems Try to Do to HSAs What They Did to Social Security Plan." *The Hill*, 8 February, 4.

Schreyögg, J. 2004. "Demographic Development and Moral Hazard: Health Insurance with Medical Savings Accounts." *Geneva Papers on Risk and Insurance* 29, 689–704.

Schuck, P. H. 1994. "Rethinking Informed Consent." *Yale Law Journal* 103, 899–960.

Schwartz, B. 2004. *The Paradox of Choice: Why More Is Less*. New York: Harper Collins.

Scitovsky, A., and Snyder, N. M. 1972. "Effects of Coinsurance on Physician Services." *Social Security Bulletin*, June, 3–19.

Seidman, L. 1977. "Medical Loans and Major-Risk National Health Insurance." *Health Services Research* 12, 123–28.

———. 1980. "Income-Related Consumer Cost Sharing: A Strategy for the Health of the Health Sector." *National Health Insurance: What Now, What Later, What Never?*, ed. M. V. Pauly. Washington: American Enterprise Institute for Public Policy Research.

———. 1981. "Consumer Choice Health Plan and the Patient Cost-Sharing Strategy: Can They Be Reconciled?" *A New Approach to the Economics of Health Care*, ed. M. Olson, 448–66. Washington: American Enterprise Institute.

Seifert, R. W., and Rukavina, M. 2006. "Bankruptcy Is the Tip of a Medical-Debt Iceberg." Health Affairs Web Exclusive, w-89–w-92.

Selden, T. M., and Gray, B. M. 2006. "Tax Subsidies for Employment-Related Health Insurance: Estimates for 2006." *Health Affairs* 25, no. 6, 1568–79.

Sen, A. 1970. *Collective Choice and Social Welfare*. San Francisco: Holden-Day.

———. 1982. *Choice, Welfare and Measurement*. Oxford: Basil Blackwell.

———. 1987. *On Ethics and Economics*. Oxford: Basil Blackwell.

Shapiro, E. 1980. "Controlling Health Care Expenditures." *Challenge* 23, no. 4, 40–44.

Shapiro, I., and Friedman, J. 2006. "New CBO Data Indicate Growth in Long-Term Income Inequality Continues." Washington: Center for Budget and Policy Priorities.

Shearer, G. 2004. "Commentary: Defined Contribution Health Plans: Attracting the Healthy and Well-Off." *Health Services Research* 39, no. 4, 1159–66.

Sheffler, R. M. 1984. "The United Mine Workers' Health Plan: An Analysis of the Cost Sharing Program." *Medical Care* 22, no. 3, 247–54.

Shen, Y., and McFeeters, J. 2006. "Out-of-Pocket Health Spending Between Low- and Higher-Income Populations." *Medical Care* 44, no. 3, 200–209.

Short, P. F. 1988. "Trends in Employee Benefits." *Health Affairs* 7, no. 3, 86–96.

Short, P. F., and Graefe, D. R. 2003. "Battery-Powered Health Insurance? Stability in Coverage of the Uninsured." *Health Affairs* 22, no. 6, 244–55.

Shryock, R. H. 1947. *The Development of Modern Medicine*. New York: Alfred A. Knopf.

Siciliani, L., and Hurst, J. 2003. *Explaining Waiting Times Variations for Elective Surgery across OECD Countries*. Paris: Organization for Economic Cooperation and Development.

Simon, H. 1979. "Rational Decision Making in Business Organizations." *American Economic Review* 69, no. 4, 493–513.

Simons, A. M., and Sinai, N. 1932. *The Way of Health Insurance*. Chicago: University of Chicago Press.

Sinai, N., Hall, M., and Homes, R. 1939. *Medical Relief Administration: Final Report of the Experience in Essex County, Ontario*. Windsor, Ont.: Essex County Medical Research.

Skinner, J. S., Staiger, D., and Fisher, E. S. 2006. "Is Technological Change in Medicine Always Worth It? The Case of Acute Myocardial Infarction." Health Affairs Web Exclusive, w34–w47.

Sloan, F., and Feldman, R. 1978. "Competition among Physicians." *Competition in the Health Care Sector: Past, Present and Future*, ed. W. Greenberg. Washington: Federal Trade Commission.

Sloan, F. A., and Hall, M. A. 2002. "Market Failures and the Evolution of State Regulation of Managed Care." *Law and Contemporary Problems* 65, no. 4, 169–206.

Slovic, P., Fischhoff, B., and Lichtenstein, S. 1982. "Facts versus Fears: Understanding Perceived Risk." *Judgment under Uncertainty: Heuristics and Biases*, ed. D. Kahneman, P. Slovic, and A. Tversky, 463–89. Cambridge: Cambridge University Press.

Somers, A. R. 1969. *Hospital Regulation: The Dilemma of Public Policy*. Princeton: Industrial Relations Section, Princeton University.

Somers, H. M., and Somers, A. R. 1961. *Doctors, Patients, and Health Insurance*. Washington: Brookings Institution.

Source Watch. 2005. "Institute of Economic Affairs," http://www.sourcewatch.org/index .php?title=Institute _ of _ Economic _ Affairs.

Spitz, B., and Abramson, J. 2005. "When Health Policy Is the Problem: A Report from the Field." *Journal of Health Politics, Policy and Law* 30, no. 3, 327–65.

Stano, M. 1981. "Individual Health Accounts: An Alternative Health Care Financing Approach." *Health Care Financing Review* 3, no. 1, 117–25.

Starr, P. 1982. *The Social Transformation of American Medicine*. New York: Basic Books.

Steuerle, E., and Hoffman, R. 1979. *Tax Expenditures for Health Care*. Washington: Office of Tax Analysis.

Stevens, R. 1989. *In Sickness and in Wealth: American Hospitals in the Twentieth Century*. New York: Basic Books.

Stevens, R., and Stevens, R. 1970. "Medicaid: Anatomy of a Dilemma." *Law and Contemporary Problems* 35, no. 2, 348–425.

Stigler, G. 1971. "The Theory of Economic Regulation." *Bell Journal of Economics* 2, no. 1, 3–21.

Stigler, G., and Becker, G. 1977. "De gustibus non est disputandum." *American Economic Review* 67, no. 2, 76–90.

Stoddart, G. L., Barer, M. L., and Evans, R. 1993. *User Charges, Snares and Delusions: Another Look at the Literature*. Vancouver: Centre for Health Services and Policy Research, University of British Columbia.

Stone, D. A. 1990. "AIDS and the Moral Economy of Insurance." *American Prospect*, March, 62–74.

———. 1993. "The Struggle for the Soul of Health Insurance." *Journal of Health Politics, Policy and Law* 18, no. 2, 287–317.

———. 2002. *Policy Paradox: The Art of Political Decision Making*, rev. edn. New York: W. W. Norton.

———. 2005. "How Market Ideology Guarantees Racial Inequality." *Healthy, Wealthy, and Fair: Health Care and the Good Society*, ed. J. A. Marone and L. R. Jacobs, 65–89. Oxford: Oxford University Press.

Strategic Policy and Research Intergovernmental Affairs. 2001. "Health Care Systems: An International Comparison," www.pnrec.org/2001papers/DaigneaultLajoie.pdf.

Sullivan, M. 2005. "Consumer-Directed Plans in Practice: Perspectives from Consumers and the Blues." Blue-Cross, Blue-Shield Association, http://bcbshealthissues.com/events/consumer.

Sutton, G. 1997. "Will You Still Need Me, Will You Still Screen Me, When I'm Past 64?" *British Medical Journal* 315, 1032–33.

Swartz, K. 2006. *Reinsuring Health: Why More Middle-Class People Are Insured and What Government Can Do*. New York: Russell Sage Foundation.

Tai-Seale, M. 2004. "Voting with Their Feet: Patient Exit and Intergroup Differences in Propensity for Switching Usual Source of Care." *Journal of Health Politics, Policy and Law* 29, 491–514.

Tamblyn, R., Laprise, R., Hanley, J. A., Abrahamowicz, M., Scott, S., Mayo, N. et al. 2001. "Adverse Events Associated with Prescription Drug Cost-Sharing among Poor and Elderly Persons." *Journal of the American Medical Association* 285, 421–29.

Taylor, A. K., and Wilensky, G. R. 1983. "The Effect of Tax Policies on Expenditures for Private Health Insurance." *Market Reforms for Health Care*, ed. J. A. Mayer, 163–84. Washington: American Enterprise Institute.

Technological Change in Health Care Research Network. 2001. "Technological Change around the World: Evidence from Heart Attack Care." *Health Affairs* 20, no. 3, 25–42.

Thomasson, M. A. 2002. "From Sickness to Health: The Twentieth Century Development of U.S. Health Insurance." *Explorations in Economic History* 39, 233–53.

———. 2003. "The Importance of Group Coverage: How Tax Policy Shaped U.S. Health Insurance." *American Economic Review* 93, no. 4, 1373–84.

Thompson, M. 1954. *Not as a Stranger*. New York: Charles Scribner's Sons.

Tollen, L. M., Ross, M., and Poor, S. 2004. "Risk Segmentation Related to the Offering of a Consumer-Directed Health Plan: A Case Study of Humana, Inc." *Health Services Research* 39, 1167–88.

"Transplant." 2004. http://www.chfpatients.com/tx/transplant.htm.

Trude, S., and Conwell, L. 2004. *Rhetoric v. Reality: Employer Views on Consumer-Driven Health Care*. Washington: Center for Studying Health System Change.

Tversky, A., and Kahneman, D. 1982. "Judgment under Uncertainty: Heuristics and Biases." *Judgment under Uncertainty: Heuristics and Biases*, ed. D. Kahneman, P. Slovic, and A. Tversky, 3–20. Cambridge: Cambridge University Press.

United Health Group. 2006. "Three-Year Study Shows Consumer-Driven Health Plans Continue to Stimulate Positive Changes in Consumer Health Behavior." Minneapolis: United Health Group.

Urban Institute / University of Maryland. 2005. *Uninsured Americans with Chronic Health Conditions*. Princeton: Robert Wood Johnson Foundation.

USA Today / Kaiser Family Foundation / Harvard School of Public Health. 2005. *Health Care Costs Survey*. Washington: Kaiser Family Foundation.

U.S. Bureau of Labor Statistics. 2005. "Economic and Employment Projections," http://www.bls.gov/news.release/ecopro.toc.htm.

U.S. Bureau of the Census. 2005. "Annual Demographic Survey, March Supplement," http://pubdb3.census.gov/macro/032005/pov/new01_000.htm.

U.S. Department of Agriculture, Food and Nutrition Service. 2001. "School Meals, the State Children's Health Insurance Program (SCHIP)."

U.S. Department of Labor. 1947. "Union Health and Welfare Plans." Bulletin no. 900. Washington: U.S. Government Printing Office.

———. 1960a. "Health and Insurance under Collective Bargaining Agreements, Hospital Insurance, Early 1959." Bulletin no. 1274. Washington: U.S. Government Printing Office.

———. 1960b. "Health and Insurance Plans under Collective Bargaining Agreements, Surgical and Medical Benefits, Late Summer 1959." Bulletin no. 1280. Washington: U.S. Government Printing Office.

———. 1961. "Health and Insurance Plans under Collective Bargaining: Major Medical Expense Benefits, Fall 1960." Bulletin no. 1293. Washington: U.S. Government Printing Office.

U.S. Department of the Treasury. 2004. "Health Savings Accounts, Additional Qs and As." Notice 2004-50.

U.S. House of Representatives, Committee on Ways and Means, Subcommittee on Health. 1976. *National Health Insurance Source Book*. Washington: U.S. Government Printing Office.

U.S. House of Representatives, Committee on Ways and Means, Subcommittee on Social Security / Subcommittee on Select Revenue Measures, 98th Congress, 2nd sess. 1984. *Hearings, Distribution and Economics of Employer-Provided Fringe Benefits*. Washington: U.S. Government Printing Office.

U.S. Senate, Committee on Labor and Public Welfare. 1951. *Health Insurance Plans in the United States*. Washington: U.S. Government Printing Office.

van Doorslaer, E., and Masseria, C. 2004. *Income-Related Inequality in the Use of Medical Care in 21 Countries*. Paris: Organization for Economic Cooperation and Development.

van Doorslaer, E., Masseria, C., and Koolman, X. 2006. "Inequalities in Access to Medical Care by Income in Developed Countries." *Canadian Medical Association Journal* 174, no. 2, 177–83.

van Doorslaer, E., Wagstaff, A., van der Burg, H., Christiansen, T., De Graeve, D., Duchesne, I., et al. 2000. "Equity in the Delivery of Health Care in Europe and the U.S." *Journal of Health Economics* 19, 553–83.

Veatch, R. M. 1981. *A Theory of Medical Ethics*. New York: Basic Books.

VHA Inc. 2003. *Consumers and Health Care: Boomers at the Gate*. Irving, Texas: VHA.

Vladeck, B. 1999. "The Political Economy of Medicare." *Health Affairs* 18, no. 1, 22–36.

———. 2003. "If Paying for Quality Is Such a Bad Idea, Why Is Everyone for It?" *Washington & Lee Law Review* 60, 1345–72.

Vogel, R. J. 1980. "The Tax Treatment of Health Insurance Premiums as a Cause of Overinsurance." *National Health Insurance: What Now, What Later, What Never?*, ed. M. V. Pauly. Washington: American Enterprise Institute for Public Policy Research.

Wagstaff, A., and van Doorslaer, E. 2000. "Equity in Health Care Finance and Delivery." *Handbook of Health Economics*, vol. 1B, ed. A. Culyer and J. Newhouse. Amsterdam: Elsevier.

Walker, J., Pan, E., Johnston, D., Adler-Milstein, J., Bates, D. W., and Middleton, B. 2005. "The Value of Health Care Information Exchange and Interoperability." Health Affairs Web Exclusive, 19 January, w5-10–w5-18.

Weisman, J. 2006. "With Insurance Policy Comes Membership." *Washington Post*, 23 July, A, 5.

White, B. 2006. "How Consumer-Driven Health Plans Will Affect Your Practice." *Family Practice Management*, March, 71–78.

White, J. 1995. *Competing Solutions: American Health Care Proposals and International Experience*. Washington: Brookings Institution Press.

Wilensky, G. 2006. "Consumer-Driven Health Plans: Early Evidence and Potential Impact on Hospitals." *Health Affairs* 25, no. 1, 174–85.

Williams, R. C. 1939. "The Medical Care Program for Farm Security Administration Borrowers." *Law and Contemporary Problems* 6, 583–94.

Wolman, D. M., and Miller, W. 2004. "The Consequences of Uninsurance for Individuals, Families, Communities and the Nation." *Journal of Law, Medicine, and Ethics* 32, 397–403.

Woolhandler, S., Campbell, T., and Himmelstein, D. U. 2003. "Costs of Health Care Administration in the United States and Canada." *New England Journal of Medicine* 349, 768–75.

Worthington, P. N. 1978. "Alternatives to Prepayment Finance for Hospital Services." *Inquiry* 15, 246–54.

Wörz, M., and Busse, R. 2005. "Analysing the Impact of Health-Care System Change in the EU Member States: Germany." *Health Economics* 14 (S1), S133–S149.

Wright, B. J., Carlson, M. J., Edlund, T., DeVoe, J., Gallia, C., and Smith, J. 2005.

"The Impact of Increased Cost Sharing on Medicaid Enrollees." *Health Affairs* 24, 1106–16.

Wynia, M. K., Cummins, D. S., VanGeest, J. B., and Wilson, I. B. 2000. "Physicians' Manipulation of Reimbursement Rules for Patients." *Journal of the American Medical Association* 283, 1858–65.

Yeager, H. 2006. "Labor Group Hits Out over Health Accounts." *Financial Times*, 1 February, 4.

Yip, W. C., and Hsiao, W. C. 1997. "Medical Savings Accounts: Lessons from China." *Health Affairs* 16, no. 6, 244–51.

Zabinski, D., Selden, T. M., Moeller, J. F., and Banthin, J. S. 1997. "Medical Savings Accounts: Microsimulation Results from a Model with Adverse Selection." *Journal of Health Economics* 18, no. 2, 195–218.

Zeldin, C., and Rukavina, M. 2007. *Borrowing to Stay Healthy: How Credit Card Debt Is Related to Medical Expenses*. Boston: Demos.

Blue Shield and, 59, 63
choice of insurer in, 14, 139
choice of provider in, 13–14
collective bargaining and, 24, 55, 61–63
consumer-driven health plans and, 24, 139–40
cost of health care affected by, 9–10
coverage expansions in, 61
declining population coverage in, 9–10, 205 n. 1 (chapter 1)
discounts for employers in, 62–63
financing of, 59, 61–62, 146, 211 n. 5
health savings accounts and, 24–25
history of, 48, 54–55, 59–64
multiemployer plans and, 61, 211 n. 15
National Labor Relations Act and, 63
National War Labor Board and, 54–55, 59–60
population covered by, 55, 61, 177–78, 211 n. 11
retiree benefits in, 206 n. 62
self-insurance and, 64, 211 n. 26
tax policy and, 38–39, 55, 60, 64, 69
unions and, 25, 55, 60, 62–63, 118, 211 n. 18
who pays for, 9, 24
See also Blue Cross; Blue Shield; employers; health insurance
EMTALA (Emergency Medical Treatment and Active Labor Act), 7, 34, 157, 209 n. 20
Enthoven, Alain, 78
Epstein, Richard, 30, 34, 208 n. 1
ERISA (Employee Retirement Income Security Act of 1974), 64
European Court of Justice, 171
European Union, 171
Evans, Robert, 89, 129, 213 n. 6
externalities, 91, 100

Farmers Security Administration, 49
Federal Employees Health Benefits Program, 18
federalism, 160, 170
fee-for-service medicine, xv, 43, 47, 98–99,

152–53, 184. *See also* health care providers
Feldstein, Martin, 29, 76, 77
fiduciary relationship, 154–55. *See also* legal issues; physicians
Finland, 180, 186
First World War, 48
Fisher, Anthony, 81
flexible spending accounts, 5, 216 n. 6
focused factories, 32
for-profit hospitals, 45, 170
framing, in behavioral psychology, 103
France, 168–69, 181
Fraser Institute, 27, 81, 166
Freedom Works, 83
Friedman, Milton, 74, 78
fringe benefits. *See* employers; employment-related health insurance

Galen Institute, ix, 27, 28
gambles, insurance vs., 103, 214 n. 18
gatekeeper systems, 170, 184
genetic medicine, 34–35
Germany, 56, 167–70, 172, 176–77, 183, 192, 197
Gingrich, Newt, 30
Glied, Sherry, 132
Golden Rule Insurance, 82–83
Goodman, John, 28, 30, 34, 39, 81–82, 114, 208 n. 4
government
    health care funded by, 10–11, 109–11, 115–16, 118, 167, 170, 172–73, 177, 182–83, 192–93
    health care role of, xi, 36–39, 52, 109–12, 117–18, 192–93
    health care system operated by, 169–70, 192
    regulation by, 18, 28, 36–37, 111–12, 160–65, 185, 208 n. 8
    research funded by, 15, 112
Great Depression, 50–51

Hall, Mark, 160, 217 n. 1
Harris, Seymour, 71

Havighurst, Clark, 30, 78
Hayek, F. A, 81
HDHPs. *See* high-deductible health plans
health care
    access to, ix, xvii–xviii, 2, 3–8, 110–
        11, 177–81, 206 n. 20. *See also*
        underinsurance; uninsureds
    advertising and, 194
    choices in, 13–15, 31–32, 97–100
    as "credence good," 97
    demand for, 75–77
    elasticity of demand for, 19, 32, 34–35,
        119–23, 130
    health and, 9, 33–34
    information and, *see* information
    innovation in, 2, 15–16, 23
    low-cost services in, 193–94
    market competition and, 17–18, 23–
        24, 42–43, 77–79, 192, 195
    market power and, 18, 37, 79, 91,
        100
    need for, 33–34, 52, 75–77, 181–82
    in other countries, *see* health care in
        comparative perspective
    payment for, *see* health care providers
    preventive, 7, 61, 33, 130, 194, 207
        n. 9
    professionals as decision makers in, 98,
        112–13
    providers, *see* health care providers
    purchasing decisions in, 19–20, 32, 79,
        93–102
    regulation of, 18, 28, 36–37, 111–12,
        160–65, 185, 205 n. 8
    research and, 15, 112, 206 n. 2
    respect for patients in, 15
    routine, 193–94
    value of, 9, 106–7, 111
    waste in, 12, 16, 35, 38, 104, 191
    See also health care costs; health insur-
        ance; health care providers; health
        care quality
health care costs, ix, 8–11, 174–77
    access affected by, 6–7, 9–10, 131–32,
        134, 145, 180–81

administrative, 108, 17, 194
affordability and, xii, 6–7, 11, 49–52,
    106–7, 145–46, 157, 180–81, 190
borrowing to pay, xiii, 6, 25, 40, 49–
    50, 79
catastrophic, xii, 19, 191–92
consumer-driven health care and, *see*
    consumer-driven health care
control in other systems of, 172–73,
    174–77
cost shifting and, 9–11, 19, 203
defensive medicine and, 220 n. 4
distribution of, xi–xii, 11, 48, 51–52,
    132, 135–40, 189
financial hardship caused by, 6–8, 11,
    131–32, 145
health planning as strategy for control-
    ling, 73–74
health savings accounts and, *see* health
    savings accounts
growth of, 51, 63–64, 68, 71–72
insurance and, 71
malpractice and, 220 n. 4
managed care and, 56, 68, 127–28, 44,
    198–99
moral hazard and, xv–xvii, xvii, 71,
    75–76, 96, 118, 191
in other countries, 6, 172–73, 174–75
resource use and, 176–77
saving to pay for, xiii, 49, 71, 79–80
as share of gross domestic product,
    175, 222 n. 21
technology's effect on, 173, 176, 185–
    86
in United States, 2, 8–11, 47–48, 51–
    52, 63–64, 172, 174–77
utilization of care affected by, 2, 73
utilization review and, 73
See also health care; health care pro-
    viders; moral hazard; Rand Health
    Insurance Experiment
health care in comparative perspective,
    161–88
    access to care, xvii, 177–80
    Beveridge model, 167–70, 172–73

legal issues (*continued*)

comparative negligence, 158, 219 n. 24

consumer fraud, 159

contributory negligence, 158, 219 n. 24

Emergency Medical Treatment and
Active Labor Act and, 7, 34, 157,
210 n 10

fiduciary relationships, 154–55

informed consent, 155–57

insurer's liability for misinformation,
165

malpractice, 28, 155, 220 n. 4

obligation to treat, 157

quasi-contract, 159

unjust enrichment, 159

libertarianism, 87, 113–14

life expectancy, 187

low-income households

consumer-driven health care and, 25,
139, 145–56

financial burden of cost sharing and,
xiv, 5–6, 123, 126–27, 136, 194,
197

malpractice, 28, 155, 220 n. 4

managed care, 1, 17, 18, 32

conflicts of interest under, 153

cost sharing and, 66–67, 161

health care costs affected by, 56, 68,
98–99, 127–28, 144

health savings accounts and, 23–24,
144, 162–64

practice of medicine under, 98–99

regulation of, 162–65

managed competition, 18, 78, 111,
171

marginal utility, 102–4

Mariner, Wendy, 30

Massachusetts Health Plan, 192

McCarran-Ferguson Act, 160

Medicaid, x, 40, 61, 68, 72, 172, 194,
197, 201, 203, 213 n. 3, 220 n. 6

choice of providers and, 14

cost sharing and, 130–37

effects of, 209 n. 10

financing of, 9–10

health savings accounts and, 21

preventive care and, 194

reasons for low take-up of, 5, 40, 209
n. 14

medical debt, xiii, 5, 6, 7, 49–50, 131. *See
also* bankruptcy; credit card debt;
health care costs: borrowing to pay
for; home equity loans

medical negligence, 28, 155, 220 n. 4

medical savings accounts (MSAs)

Balanced Budget Act and, 20

Health Insurance Portability and
Accountability Act and, 20, 83–84,
132, 207 n. 6

history of, 20, 79–84, 132

Medicare and, x, 20

in Singapore, xvi, 120, 147–48

in South Africa, xvi, 120, 148

medical service bureaus, 50

Medicare, 61, 68, 72, 116, 127, 173, 194,
197, 203

choice of providers and, 13

financing of, 10

Medicare Advantage (managed care),
18, 111

Medicare Part D (prescription drug
program), 192, 221 n. 6, 222 n. 12

MSAs and, x, 20

Medicare Modernization Act (MMA)

HSA tax subsidies and, 20–21, 84

state insurance mandates and, 160

medisave accounts, xvi, 120, 147–48, 167,
186

Moffitt, Robert, 28, 167

moral hazard, xv–xvii, 18, 96, 103–5,
120, 191, 215 n. 20

defined, xv–xvii

ex ante, xv, 33–34, 36, 128

history of concept of, 70–85

as moral issue, 72, 75

Nyman's theory of, 103

Pauly's theory of, 75–76

physician-induced demand as, xv–xvii

in public insurance systems, 38, 70

Timothy Stoltzfus Jost is the Robert L. Willett Family Professor of Law at Washington and Lee University.

Library of Congress Cataloging-in-Publication Data
Jost, Timothy S.
Health care at risk : a critique of the consumer-driven movement / Timothy Stoltzfus Jost.
p. ; cm.
Includes bibliographical references and index.
ISBN-13: 978-0-8223-4101-7 (cloth : alk. paper)
ISBN-13: 978-0-8223-4124-6 (pbk. : alk. paper)
1. Health planning — United States — Citizen participation. 2. Medical care — United
States — Cost control. 3. Medical care, Cost of — United States. 4. Health care
reform — United States. I. Title.
[DNLM: 1. Delivery of Health Care — United States. 2. Consumer Participation —
United States. 3. Cost Sharing — United States. 4. Health Care Reform — United States.
W 84 AA1 J84H 2007]
RA394.J67 2007
362.10973 — dc22   2007007937